CANCER RISK

Assessing and Reducing the Dangers in Our Society

Also of Interest

† *Genetic Technology: A New Frontier*, Office of Technology Assessment

† *Science, Technology, and the Issues of the Eighties: Policy Outlook*, edited by Albert H. Teich and Ray Thornton for the American Association for the Advancement of Science

† *Politics, Science and Cancer: The Laetrile Phenomenon*, edited by Gerald E. Markle and James C. Petersen

Risk in the Technological Society, edited by Christoph Hohenemser and Jeanne X. Kasperson

† *Accident at Three Mile Island: The Human Dimensions*, edited by David L. Sills, C. P. Wolf, and Vivien B. Shelanski

Patterns and Effects of Diet and Disease Today, edited by John A. Hefferren, Mary L. Moller, and Henry M. Koehler

† Available in hardcover and paperback.

A Westview Special Study

Cancer Risk: Assessing and Reducing the Dangers in Our Society
Office of Technology Assessment

Cancer strikes one out of four Americans, kills one out of five. It accounts for about 10 percent of the nation's total cost of illness, perhaps more. These numbers are distressing, but the impact of cancer extends beyond the numbers of lives taken and dollars spent. The human suffering it causes touches almost everyone.

Cancer is a collection of 200 diseases grouped together because of their similar growth processes. Each cancer, regardless of the part of the body it affects, is believed to originate from a single "transformed" cell—one unresponsive to normal controls over growth and whose progeny may grow and multiply to produce a tumor. Studies over the last two decades have led to the widespread conclusion that 60 to 90 percent of all cancer is associated with the environment—that is, anything that interacts with humans, including substances eaten, drunk, and smoked; natural and medical radiation; workplace exposures; drugs; aspects of sexual behavior; and substances present in the air, water, and soil. Preventing interactions between cancer-causing substances (carcinogens) and humans theoretically could reduce cancer's toll.

Relating specific exposures and behaviors to the occurrence of cancer is clearly a first step toward prevention; once carcinogenic influences are identified, efforts to control them can be undertaken. This book illuminates the debates about the importance of environmental factors in cancer occurrence and the laws that require actions to reduce exposures to cancer-causing substances. It describes what is known about the occurrence of cancer and death from cancer in the United States; methods to identify cancer-causing substances, exposures, and behaviors and to estimate the amount of cancer that may result from a particular behavior or exposure; federal laws that provide for control of exposures to carcinogens; and future legislative options.

The Office of Technology Assessment was created in 1972 as an advisory arm of the U.S. Congress. OTA's basic function is to help legislative policymakers anticipate and plan for the consequences of technological changes and to examine the many ways, expected and unexpected, in which technology affects people's lives. The assessment of technology calls for exploration of the physical, biological, economic, social, and political impacts that can result from applications of scientific knowledge. OTA provides Congress with independent and timely information about the potential effects—both beneficial and harmful—of technological applications.

CANCER RISK

Assessing and Reducing the Dangers in Our Society

Office of Technology Assessment

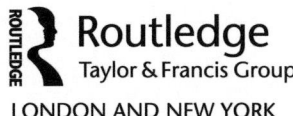

Routledge
Taylor & Francis Group

LONDON AND NEW YORK

First published 1982 by Westview Press, Inc.

Published 2018 by Routledge
52 Vanderbilt Avenue, New York, NY 10017
2 Park Square, Milton Park, Abingdon, Oxon OX14 4RN

Routledge is an imprint of the Taylor & Francis Group, an informa business

Copyright © 1982 Taylor & Francis

Library of Congress Cataloging in Publication Data
Main entry under title:
Cancer risk, assessing and reducing the
    dangers in our society.
    (A Westview special study)
    Bibliography: p.
    1. Cancer—United States—Prevention.   2. Environmentally induced diseases—United States.
I. United States. Congresses. Office of Technology Assessment. [DNLM: 1. Data collection.
2. Neoplasms—Etiology.   3. Risk. QZ 202 C215]
RC276.C275   616.99′4071   82-2633
ISBN 13: 978-0-367-01932-7 (hbk)   AACR2
ISBN 13: 978-0-367-16919-0 (pbk)

OTA Project Staff

Joyce C. Lashof, *Assistant Director, OTA*
Health and Life Sciences Division

H. David Banta, *Health Program Manager*

Michael Gough, *Project Director*

Robert J. Fensterheim,* *Research Associate*

Hellen Gelband,* *Research Associate*

Virginia Cwalina, *Administrative Assistant*
Shirley Ann Gayheart, *Secretary*
Nancy L. Kenney, *Secretary*
Martha Ingram Finney,* *Editor*

Other Contributing Staff

Barbara Lausche, *Senior Analyst*
Elizabeth Williams, *Senior Analyst*

Contractors

Richard Doll, *Oxford University*
Richard Peto, *Oxford University*
Michael Baram, *Bracken and Baram, Boston, Mass.*
Roy Albert, *New York University Medical School*
William Rowe, *American University*
Clement Associates, Inc., *Washington, D.C.*

OTA Publishing Staff

John C. Holmes, *Publishing Officer*

John Bergling   Kathie S. Boss   Debra M. Datcher   Joe Henson

*OTA contract personnel.

Advisory Panel

Norton Nelson, *Panel Chairman*
Department of Environmental Medicine, New York University Medical School

David Axelrod
Commissioner of Health
State of New York

Peter A. A. Berle
Berle, Butzel, Kass, and Case

Theodore L. Cairns
E. I. DuPont de Nemours & Co.,
Inc. (retired)

Paul F. Deisler, Jr.
Vice President, Health, Safety
and Environment
Shell Oil Co.

George S. Dominguez
Director of Government
Relations
CIBA-Geigy

David Doniger
Natural Resources Defense
Council

A. Myrick Freeman
Professor of Economics
Bowdoin College

Robert Harris
Environmental Defense Fund

Priscilla W. Laws
Professor of Physics
Dickinson College

Mark Lepper
Vice President for Evaluation
Rush-Presbyterian Medical
School, St.Lukes Medical Center

Brian MacMahon
Chairman, Epidemiology
Department
Harvard University School of Public Health

Robert A. Neal
President
Chemical Industry Institute
of Toxicology

Vaun A. Newill
Director, Research and
Environmental Health Division
Exxon Corp.

William J. Nicholson
Department of Community
Medicine
Mt. Sinai School of Medicine

R. Talbot Page
California Institute of
Technology

Margaret Seminario
Department of Occupational
Safety and Health
American Federation of Labor/
Congress of Industrial
Organizations

Alice S. Whittemore
Division of Epidemiology
Stanford University School of
Medicine

Michael Wright
Safety and Health Department
United Steelworkers of America

Foreword

Congressional interest in cancer is long standing and continuing. Programs in basic cancer research, and in treatment and prevention of the disease are now complemented by some two dozen laws directed at reducing exposures to cancer-causing substances. This report examines the technologies used to gather and analyze information about cancer in our society, as well as the ways in which those technologies affect and are affected by the public health and environmental legislative mandates.

The report discusses the strengths and weaknesses of data sources used for determining trends in cancer occurrence and mortality, and reviews estimates of the contribution of various factors—behaviors and exposures—associated with cancer in this country. Evidence linking today's cancers with past carcinogenic influences has come mainly from epidemiology, which continues to scrutinize aspects of the American lifestyle, for possible associations with cancer.

Congressional mandates intended to shield people from new and already-present carcinogens have heightened the need for methods to identify such harmful agents before they have an impact on human health. Laboratory testing technologies currently used to determine the carcinogenicity of substances, and technologies that may become important in the near future are discussed and evaluated. The assessment examines the use of extrapolation techniques for estimating human carcinogenic risks from test-derived data; the advantages and disadvantages of the available extrapolation models; and the ultimate use of these techniques in setting standards for controlling exposures under diverse legislation. The report then looks at the problems of decisionmaking in the face of the often-great uncertainties accompanying scientific findings and the proposals for regulatory reform that have grown out of concern for these issues.

In preparing the full report, OTA staff consulted with members of the advisory panel for the study, with contractors who prepared material for the assessment, and with other knowledgeable persons in environmental organizations, Government, industry, labor organizations, research institutions, and universities.

A draft of the final report was reviewed by the advisory panel, chaired by Dr. Norton Nelson, the OTA Health Program Advisory Committee, chaired by Dr. Sidney S. Lee, and by approximately 80 other individuals and groups. We are grateful for their assistance and that of many other people who assisted and advised in the preparation of this report.

JOHN H. GIBBONS
Director

Contents

1.
Summary

Contents

LIST OF TABLES

1.
Summary

Cancer occupies center stage in American concern about disease because of its toll in lives, suffering, and dollars. It strikes one out of four Americans, kills one out of five, and as the second-leading cause of death, following heart disease, killed over 400,000 people in the United States in 1979. According to estimates from the National Center for Health Statistics (NCHS), cancer accounted for about 10 percent of the Nation's total cost of illness in 1977. These numbers are distressing, but the impacts of cancer extend beyond the numbers of lives taken and dollars spent. The human suffering it causes touches almost everyone.

Cancer is a collection of about 200 diseases grouped together because of their similar growth processes. Each cancer, regardless of the part of the body it affects, is believed to originate from a single "transformed" cell. A transformed cell is unresponsive to normal controls over growth, and its progeny may grow and multiply to produce a tumor. Studies in human populations and in laboratory animals have linked exposures to certain substances with cancer. This knowledge of cancer's origins has led to the conclusion that preventing interactions between cancer-causing substances and humans can reduce cancer's toll.

CANCER AND "ENVIRONMENT"

Studies over the last two decades yielded a variety of statements that 60 to 90 percent of cancer is associated with the environment and therefore is theoretically preventable. As it was used in those statements and is used in this report, "environment" encompasses anything that interacts with humans, including substances eaten, drunk, and smoked, natural and medical radiation, workplace exposures, drugs, aspects of sexual behavior, and substances present in the air, water, and soil. Unfortunately, the statements were sometimes repeated with "environment" used to mean only air, water, and soil pollution.

Relating exposures and behaviors to cancer occurrence is a first step in cancer prevention. Once carcinogenic influences are identified, efforts to control them can be undertaken toward

the goal of reducing cancer. This study is intended to illuminate the debates about the importance of environmental factors in cancer occurrence, the laws that require actions to reduce exposures to cancer-causing substances (carcinogens), and describes:

- what is known about the occurrence of cancer and death from cancer in the United States;
- methods to identify cancer-causing substances, exposures, and behaviors;
- methods to estimate the amount of cancer which may result from a particular behavior or exposure;
- Federal laws that provide for regulatory control of carcinogenic exposures; and
- options for Congress.

CANCER MORTALITY AND INCIDENCE

Nationwide mortality data are used to answer questions about the number of deaths caused by cancer in the United States. Without

doubt, the number of Americans dying from cancer has increased during the last century. Paradoxically, a major part of this increase resulted from improvements in public health and medical care. In years past, infectious diseases killed large numbers of people in infancy and during childhood. Now that improved health care has softened the impact of those diseases, many more people live to old ages when cancer causes significant mortality.

Cancer deaths are not evenly distributed among all body sites, the lung, colon, and breast accounting for over 40 percent of the total (see table 1). Changes in cancer rates over time also vary by body site. For this reason, discussion of cancer rates at particular body sites is more revealing than discussion of overall trends which mask changes at individual sites. Moreover, because some cancer-causing substances act at specific sites, more information about oppotunities for prevention is obtained from the analysis of particular sites.

To permit the examination of cancer rates over time, standardization, a statistical technique, is applied to make allowances for a changing population structure. Standardization allows the direct comparison of single, summary statistics, e.g., the mortality rates from lung cancer for the entire population in 1950 and 1981. In this report, mortality rates are standardized to the age and racial structure of the 1970 U.S. census, unless otherwise specified.

Age-specific rates are also used extensively for examining trends. These rates measure the

proportion of people in defined age classes who have developed or died from cancer, and are unaffected by changes in the age structure of the population. Of greatest importance in detecting and identifying carcinogens, changes over time in younger age groups often presage future, larger changes in that group of people as they enter older age groups.

In general, cancer mortality rates are higher among nonwhite males than among white males. Differences between nonwhite and white females are less pronounced. The observed greater fluctuations in rates from year to year for nonwhites is consistent with the conclusion that reporting of vital statistics is poorer for nonwhites than for whites.

Greatest concern is expressed about the increasing trends. The largest increases since 1950 are in respiratory cancers (mainly of the lung, larynx, pharynx, trachea), which are largely ascribed to the effects of smoking. Male respiratory cancer rates began to rise about 25 years earlier than female rates, which reflects the difference in time when the two sexes adopted smoking. Further evidence for the importance of smoking in lung cancer is the recent decrease in lung cancer mortality among males younger than 50. The percentage of males who smoke is known to have decreased during the last 20 years, and studies have shown that smoking cessation reduces lung cancer occurrence. Addi-

Table 1.—Mortality From Major Cancer Sites in the United States, 1978, All Races

Anatomic site	Number of deaths			Percentage of total		
	Male	Female	Total	Male	Female	Total
All malignant neoplasms	215,997	180,995	396,992	100%	100%	100%
Lung, trachea, and bronchus	71,006	24,080	95,086	32.9	13.3	24.0
Colon	20,694	23,484	44,178	9.6	13.0	11.1
Breast	280	34,329	34,609	0.13	19.0	8.7
Prostate	21,674	—	21,674	10.0	—	5.5
Pancreas	11,010	9,767	20,777	5.1	5.4	5.2
Blood (leukemia)	8,683	6,708	15,391	4.0	3.7	3.9
Uterus	—	10,872	10,872	—	6.0	2.7
Ovary, fallopian tubes, and broad ligament	—	10,803	10,803	—	6.0	2.7
Bladder	6,771	3,078	9,849	3.1	1.7	2.5
Brain and other parts of nervous system	5,373	4,362	9,735	2.5	2.4	2.5
Rectum	5,002	4,089	9,091	2.3	2.3	2.3
Oral: Buccal cavity and pharynx	5,821	2,520	8,341	2.7	1.4	2.1
Kidney and other urinary organs	4,809	2,916	7,725	2.2	1.6	1.9
Esophagus	5,552	2,030	7,582	2.6	1.1	1.9
Skin	3,537	2,511	6,048	1.6	1.4	1.5
All other	45,785	39,446	85,231	21.2	21.8	21.5

SOURCE: Office of Technology Assessment.

tionally, changes in cigarette composition are thought to contribute to a reduced risk of lung cancer. Decreases among men now over 50 are not expected because those populations include a large proportion of long-time smokers who remain at high risk.

Death rates from prostate and kidney cancers among males have risen somewhat, and mortality rates from malignant skin tumors (melanomas) have increased in white males and females. Mortality from breast cancer, the number one cancer killer of women, has remained relatively constant. Overall mortality from nonrespiratory cancers (i.e., excluding most cancers generally associated with smoking) has decreased in females and remained constant in males during the last 30 years.

The more satisfying trends are those that are decreasing. The most striking, among both men and women, has been the great decrease in stomach cancer since 1930. Although generally ascribed to changes in diet, the reasons for the decrease are not known with any certainty. A decrease in uterine cancer within the last few decades is attributed to higher living standards, better screening tests for early cancer, and an increase in hysterectomies, which reduces the number of women at risk.

In general, mortality data (numbers of deaths) are considered more reliable for deciding about trends in cancer occurrence than are data about cancer incidence (numbers of new cases). This is largely because nationwide mortality data have been collected on a regular basis for almost 50 years. In contrast, incidence data for a sample of the entire country have been collected systematically only since 1973 by the National Cancer Institute's (NCI's) Surveillance, Epidemiology, and End Results (SEER) program. Before that, incidence data are available only for three points in time since 1937. The 10-percent sample of the population included in the SEER areas is not representative of the entire population. Some groups—orientals—are overrepresented in the data collected, and some groups—rural blacks—are underrepresented. Incidence rates for nonwhites, at least during the first 4 years of the SEER program, were considered too unreliable for meaningful analysis.

Incidence data are important because they provide information not captured in mortality data. They record each new case of cancer whether the person dies from cancer, is cured, or dies from other causes.

Followup studies of SEER program participants have provided information about survival from the various types and stages of cancer. A problem encountered in such studies was that people who move from the registration area after treatment are sometimes lost to further study, making it difficult to ascertain whether they eventually succumb to cancer or if treatment cured them. Use of the newly established (1981) National Death Index, by which deaths can be identified through a single query to NCHS rather than through a request to every State, is expected to facilitate SEER program followup studies. If this expectation is realized, information from the "End Results" component of SEER should be improved.

Data collected in the SEER program (1973-76), in combination with data from the Third National Cancer Survey (TNCS), carried out from 1969 through 1971, have been interpreted as showing an increase of more than 10 percent in cancer incidence during the last decade. The major changes seen in the incidence data parallel those seen in mortality data—increases in lung cancer and decreases in stomach and uterine cancers. However, publication of this analysis sparked a controversy about the true nature of incidence trends, since only 2 years earlier an analysis of data from the three national cancer surveys had shown an overall decrease of about 4 percent between 1947 and 1970. Some observers are concerned about the possibility that, after at least half a century of stable or declining rates, cancer incidence has gone up and that the increase might result from newly introduced chemical carcinogens. Those who dispute the importance of the observed increase contend that it reflects changes in the reporting of cancer incidence between TNCS and SEER (1973 through 1976), and not real changes in cancer incidence. As more data are collected during the next few years, a clearer picture of incidence trends may emerge.

INITIATION, PROMOTION, AND SYNERGISM

Cancer causation is thought to involve at least two steps: an early initiation step and a later promotion effect. A single agent may cause both events, or two or more separate agents working in the proper sequence may be necessary. Initiation is generally thought to involve a genetic change in the cell, but that change is not expressed and does not result in a tumor unless a promotion event follows it. The latent period of most cancers—the time between exposure to an initiator and appearance of the disease—is often 20 years or more. This long latent period is the cause of a great deal of apprehension among policymakers, scientists, and the general public because new substances and living habits are continually introduced, and today's harmful exposures may not cause ill effects for years.

The time between exposure to a promoter, after initiation has occurred, and the appearance of cancer, can be much shorter. "Initiated cells" may lie quiescent if they are not "turned on" by a promoter, and cancer may never develop if sufficient exposures to promoters do not occur. The practical importance of this property of promoters is illustrated by the change in cancer risk experienced by ex-smokers of cigarettes. Smoking is thought to play both an initiation and promotion role in cancer causation. Because of smoking's promotional properties, the risk of cancer falls off rapidly after a smoker quits.

Synergism, another form of interaction, occurs when two or more substances potentiate each other's effects, producing more cancers than can be accounted for by adding the effects of each. The multiplicative effects of cigarette smoking and exposure to asbestos and smoking and exposure to radiation are well-known examples of synergism.

Unfortunately, relatively little is understood about interacting agents—either synergisms or initiation and promotion. In particular, promoters have not received as much experimental attention as have initiators or complete carcinogens, which both initiate and promote.

FACTORS ASSOCIATED WITH CANCER

The possibility that cancers may be prevented by eliminating or modifying behaviors or exposures has stimulated the continued search for factors important in cancer causation. Importantly for prevention efforts, studies of agents that interact in causing cancer have shown that altering exposure to a single factor may eliminate or greatly reduce the risk of cancer.

Evidence for the associations between various "factors" and cancer ranges from very strong to very weak. Regardless of the strength of the association, the estimated magnitude of the amount of cancer associated with factors also varies. For instance, the strongest associations include those between smoking tobacco and respiratory cancers, between asbestos and cancer of the lung and other sites, and between ionizing radiation and cancer at many sites. While each of the three associations is strong, the percentage of cancer associated with each is different. Smoking is associated with more than 20 percent of cancer, asbestos with between 3 and 18 percent, and natural radiation with less than 1 to 3 percent.

Table 2 (pp. 8-9) presents information about associations between several factors and cancer. The associations between some aspects of human biology and reproduction and a proportion of cancer, especially in women, are well-established, as is the association of a small percentage of cancer with medical drugs. The specifics of the association between human diet and cancer are not understood, but diet is generally considered to be associated with a large percentage of cancer. Infection, especially viral infection, is associated with particular tumors that occur mainly in people in other parts of the world, and is also thought to be associated with some urogenital cancers in the United States.

The magnitude of associations between air and water pollution and cancer are argued and studies to examine the associations are difficult to design and execute. The same is true of associations between consumer products and cancer.

There is no disputing that occupational exposures to asbestos and some chemicals have caused human cancer, and table 2 presents estimates both for asbestos-caused cancer and total occupationally associated cancer. As the data in the table show, there is significant disagreement about how much current cancer and cancer in the near future is to be associated with occupational exposures.

Associating a high or low percentage of cancer with a factor does not reflect the present-day opportunities for prevention. For instance, diet is considered very important, but because associations with specific elements and cancer are poorly understood, there are few practical preventive measures now available.

The opportunities for prevention of occupation-related cancers at this time are better. Identification of a cancer-causing substance in the workplace can lead to reductions in exposure either by regulation or through voluntary activities on the part of industry. While reducing or eliminating occupational exposures to carcinogens might only slightly reduce the overall cancer toll, it could have a profound effect on the amount of cancer among workers who may now be at risk. A reduction of only 1 percent in cancer mortality means 4,000 fewer cancer deaths each year, so that even small reductions translate into relatively large numbers.

IDENTIFICATION OF CARCINOGENS

The Federal Government has centered efforts to control cancer on reducing exposures to chemical and physical carcinogens.

Carcinogens can be identified through epidemiology—the study of diseases and their determinants in human populations—and through various laboratory tests. Currently 18 chemicals and chemical processes are listed as human carcinogens and an additional 18 listed as probable human carcinogens by the International Agency for Research on Cancer (IARC), a World Health Organization agency. IARC conclusions, based on reviews of the worldwide literature, are accepted as authoritative by government agencies and many other organizations.

In the United States, Congress has directed the National Toxicology Program (NTP) to produce an annual list of carcinogens. The first list, published in 1980, was composed of the substances identified as human carcinogens by IARC. The next publication is to be considerably expanded and will include usage and exposure data and information on the regulatory status of over 100 chemicals either considered to be carcinogens or regulated by the Federal Government because of carcinogenicity.

Cancer epidemiology established the associations between the 36 substances and human cancer listed by IARC as well as the carcinogenicity of smoking, alcohol consumption, and radiation. However, **epidemiology is limited as a technique for identifying carcinogens because cancers typically appear years or decades after exposure.** If a carcinogen were identified 20 years after its widespread use began, many people might develop cancer from it even though its use is then immediately discontinued. Certainly, those people who were identified in the study as having had their cancer caused by the substance would have been irreparably harmed. Epidemiology is complicated because people are difficult to study; people move from place to place, change their type of work, change their habits, and it is hard to locate them and to estimate their past exposures to suspect agents.

Laboratory tests, which do not depend on human illness and death to produce data, have been developed to identify carcinogens. Currently, the testing of suspect chemicals in laboratory animals, generally rats and mice, is the backbone of carcinogen identification. The suspect chemical is administered to the animals

Table 2.—Summary of Cancer-Associated Environmental Factors[a]

Factor[b]	Sites considered in drawing the estimates	Range of estimates associated with factor
Diet	*Digestive tract, breast, endometrium, ovary*	*35–50 percent*

Associations between diet and cancer are suggested by epidemiologic and experimental laboratory studies. Significant differences in cancer rates are observed between different population groups with varying eating habits. Dietary components, such as high-fat and low-fiber content, and nutritional habits that affect hormonal and metabolic balances are believed more important than additives and contaminants. The magnitude of the estimates reflect observed relationships between diet and prominent cancer sites, e.g., breast and colon.

Tobacco	*Upper respiratory tract, bladder, esophagus, kidney, pancreas*	*22–30 percent*

Tobacco is associated with cancer at many anatomical sites, principally the lung. Many estimates of the proportion of overall cancer mortality associated with tobacco smoking are firmly based on epidemiologic studies that compared cancer mortality among individuals with varying smoking habits. Several carcinogens act synergistically with tobacco, e.g., asbestos, alcohol, radiation.

Occupation, asbestos	*Upper respiratory tract, others*	*3–18 percent*

Several occupational exposures are firmly linked to cancer occurrence, the most important of these is asbestos. Estimates for the contribution of asbestos to current cancer deaths and cancers in the near future range from 3 percent (1.4–4.4 percent) to an upper estimate of 13–18 percent. Most estimates lie toward the lower end of the range. The exposures responsible for these cancers occurred primarily in the 1940's and 1950's and the resultant cancers are expected to peak in the early to mid-1980's.

Occupation, all exposures	*Upper respiratory tract, others*	*4–38 percent*

Estimates of the proportion of cancer associated with all occupational exposures range from 4 percent (2–10 percent) to a high of 23–38 percent. The higher estimates are from a paper that estimated that asbestos is associated with 13–18 percent of all cancer and added to that estimates of cancer associated with five other occupational exposures. Almost all other estimates are near the lower end of the range.

Alcohol	*Upper digestive tract, larynx, liver*	*3–5 percent*

Alcohol consumption is associated with cancer in the upper digestive tract and in the liver. The digestive tract cancers occur more frequently in smokers than nonsmokers, and therefore many of these cancers could be prevented if either tobacco or alcohol were discontinued. The majority of reliable estimates are based on apportioning a percentage of the cancers at the alcohol-related sites to alcohol, and the numerical estimates are very similar.

Infection	*Uterine cervix, prostate, and other sites*	*1–15 percent*

Epidemiologic data strongly suggest an association between a virus and cervical cancer, and cancer at that site accounts for the lower numerical estimate. The higher estimate is much more tentative and associates all urogenital cancers in both sexes with infections of venereal origin. Some other cancers which occur commonly in other parts of the world are strongly associated with viral infection. They are rare in the United States.

Sexual development, reproductive patterns, and sexual practices	*Breast, endometrium, ovary, cervix, testis*	*1–13 percent[c]*

All of the hormonally related cancers in women, breast, endometrial, and ovarian are believed associated with sexual development and reproductive patterns. The important characteristics are: 1) age at sexual maturity; 2) age at birth of first child; 3) age at menopause. The higher numerical estimate includes the large number of breast cancers. Testicular cancers are associated with developmental and hormonal abnormalities.

Pollution	*Lung, bladder, rectum*	*Less than 5 percent*

Air pollution: Several epidemiologic studies of the effects of air pollution demonstrate an increased risk of lung cancer in heavily polluted areas, but these conclusions are weakened because smoking and occupational exposures were not always taken into account. The most important carcinogens are believed to be combustion products of fossil fuels. There is continued concern that chlorofluorocarbons introduced into the atmosphere may deplete the ozone layer. This would result in more ultraviolet light reaching the surface of the Earth and increase the number of cases of skin cancer.

Drinking water pollution: Many carcinogenic chemicals have been identified in drinking water but the extent to which past and present levels contribute to the overall cancer rate is uncertain. Several descriptive epidemiologic studies have suggested an association with an increased risk of cancer but the studies are plagued by confounding variables. A soon to be released NCI epidemiologic study is expected to provide more definitive evidence regarding the association between quality of drinking water and bladder cancer.

Medical drugs and radiation	*Breast, endometrium, ovary, thyroid, bone, lung, blood (leukemia)*	*1–4 percent*

Drugs known to be carcinogenic are used in the treatment of diseases, including some cancers. In addition, hormonal therapies, particularly the estrogens, are firmly linked to an increased cancer risk. Medical radiation exposures are known to have caused cancer and while dosage levels can be estimated, the level of risk from present day exposures is uncertain.

Table 2.—Summary of Cancer-Associated Environmental Factorsa—Continued

Factorb	Sites considered in drawing the estimates	Range of estimates associated with factor
Natural radiation	*Skin, breast, thyroid, lung, bone, blood (leukemia)*	*Less than 1–3 percent*

There is no doubt that natural radiation, consisting of ionizing radiation from cosmic rays and radioactive materials, can cause cancer. While disagreements persist regarding the amount of risk associated with low-level ionizing radiation, the estimates generally agree within one order of magnitude. Ultraviolet radiation from the Sun is believed responsible for most of the 400,000 nonmelanoma skin cancers. These tumors are not usually included in quantitative estimates of cancer rates because they are poorly recorded and generally curable. They are not included here.

Consumer products	*Possibly all sites*	*Less than 1–2 percent*

Substances known to be carcinogenic are present in consumer products at usually very low levels. The extent to which they contribute to the overall cancer rate is uncertain.

Unknown associations	*All sites*	*(?)*

Many substances have not been tested for carcinogenicity and associations between some of those substances and cancer may exist. Furthermore, substances newly introduced into the environment may have an impact in the future. In particular, there is concern that point sources of pollutants, such as dumps, may be contributing to cancer. Because the associations are unknown, the estimate is uncertain but it is certainly not zero. Additionally, stress, which may be manifested by overeating, smoking, or in other ways, probably plays a role in cancer causation.

aMany cancers may be associated with more than one factor. Factors are not mutually exclusive, and the total, if all associations were known, would add to much more than 100 percent.
bEstimates are listed under the factors that most closely approximate the description published with them. The estimates are detailed and their sources referenced in ch. 3.
cRange of single estimate.
SOURCE: Office of Technology Assessment.

either in their food, water, air, or (less frequently) by force feeding, skin painting, or injection. As the animals die, or when the survivors are killed at the end of the exposure period (which is generally the lifespan of the animal), a pathologist examines them for tumors. The number of tumors in the exposed animals is then compared with the number in a group of "control" animals. The controls are treated exactly as the experimentals except that they are not exposed to the chemical under test. The finding of a significant excess of tumors in the exposed animals compared with the number found in controls in a well-designed, well-executed animal test for carcinogenicity leads to a conclusion that the chemical is a carcinogen in that species.

IARC has reviewed the literature concerning 362 substances which have been tested in animals and considers the data "sufficient" to conclude that 121 are carcinogens. For about 100 others, there was "limited" evidence of carcinogenicity, indicating that further information is desirable, but that the available evidence produces a strong warning about carcinogenicity. Data were "insufficient" to make decisions about the carcinogenicity of the remaining substances. The IARC review program is active and continuing and updates it findings periodically.

The reliability of animal tests, bioassays, depends on their design and execution. NCI published guidelines for bioassays in 1976. Bioassays now cost between $400,000 and $1 million and require up to 5 years to complete. Clearly such expensive tools should be used only to test highly suspect chemicals, and much effort is devoted to selecting chemicals for testing.

Molecular structure analysis and examination of basic chemical and physical properties are used to make preliminary decisions about the likelihood of a chemical being a carcinogen and whether or not to test it. For instance, greater suspicion is attached to chemicals that share common features with identified carcinogens. Unfortunately, not all members of a structural class behave similarly, which places limits on this approach. In making decisions about whether chemicals should be tested further, scientists consider other data, including any available toxicological information. These preliminary decisions may be critical, because if a decision is made not to test a substance, nothing more may be learned about its toxicity. The wrong decision might result in a carcinogen entering the environment and being ignored until it causes disease in a large number of people.

The most exciting new developments in testing are the short-term tests, which cost from a few hundred to a few thousand dollars and require a few days to months to complete. Such tests have been under development for about 15 years, and most depend on biologically measuring interactions between the suspect chemical and the genetic material, deoxyribonucleic acid (DNA). The best-known test, the "Ames test," measures mutagenicity (capacity to cause genetic changes) in bacteria. Other short-term tests use micro-organisms, nonmammalian laboratory animals, and cultured human and animal cells. Some measure mutagenicity and some the capacity of a chemical to alter DNA metabolism or to transform a normal cell into a cell exhibiting abnormal growth characteristics.

Many chemicals that have already been identified as carcinogens or noncarcinogens in bioassays have also been assayed in short-term tests to measure congruence between the two types of tests. Results from these "validation" studies vary, but up to 90 percent of both carcinogens and noncarcinogens were correctly classified by short-term tests. These figures are sometimes questioned because they were derived from studies that excluded classes of chemicals known to be difficult to classify by

the short-term tests being evaluated. However, the International Program for the Evaluation of Short-Term Tests for Carcinogenicity concluded that the Ames test, in combination with other tests, correctly identified about 80 percent of the tested carcinogens and noncarcinogens. That study purposefully included some chemicals known to be difficult to classify by short-term tests, and it further demonstrates the promise of short-term tests.

Short-term tests now play an important role in "screening" substances to aid in making decisions about whether or not to test them in animals. The role of short-term tests is expected to increase in the future as more such tests are developed and validated. However, the eventual replacement of animal tests by short-term tests is probably some time away.

One factor likely to retard replacement of animal tests by short-term tests is the poor quantitative agreement between the two kinds of tests. Qualitative agreement, as measured in validation studies, is good—i.e., a mutagen is very likely to be a carcinogen—but poor quantitative agreement means that a powerful mutagen may be a weak carcinogen or the other way around. Additionally, because there is some evidence to support the idea that the potency of a carcinogen in animals is predictive of its potency in humans, the poor agreement about potency between animal and short-term tests may inhibit wider use of the latter tests.

PROGRAMS TO IDENTIFY CARCINOGENS

Government Programs

The most important recent development in governmental management of test development and implementation is the establishment of NTP by the Department of Health, Education, and Welfare in 1978. The program encompasses the short-term and bioassay testing activities of the Department of Health and Human Services (DHHS) but not the testing programs that exist in other executive branch departments. Other agencies with a stake in carcinogen testing, the Environmental Protection Agency (EPA), the

Consumer Product Safety Commission (CPSC), and the Occupational Safety and Health Administration (OSHA), participate in the selection of substances to be tested by NTP. Each of these agencies retains responsibility for development of policies and guidelines for testing and interpretation of results under the laws that they administer.

NTP has assumed the management of the carcinogen bioassay program that was formerly located at NCI. This is the largest single test program, and began the testing of about 50 chemicals in fiscal year 1980; the number will drop to about 30 in fiscal year 1981 because of budgetary limitations.

Government-sponsored cancer epidemiology is supported principally by the National Institutes of Health, with the National Institute of Occupational Safety and Health, and other agencies carrying out some research. Epidemiologic research is marked by flexibility in experimental design, and it has not been placed under an umbrella organization like NTP.

Nongovernment Programs

Many chemical, drug, and petroleum companies have large, active, inhouse toxicology and epidemiology units. These resources are employed to develop information about substances of concern to the companies and also to supply data to Federal regulatory agencies. One of the most modern toxicology laboratories is that of the Chemical Industry Institute of Toxicology (CIIT). This laboratory recently completed extensive testing of formaldehyde, which demonstrated that the chemical causes nasal cancer in rats. CPSC and other agencies have proposed regulations to curtail exposures to formaldehyde based on information from CIIT studies.

Many epidemiologic studies and much of the development of test procedures take place in academic institutions. Funding for these activities comes from both Federal and non-Federal sources, and these institutions have been important in gaining knowledge and improving techniques.

ANALYSES OF TEST RESULTS

Results from tests are conveniently discussed as being "positive," "negative," or "inconclusive." A "positive" test is sufficient to convince all (or most) experts that the tested substance causes the measured effect—e.g., cancer in bioassay. Similarly, a "negative" result is one that convinces all (or most) experts that the tested substance does not exert the effect measured in the test. "Inconclusive" means that no conclusion can be drawn from the test. Test results are analyzed initially by the scientists who conduct the tests. Their conclusions may be reviewed by other experts later on, and such peer review is important for the acceptance or rejection of the conclusions.

Positive epidemiologic results show an association between an exposure or behavior and human cancer. When they are available and based on a valid study, they tend to dominate any decision to be made about carcinogenicity. When no or limited epidemiologic data are available, bioassays which measure carcinogenicity in intact animals are the most important source of information. The last decade saw Government organizations, Congress, executive agencies, and the courts, as well as private sector organizations endorse bioassays and agree that they can be used to identify potential human carcinogens. For instance, IARC concluded:

> . . . it is reasonable, for practical purposes, to regard chemicals for which there is sufficient evidence of carcinogenicity . . . in animals as if they presented a carcinogenic risk for humans.

The use of short-term test results varies depending on whether the substance being tested is *in use* or *new*. When making decisions about currently used chemicals, short-term test results are used to decide whether or not to proceed to a bioassay, and they are accorded a supporting role in making decisions about carcinogenicity.

In industry, short-term tests play a role in making decisions about whether or not to proceed with *development* of a new chemical. A positive result, indicating that the cost of developing the chemical for market might have to include extensive and expensive toxicological testing, may be factored into a manufacturer's decision to develop or not to develop a chemical. A risky chemical may be dropped from consideration for further development.

A problem that bedevils decisionmaking is the existence of both "positive" and "negative" results from tests of the same substance. Careful analysis of the design and execution of the "positive" and "negative" tests sometimes resolves the discrepancies and allows reconciliation of the results. When the conflicting results cannot be explained, more importance is attached to the positive results.

It is not possible to say how many of the 55,000 chemicals in commerce are carcinogens. About 7,000 have been tested in bioassay, and 10 to 16 percent were "positive." However, this percentage has little meaning when discussing all chemicals. There is a strong bias toward testing risky chemicals, as is shown by the fact that about half of 190 chemicals tested in NCI's bioassay program were reported to be positive. On the other hand, many tests done years ago are insensitive by today's standards and that would tend to decrease the percentage of substances detected as carcinogens.

The IARC list of 18 human carcinogens, plus tobacco smoke, alcohol, radiation, and the 18 probable human carcinogens, provide a minimal answer to the question of how many substances are known to cause or probably cause human cancer. The IARC list of 121 substances that produced "sufficient" evidence for carcinogenicity in animals expands the number of substances that must be considered as carcinogenic hazards for humans. These two lists add up to the "rock-bottom" number of about 160 substances. How many more carcinogens will be identified is uncertain, and what is known about the tested chemicals may be overshadowed by what is unknown both about untested chemicals and about complex human exposures and behaviors that are not amenable to laboratory testing.

EXTRAPOLATION FROM TEST RESULTS TO ESTIMATES OF HUMAN CANCER INCIDENCE

Extrapolation techniques are used to estimate the probability of human cancer from study-derived data. Extrapolation can be divided into two parts. "Biologic extrapolation" involves the use of scaling factors to make adjustments between biologic effects in small, short-lived laboratory animals and in humans. "Numeric extrapolation" models are used to estimate the probability of cancer at doses below those administered to animals in a test and to estimate cancer incidence at exposure levels other than those measured in epidemiologic studies.

Some extrapolation models assume a "threshold" dose, a nonzero dose below which exposures are "safe" and not associated with risk. Individual thresholds may exist, because not all individuals exposed to similar levels of carcinogens develop cancer, but such differences in sensitivity may also be explained by differences in luck rather than in biology. However, it is generally accepted that a population threshold which would define a "risk-free" dose for a group of people composed of diverse individuals, if it exists, cannot now be demonstrated. Federal agencies do not accept the idea of thresholds in making decisions about carcinogenic risks.

Numeric extrapolation models differ in the incidence of cancer that they predict from a given exposure. Extrapolation models which assume that incidence at low-exposure levels is directly proportional to dose generally estimate higher incidences. Such "linear" models are "conservative" in that, if they err, they overestimate the amount of disease to be expected. All governmental agencies that use extrapolation employ linear models for predicting cancer incidence. Other models project risks that decrease more rapidly than dose, and they are advanced as alternatives to the linear model. The choice of a model is important because, if an acceptable level of risk were decided on, almost any other model would allow higher exposures than do linear models.

Opinions differ about whether and how extrapolation methods should be used in estimating the amount of human cancer that might be caused by exposure to a carcinogen:

- Some individuals object to any use of numeric extrapolation. For them, identification of a substance as a carcinogen is enough to justify efforts to reduce or to eliminate exposure.
- Other people see extrapolation as useful to separate more risky from less risky substances.
- The most extensive use of extrapolation is recommended by people who urge that extrapolation methods be used to estimate quantitatively the amount of human cancer likely to result from exposures. Such estimates are seen as necessary by those who wish to compare quantitatively the risks and benefits from carcinogens.

The disagreements among the groups who hold different opinions about use of extrapolation are vocal and current. A particular problem in quantitative extrapolation arises from the fact that different extrapolation models produce estimates of cancer incidence that differ by factors of 1,000 or more at levels of human exposure. Given such uncertainty, some labor and environmental organizations and many individuals refuse to choose one model or another for estimating the impact of a carcinogen on humans, and oppose the use of quantitative extrapolation. Fewer objections are raised against choosing a model to order carcinogens on the basis of their likelihood of causing cancer. Regardless of which particular model is chosen,

it should produce approximately the same relative ranking as any other.

Proponents of quantitative extrapolation argue that careful attention to the available data aids in choosing the correct model and reduces chances for error. Arguments about the applicability of these techniques will continue, especially because efforts to apply cost-benefit analysis to making decisions about carcinogens will require quantitative estimates of cancer incidence.

There are now no convincing data to dictate which extrapolation model is best for estimating human cancer incidence, whether from epidemiologic data or animal data, or even that one model will be consistently better than all others. However, one particular model for estimating human incidence from animal data (linear, no threshold extrapolation and relating animal and humans on the basis of total lifetime exposure divided by body weight) has been reported to estimate human cancer incidence within a factor of 10 to 100 when compared to incidence measured by epidemiologic studies. While this agreement is gratifyingly good, data exist to make these comparisons for fewer than 20 substances.

STATUTORY AND REGULATORY DEFINITIONS OF "CARCINOGEN"

Regulation of carcinogens has been marked by repeated arguments about the amount and kind of evidence necessary to make decisions to regulate substances as carcinogens. Several Federal documents describe the types of tests agencies will consider and the criteria they will apply to make such decisions. Statements of regulatory agency policy are found in EPA's Interim Guideline for Carcinogenic Risk Assessment, EPA's air carcinogen policy statement, OSHA's generic cancer policy, and the Regulatory Council's policy statement, which drew heavily on

recommendations of the Interagency Regulatory Liaison Group (IRLG). IRLG now coordinates Federal regulatory agency discussion about identifying and characterizing toxic substances, including carcinogens.

All Federal agencies accept positive epidemiologic studies as strong evidence for carcinogenicity, and a positive bioassay result in a single species as evidence that the substance is a potential human carcinogen. All relegate short-term tests to a supporting role. Trade associations, such as the American Industrial Health Council (AIHC), fault the regulatory agency policies. AIHC insists that positive bioassays in two different species should be required to define a carcinogen.

The importance of the dispute about whether a positive test in only one of two test species or positive tests in both species is necessary to reach a conclusion about potential human carcinogenicity is illustrated by an analysis of NCI bioassay data. Of 190 chemicals tested, 98 were judged positive in either one or two species. While 44 were positive in both species, 54 were positive in either the rat or the mouse, but not both. Although different analytical techniques can reduce the number of discrepant results, there is now no resolution to the arguments raised by one positive result in a two-species test. The agencies take the position that public health considerations require that results from the more sensitive animal be taken as indicating the substance is a potential human carcinogen, and others disagree.

An epidemiologic study that is not positive demonstrates that no excess cancer was detected in that study. Clearly a study that examines large numbers of people over a long period of time is more likely to detect carcinogenic risks than a smaller, shorter study. In general, epidemiology cannot detect risks at the level predicted from animal tests, and agencies specify stringent requirements under which they would weigh negative epidemiologic data against positive animal data. Judicial decisions have supported the prominent role given to "positive" animal tests.

AIHC urges that all epidemiologic evidence be considered because of uncertainties in extrapolating from animals to humans, and because human response may differ from that of test animals. Furthermore, AIHC sees epidemiologic studies as useful for putting a limit on the amount of risk associated with a substance.

FEDERAL GOVERNMENT DECISIONMAKING ABOUT CARCINOGENICITY

Scientists in each regulatory agency review study designs and results to decide for their own agency whether or not a substance is a carcinogen and, in some cases, to estimate the number of cancers it may cause.

Suggestions have been made by the various groups to change the process used in deciding whether or not a substance is a potential human carcinogen for regulatory purposes. The suggestions propose that a single panel of scientists evaluate study results for all Government agencies. A panel, depending on the particular proposal, might be composed of Federal scientists, non-Federal scientists, or both. The panel would report its finding to all regulatory agencies. These proposals separate the "scientific" decisions about the toxicity of the substance and its possible impact on humans from the "policy"

decision about how to reduce risks it may pose to humans. Policy actions to be taken on the results of the scientific decision would remain the responsibility of the regulatory agencies.

Proponents claim a panel would improve the efficiency of the regulatory process. It would make technical decisions for all the agencies, rather than each agency making its own. Secondly, a time limit could be imposed on panel deliberations to ensure that its work is completed quickly. Finally, under some proposals, a regulatory agency would initiate the panel review of data about a suspect substance, and therefore the review could take place when it best fits the agency schedule.

Public interest, labor, environmental organizations, and Federal regulatory agencies oppose these suggestions. They see the regulatory agencies as the appropriate and lawful locations for making decisions about risk. In general, they see a science panel as another layer of bureaucracy that might hinder regulatory activities, and worry that a single panel might be more sensitive to pressure from interested parties. Furthermore, they see the division between "science" and "policy" in decisions about cancer as illusionary. They argue that such a panel might have the power to delay decisions by imposing a higher standard of proof that a substance is a carcinogen than is required by law. This, they say, would stymie preventive "precautionary" governmental action that they view as necessary to protect lives and health when certainty cannot be achieved.

The number of proposals for risk-determination panels almost guarantees that the panels will remain an issue in Federal policy about carcinogens. Establishment of such a panel would represent a significant change in how the Federal Government makes decisions about health risks and would probably require specific legislation. In November 1980, Congress provided $0.5 million to the Food and Drug Administration (FDA) to place a contract to investigate the feasibility of a panel. The report from the study is expected by the end of 1982.

REGULATED CARCINOGENS

Approximately 96 substances have been regulated as carcinogens or suspect carcinogens, and an additional 49 toxic chemicals which have been identified as carcinogens by EPA are required to be considered for regulation under the 1977 Clean Water Act Amendments. When overlaps between the list of already regulated substances and those required for regulation are taken into account, there is a total of approximately 102 substances. Fifty-seven of those substances are regulated under more than one law. This is expected because exposures to a carcinogen may occur in air, in water, from solid waste on land, and in the workplace so a carcinogen may be regulated under several statutes. Twenty-one of the substances that are regulated under a single law are FDA-regulated components of food.

COLLECTION AND COORDINATION OF EXPOSURE AND HEALTH DATA

Congress has enacted several pieces of legislation that require Federal agencies to control carcinogenic chemicals. OSHA is responsible for the occupational setting; CPSC, consumer products; FDA, some food, drugs, and cosmetics; EPA, the "environment" (air, water, and soil); and the Department of Agriculture, food. In order to meet their responsibilities, agencies must collect information and assess risks.

Data about exposure histories and health status are useful in assessing associations between the environment and cancer. Both types of information are collected by Federal agencies but often in separate data systems in different agencies. Because of privacy and confidentiality restrictions, these records can seldom be brought together to "link" information pertaining to an individual. In general, these records either cannot be made available to researchers or can be made available only without personal identifiers, which makes linkage impossible. Efforts to ease these restrictions are being pursued.

Federal, State, and local groups collect environmental data for a multitude of reasons, and individual programs periodically review their monitoring capabilities and directions. However, there is no federally coordinated focus to review the quality and quantity of data that are collected. Thus, there is no assurance that adequate exposure data are collected for identifying and estimating carcinogenic risks.

The Toxic Substances Control Act (TSCA) of 1976 was designed to strengthen the ability of the Federal Government to accumulate information on potentially hazardous substances and to protect the public from their risks. TSCA required establishment of new programs at EPA, and, not unexpectedly, there have been difficulties. A 1980 General Accounting Office (GAO) review concluded that EPA's "disappointing" progress in implementing TSCA was partly because of too few staff members and recruitment problems.

TSCA's authority for acquiring information to assess carcinogenic risks differs, depending on whether chemicals are "new" or "existing" in commerce. Companies must notify EPA in a "premanufacture notice" (PMN) of their intention to manufacture or import a new substance at least 90 days in advance. Based upon information submitted by industry, EPA then decides if the new substance "may present an unreasonable risk" to health or the environment. If EPA concludes such a risk may exist, it can require additional information before allowing manufacture.

EPA has been hampered in evaluating PMNs because more than 60 percent of the first 199 PMNs contained no toxicity data. EPA has had to rely on molecular-structure analysis and, when available, short-term test results to make premanufacture decisions. EPA has twice asked for additional information that was not included on the PMN, and each time the company decided not to generate the data and not to manufacture. To improve the availability of data, EPA is considering following the lead of the Organization for Economic Cooperation and Development and requiring submission of a base set of data including short-term test results before it will permit manufacture. However, requiring testing of chemicals simply because they are "new" is not now possible, and TSCA would have to be amended to permit it.

If EPA does not take regulatory action on a PMN, the substance may be produced and used as desired. However, it does not mean that the substance is safe or approved. Once production of the chemical is initiated, it is no longer classified as new, and EPA can require testing under the provisions for existing chemicals. EPA can also issue a "significant new use rule" (SNUR) for a new chemical when there is concern that specific uses of the chemical, other than those specified in the PMN, might pose a risk. An SNUR requires that EPA be notified before the substance is used in a manner covered by the SNUR. To date, one SNUR has been proposed, and EPA is considering SNURs on more than 40 chemicals for which PMNs were received.

One of TSCA's first activities related to existing chemicals was the compilation of an inventory of chemical substances manufactured in the United States. The initial inventory, published 18 months late in June 1979 and updated in July 1980, lists about 55,000 chemicals. EPA can, by rule, require industry testing of potentially harmful chemicals present in commerce if the available information, while insufficient for an evaluation of risk, supports the finding that the chemicals "may present an unreasonable risk" or may result in substantial or significant exposure. Screening all chemicals in commerce to choose those few most needing testing is a large task, and TSCA established the Interagency Testing Committee (ITC) to make recommendations about which chemicals should be tested. ITC has recommended about 50 chemicals to EPA, but EPA has been unsuccessful in meeting deadlines for ordering tests to be done. EPA was sued by the Natural Resources Defense Council because it failed to meet TSCA-specified deadlines, and it is now developing test rules under a schedule that was produced in response to a court order.

A 1980 GAO report estimated that the initiation of a rule to require testing can take as long as 5 years, and up to 54 months is then allowed to complete a chronic bioassay for carcinogenicity. Hence, 9 years or more may elapse before information about a chemical's potential carcinogenicity is available under the testing provisions of TSCA.

Environmental groups are critical of EPA's slow progress in test-rule development and argue that EPA could move more quickly. In particular, they cite EPA's exhaustive review of the literature about a substance as being unnecessarily thorough for test-rule development. EPA cites problems that it anticipates if its literature reviews are not so complete, as well as problems it has faced in establishing the new program, as reasons for its slow progress. From the other side, industry objects to some EPA procedures, including the agency's intention to require testing of some chemicals as representative of "chemical categories." Industry suggests that identifying members of a category as carcinogens will falsely prejudice attitudes towards other members of that category. EPA counters that testing certain representative members of categories will be more efficient than testing chemicals on a one-by-one basis and that the public is better served by testing the wider range of chemicals that can be accomplished under a category approach. EPA's first proposed test rule specified testing of 5 chemicals from a category that included 11 chemicals.

LAWS THAT PROVIDE FOR THE REGULATION OF CARCINOGENIC RISKS

Reflecting public concern about cancer, Congress has enacted laws to regulate exposures to carcinogens in order to protect public health. The laws were written at different times by different Congresses and are directed at controlling exposures from different sources. Not unexpectedly, the laws differ in the amount and type of evidence they require, and some do and some do not require that benefits of the carcinogen be balanced against its risks in making decisions about regulation. "Zero-risk" laws, such as the Delaney clause of the Food, Drug, and Cosmetic Act, and the Resource Conservation and Recovery Act, direct regulatory agencies to eliminate risks without consideration of other factors. Because the Federal Government does not accept a threshold level for carcinogens, a strict interpretation of these laws would require that risk be entirely eliminated. Proponents of these laws point to the limited benefits associated with food additives or pollutants escaping from dumps and argue for allowing no risk from such exposures. The opponents suggest that consumers might choose an additive in spite of its risks and that reducing low-level risks from dumps may cost too much.

The "technology-based" laws, such as the Clean Water Act, direct EPA to impose specific levels of control, considering technical and economic feasibility. The Clean Air Act and the Occupational Safety and Health Act are also largely technology based. In practice, regulations from these laws direct that pollutants or exposures be controlled by installation of specified control devices.

The "balancing" laws, the Federal Insecticide, Fungicide, and Rodenticide Act, TSCA, and the Consumer Product Safety Act direct agencies to consider other factors in addition to health risk in promulgating regulations. For instance, TSCA directs EPA to control "unreasonable risks" and gives the agency some leeway in deciding what to regulate and how stringently to regulate.

An example of the complexity of the laws and of regulations based on them is provided by the Clean Air Act. The section of the Act providing for the regulation of airborne toxic substances from stationary sources was written as "zero-risk." However, EPA's proposed airborne carcinogen policy concluded that such stringent control was not always feasible because elimination of exposure to some carcinogens might cause too much economic disruption. EPA has proposed that it will first apply a technology-based standard for control and then, if necessary, balance risks and other factors in making a decision about whether any residual risk is "unreasonable" and requires further regulation. The "unreasonable-risk" decision is analogous to EPA requirements under TSCA. The Clean Air Act, then, was written as zero-risk, but regulations from it are first technology based and then balancing.

Congress, reflecting the difficulties inherent in regulating when risks and benefits are uncertain and difficult to quantify, delegated to the agencies the task of operationally defining certain key balancing terms. Words in the laws, for instance, those requiring EPA to regulate "unreasonable risks" under TSCA, were purposefully left undefined. The agencies and the courts, by their decisions, are now defining those terms.

Some regulatory agency lawyers have been asked about the ability of the agencies to work within the confines of the present laws. They expressed confidence that the agencies can administer the balancing laws (such as TSCA) and apparently appreciate the flexibility of the laws as they are now written.

Other observers are of the opinion that greater attention to the balancing terms in the law would improve the regulatory processes. To some extent, defining a balance may mean accepting a specified risk, and Congress, composed of elected representatives, is most often seen as the body to decide on such a level. Congress already avails itself of opportunities during oversight and reauthorization hearings to question agencies and other organizations about difficulties in implementing the laws. Continuation of these activities may be sufficient to satisfy Congress that the language of the laws does or does not present a problem that can be rectified by congressional action.

BALANCING RISKS, COSTS, AND BENEFITS IN DECISIONS ABOUT REGULATING CARCINOGENS

Beyond the technical level of deciding whether or not a substance is a carcinogen and estimating the amount of human cancer it may cause is any decision that requires weighing risks against the benefits of its continued use. The decision is complicated by equity considerations. The people who most directly bear risks from exposures to carcinogens are not necessarily the people who most directly benefit from the activities that produce the risk. Depending on conditions, either the risks or the benefits may be accorded greater quantitative importance.

Numerous surveys show that society wants protection from health risks and is willing to pay for it. At the same time, economic and other considerations cause society to attempt to spend no more than is necessary. Uncertainties attached to estimates of health risks and economic benefits complicate regulatory decisionmaking. Improvements in cancer risk identification and measurement will reduce the uncertainty, but balancing health risks against costs of control and the benefits of the regulated substance will remain a difficult value judgment.

REGULATORY REFORM

Concern about increasing regulatory costs and burdens in recent years has produced a push for changes in regulatory decisionmaking. Charges of overregulation or untimely regulation have been leveled at many programs, including those that regulate exposures to carcinogens.

Current procedural reform proposals include:

- more emphasis on regulatory benefit-cost analysis;

- more systematic regulatory review;
- more flexibility in rulemaking;
- appointment of additional administrative law judges and greater involvement of the Administrative Conference; and
- providing financial assistance to public intervenors who are seen to be at a disadvantage when opposed by resources of industry or agencies.

Each of these proposals is directed at improving regulatory decisionmaking, but not all would have the same effect. Increased emphasis on benefit-cost analysis will impose an additional hurdle for proposed regulations and reduce the number and the cost of regulations. Opponents of this proposal cite problems with the quantification of costs and benefits and its ignoring of equity considerations. They object to it as another barrier against regulations that they see as necessary to protect health and environment.

Systematic regulatory review, whether by the President, Congress, or courts, is also designed to reduce the number and cost of regulations. Opponents again object to the imposition of an additional hurdle to the promulgation of what they see as desirable regulations. Additionally, they see the review as stripping the agencies of some of the authority delegated to them by Congress and putting technical decisions into organizations which lack the necessary experience and knowledge to deal with them.

More flexibility in rulemaking would alter agency regulatory proceedings. The first stage of proceedings might be conducted as an informal hearing, without employing trial-type procedures. The right of cross-examination and use of the full adversary process would be reserved only for those issues which warranted further proceedings, as determined by the presiding hearing officer. Such increased flexibility might significantly expedite the entire administrative decisionmaking process.

Appointment of more administrative law judges and greater involvement of the Administrative Conference in reviewing judicial performance is intended to make the current regulatory process more responsive. Systematic regulatory review by the courts might increase the need for administrative law judges.

Public intervenors from consumer, environmental, or other groups often have interest in regulations. They are sometimes hampered in their efforts to participate in regulatory hearings because of lack of finances. Providing such groups with financial assistance would allow them to be heard. This proposal is opposed by those who believe public financing should not be provided to private "public interest" groups.

The regulatory reform proposals reach to the heart of the Federal Government's role in protecting the health and the economic interests of the public, both as a whole, and as composed of diverse groups, such as labor and industry. The decision that its current activities are appropriate and sufficient or that they should be curtailed or expanded will involve profound and basic social, political, and equity considerations. Cancer may be the focus for such debates about health regulation. Its toll in death and suffering is large, it is widely feared, efforts to gain knowledge of its causes often depend on measures with wide margins of error, and payoffs from reduced exposures may be years or even decades away. The debate will involve more than technical issues.

OPTIONS

Options for improving technologies for determining cancer risks from the environment are divided into four groups. The first group (options 1 through 4) is concerned with gathering information about the occurrence and distribution of cancer in the population and carcinogenic risks in the environment. The second group (options 5 through 7) is related to testing substances for carcinogenicity. Options 8 through 10 relate to TSCA and its implementation. The final option is concerned with possible changes in the process used by regulatory agencies in making technical decisions about carcinogens.

Methods for obtaining better information about the occurrence, distribution, and outcome of cancer.

These four options are discussed separately and can be considered for implementation separately. Adoption of any or all of the options would improve the quality and quantity of data available to draw conclusions about the occurrence and distribution of cancer. This information would allow more precise estimates to be made about the incidence of cancer and therefore allow accurate monitoring of cancer trends. Results from the specific studies in option 3 might clarify many questions about relationships between particular exposures and behaviors and cancer. They would be immediately useful for prevention programs.

OPTION 1

Expand the operation of NCI's SEER program to collect cancer incidence and survival data representative of the entire country and design programs to assess validity of collected data.

The SEER program, which started in 1973, is the first continuous cancer incidence reporting program in the United States and provides an approximation of cancer incidence and survival rates for the country as a whole. The SEER program has been and should continue to be a useful source of identified cancer cases which greatly facilitates studies about the disease. Detailed diagnostic information is available on each case recorded by the SEER program, and patients, family members, and friends can be queried to learn more about exposures, behaviors, and occurrence of cancer.

SEER program data are collected from about 10 percent of the total population, but the geographical regions covered by the SEER program do not closely represent the demographic makeup of the entire country. A slightly expanded SEER program could encompass more of the country and be constructed so as to collect data representative of the entire population. Expanded coverage would generate data for a more careful and detailed examination of cancer rates over time than what is now possible. An important component of an expanded SEER program could be rigorous examination of the validity of the collected data. For instance, the accuracy of diagnoses and transfer of the diagnosis information to the SEER program data could be monitored to reduce uncertainties about data. Such attention to data reliability would make conclusions drawn from the data more convincing and accepted.

The current SEER program costs about $10 million annually out of the total NCI budget of about $1 billion. Expanding the program would cost more money and would also require cooperation of additional local medical organizations to establish new SEER data collection areas. Balanced against these costs are opportunities to gather incidence and survival data representative of the whole country and to learn more about cancer in the U.S. population.

OPTION 2

Establish a National Cancer Registry (NCR) to record all new cases of cancer in the United States.

An NCR would provide the most comprehensive data possible on cancer incidence in this country. With a national registry, cancer would become a reportable disease, as are some infectious diseases. This data base would be useful for trend analysis and for identifying cancer cases for epidemiologic study. The NCR would record the date on which cancer was diagnosed and could be used in conjunction with the National Death Index to generate information about survival.

An NCR would collect less detailed information on each case than is now collected by the SEER program, but would record on the order of ten times more cases. Establishing an NCR would not reduce the need for the SEER program, but rather would add to the cancer incidence data base.

About 30 States presently have enacted regulations or laws requiring that cancer cases be reported to a central authority, but most of those States have not yet initiated programs to implement the laws. Establishment of an NCR which would invite States to participate might provide incentive for States to implement their own programs. At the Federal level, the Centers for Disease Control, or another appropriate organization, might serve as the agency for receiving, storing, and disseminating registry data.

The establishment of a well-structured NCR might become a seed project for a comprehensive registry for many chronic diseases of national importance. The interrelationships and multifactorial nature of chronic diseases make this a worthwhile step towards the goal of understanding major public health problems.

As a new venture, NCR would require much money and, perhaps, a long time before it became useful for truly national studies. However, it would be immediately useful in identifying cancer cases for study. The percentage of cases reported to it, if the experience of other registries is an accurate indication, would increase with time. This increase might produce an artifactual "cancer epidemic" as better reporting showed an increase in cases regardless of actual trends, but such a development can be anticipated.

OPTION 3

Encourage epidemiologic studies to answer specific questions. Three such studies might be:

- study of workplace-related cancers;
- study of cancer and dietary habits; and
- study of respiratory cancer.

Study of Workplace-Related Cancers.—There is a controversy over the amount of cancer associated with occupational exposures. Many currently available study results lend themselves to various interpretations. Additional studies might help resolve the existing controversies and, more importantly, might pinpoint opportunities for regulatory and voluntary reduction in exposures. The National Institute of Occupational Safety and Health now conducts workplace carcinogenicity studies and continuing its support is one mechanism to obtain more information.

Cohort studies identify and follow healthy people with a common characteristic or exposure to look for associations with subsequent cancer occurrence. Such studies could be initiated to examine the cancer risk posed by occupational exposures to chemicals now identified as carcinogens in laboratory tests or suspect for other reasons. Priority consideration might be given to those chemicals perceived to have a higher degree of risk, to which many people are exposed, and for which means of control exist.

Study of cancer incidence and mortality at body sites known or thought to be associated with occupational exposures could be examined in case-control studies, which compare exposures and behavioral histories of people afflicted with cancer (cases) with those of unafflicted persons (controls). Lung cancer is the most common occupationally related cancer. Other types, including nasopharyngeal carcinoma, melanoma, bladder and brain cancers are worthy of study, because of past associations with occupational factors, but no site is free of suspected occupational associations.

The availability of exposure data is a particularly acute problem to be addressed in designing any occupational study. Monitoring in the workplace is now required only for a few chemicals already regulated by OSHA, and although some companies monitor levels of suspect substances, no information is routinely available for many other chemicals. However, OSHA now requires that a company retain all exposure records that it collects and any collected data can be made available for study. For cohort studies, it may be necessary to initiate and continue monitoring for many years before results are obtainable. Results from such studies are considered very powerful.

Studies of Cancer and Dietary Habits.—Diet is generally considered an important factor in cancer causation, but few specifics are known. Long-term cohort studies could be designed to investigate relationships between dietary variables and cancer. For example, different ethnic populations with distinct eating habits could be followed and their cancer incidence ascertained over the years. Such studies are expensive and time-consuming, but they may provide otherwise unobtainable information about risk factors and protective agents in food.

Large-scale case-control studies also could investigate hypotheses relating diet and particular cancer sites. Congress mandated one such study to investigate whether or not nonnutritive sweeteners cause human bladder cancer. The study involved questioning of 3,000 persons with bladder cancer (cases) and 6,000 others without bladder cancer (controls). The study showed "that past artificial sweetener use has had a minimal effect, if any, on bladder cancer rates." The same study was used to investigate possible links between water quality and bladder cancer. Results from that part of the study are expected to be published in 1981. Case-control studies might also associate particular diets with reduced cancer risks which would provide information immediately useful for prevention.

The long latent period between exposures associated with cancer and manifestation of the disease makes associations between them difficult to determine. One possible way to improve this situation, especially for diet-related cancer research, might be to establish a Biological Samples Bank. Such a bank would store samples of urine, hair, blood, feces, and perhaps tissues, as well as answers to questions about diet, recreation, and work from as many as a quarter-million people. An additional activity of the bank would be to obtain a copy of the death certificate for each person represented in the bank. The certificate would be included in the individual record. The data could be stored on microfiche, and the biological samples would be stored under the best possible conditions. No additional processing of the sample and data would be undertaken by the bank, but they would be held until requested by researchers. A researcher investigating a particular illness or cause of death could request questionnaire data and biological samples collected from people who became sick with or who died from that disease. The same information and samples obtained from people who were not afflicted would provide control data.

The Biological Samples Bank would have some of the advantages of large-scale cohort studies but at lower cost. Money would not be expended in following individuals for long periods of time or in carrying out analyses that would not be utilized, and a charge levied for each sample provided to a researcher would offset some of the costs of the program. The bank would allow both Government and non-Government scientists to test hypotheses in a wide range of areas. The program would be far larger than anything like it ever attempted, and its management would have to be carefully

planned or access to samples might be so cumbersome that the bank would be unusable.

Studies of Respiratory Cancer.—Cancers of the respiratory tract, breast, and colon account for the majority of cancer cases and deaths. Studies which could relate exposures and behaviors with cancer at these sites might produce important information for prevention. In particular, a large case-control study of respiratory cancer would answer several important questions. A sufficiently large study should include on the order of 10,000 cases, about one-tenth of 1 year's total respiratory cancers, and ideally, twice that number of controls. Each case and control would be interviewed to determine smoking habits, place of residence, types of jobs, and eating habits. Case finding and selection of controls could be carried out in a fashion similar to the congressionally mandated study of the effects of nonnutritive sweeteners, which focused on bladder cancer.

This size study should be sensitive enough to detect all numerically important influences in respiratory cancer causation. The major goals of the study, which could be completed in 2 or 3 years, would be to:

- generate an estimate of the contribution of occupational factors and cigarette smoking to respiratory cancer;
- identify hitherto unrecognized occupational respiratory tract carcinogens;
- determine more accurately the effects of "passive smoking" on nonsmoking spouses and children;
- generate a direct estimate of respiratory cancer onset rates in those not exposed to tobacco, either through smoking or passive smoking; and
- obtain direct evidence about different types of cigarettes, including the various low-tar brands, on carcinogenesis.

OPTION 4

Consider for implementation the recommendations made by congressionally mandated commissions and studies for the improvement of Federal environmental health data collection activities.

Congressional and executive branch concern about the adequacy of environmental health data has resulted in the establishment of several advisory groups and studies. Although relatively new, they have already made numerous recommendations for improving Federal environmental health data collection and management. In particular, consideration might be given to recent recommendations made by the Task Force on Environmental Cancer and Heart and Lung Disease and in the NCHS report, *Environmental Health.*

The Task Force recommended:

1. Additional research on methodology to achieve less expensive study design and to improve the collection and evaluation of scientific data.
2. Research on the relative contribution to disease made by substances in air, water, and soil, in order to quantify the toxicological effects and the risks to human health, and to develop strategies for control.
3. Support for environmental and occupational health education and development of career opportunities in primary, secondary, and vocational schools, and better coordination of these activities.

NCHS suggested:

1. Several recommendations concerned with developing interagency data systems and other data-linkage activities to improve epidemiologic study capacity.
2. Procedures and legislation to facilitate the sharing of data among Federal agencies while safeguarding the rights of all individuals.
3. Establishing a mechanism for evaluating priorities in Federal environmental health activities.

Additional recommendations for improved data collection are contained in a report of the Institute of Medicine to DHHS. This planning document on the *Costs of Environment-Related Health Effects* will serve to guide DHHS in its ongoing study mandated by the Health Services Research, Health Statistics, and Health Care Technology act of 1978.

Specific comments about the effects of the Privacy Act and the Tax Reform Act of 1976 on epidemiologic research are to be found in the Report of the Work Group on Records and Privacy of the DHEW Interagency Task Force on the Health Effects of Ionizing Radiation. In addition to suggesting changes in those two acts, the Work Group also discussed changes in the medical records law and the advantages of extending the National Death Index back in time to include deaths that occurred before 1979. Although the report was concerned with radiation risks, its recommendations are applicable to cancer epidemiology in general.

One means of centralizing environmental health data collection activities is to establish a center to coordinate the data collection activities of the Federal Government. With representation from various research and regulatory agencies, the center could provide a mechanism for setting national monitoring priorities. The center would also be in an ideal position for directing research to improve technologies for measuring exposure to environmental agents and to reduce information gaps and duplicative efforts.

The congressionally mandated coordination and review efforts have already been productive, and continuing them has the advantage of building on a base of experience. Congress requires periodic reports from them, and through those and its other oversight responsibilities, Congress can monitor the performance of the advisory groups and studies.

Alternatives for fostering development of short-term tests and an option to expand support of NTP.

OPTION 5

Encourage NTP to pursue the development of tests to replace the long-term carcinogenicity bioassay in small mammals.

Improvements in the design and execution of carcinogenicity bioassay in small laboratory animals have been accompanied by increased acceptance of the results as being predictive for human effects. The tests are used worldwide, scientists continue to discuss and refine them, and in the United States, NTP has improved the management of the Government test program. Despite all this progress, no improvements are expected in two aspects of the tests: they are expensive (up to $1.0 million for each substance tested) and they require a great length of time (from 3 to 5 years).

In its first annual plan (1979), NTP identified the development and validation of less expensive, quicker tests as a priority goal. NTP has outlined a testing scheme involving both short-term and long-term tests and is working to decide which short-term tests work best for identifying a number of toxics, including carcinogens. The attention paid to short-term tests by NTP promises that progress will be made. The concentration of DHHS toxicological expertise in NTP and the development of NTP's working relationships with agencies outside DHHS assure that the program can call on the appropriate people in pursuing the goal of new tests.

Congress might encourage short-term test development and validation in its oversight activities, and it might consider additional funding for the programs. There is currently a great deal of interest in the short-term tests and additional congressional support might have a profound effect on their development.

A potential disadvantage of relying on NTP for guiding and directing this research and development effort is that NTP has many other responsibilities. As discussed in this assessment and in option 7 below, NTP also is responsible for the management of large animal test programs. As a part of a multipurpose program, short-term test development has to compete for resources with other parts of the NTP. If it were decided that short-term tests are sufficiently important to be set apart from other NTP activities, the following option might be considered.

OPTION 6

Establish a commission to advise the Federal Government about optimal methods for development of short-term tests.

A commission, composed of experts from academe, industry, public interest groups, and Government agencies could be established to make recommendations about short-term tests. This would have the advantage of concentrating the talents of diverse people on test development and bringing increased attention to the tests.

The existence of a commission would probably result in short-term tests being given higher priority in NTP. The exact tasks of the commission would be decided by NTP and other parties with interest in the tests. However, one task might be the serious consideration of which, if any, tests offer promise as substitutes for long-term animal carcinogenicity bioassays when making regulatory decisions. The establishment of criteria that a single test or a combination of tests would have to meet to be considered for regulatory decisionmaking would be a spur and a guide to test development. The possible disadvantage of a commission is that it may provide nothing different from what NTP (as in the previous option) might provide.

The commission could focus attention on the tests, the most likely ways for their employment and what criteria they must meet. Adoption of this option would reinforce the conclusions already reached by many experts that the short-term tests show great promise. In a major way, the commission might answer the question "promising for what?"

OPTION 7

Expand support of the National Toxicology Program.

NTP has made a promising start at managing DHHS' short-term testing and animal toxicology programs. As mentioned above, it has identified the desirability of obtaining alternatives to the current carcinogenicity bioassay, and whether the direction of that effort remains within NTP (option 5) or is shared with a commission (option 6), NTP personnel will continue to be involved in test development. In addition to short-term test research, NTP administers the largest animal test program for carcinogenicity. Those expensive and time-consuming tests are used for two general purposes: to test substances that are of interest to regulatory agencies and to provide information useful in developing and validating possible new tests.

NTP has been successful in organizing expert advice for its programs. It has assembled a board of non-Government scientists to advise the overall program, a panel of regulatory agency representatives to aid in selecting chemicals for animal carcingencity bioassay, and, most recently, a panel of nongovernmental experts to review the results of animal tests for carcinogenicity. Each of these efforts increases the sources of advice for NTP, and assures NTP higher visibility.

Arguments for encouraging and expanding NTP center on its promising start, its attention to immediate testing needs through the bioassay program, and from the possibility of future payoffs from new test development. Its establishment of advisory committees of Government and private sector representatives helps assure that it will remain responsive to national needs. A possible disadvantage of NTP is that its wide purview and efforts both to develop test methods and to serve the needs of the regulatory agencies may stretch it too thin. Continued congressional interest and oversight can help avoid this possibility.

Options concerned with EPA's implementation of TSCA:

The following three options discuss collection of sufficient information to protect the public from unreasonable risks, as required by TSCA. The first option is to provide additional support to EPA. The second and third options consider changes in TSCA.

OPTION 8

Increase the resources available to EPA to enable it to assess more effectively potential risks from substances before they are introduced into commerce and from substances already present in commerce.

One of the most important tools for protecting the public from toxic substances is provided in the sections of TSCA which enable EPA to gather information about substances before they are introduced into commerce. The mechanism for obtaining this information is the PMN which must be submitted to EPA 90 days before a manufacturer or processor can *produce* or import a substance. EPA must then evaluate the PMN to determine whether or not the submitted information supports a conclusion that the substance "may present an unreasonable risk." If the decision is made that a substance may present such a risk, EPA can then require submission of additional information before allowing introduction of the substance into commerce.

EPA, which bears responsibility for evaluation of PMNs, is overburdened. EPA estimated that 1,500 people were necessary for the program in fiscal year 1979; 382 permanent positions were authorized; 313 were filled.

A GAO report characterized EPA's progress in implementing TSCA as "disappointing," and drew attention to too few staff members as part of the problem. If more resources are not made available, review of PMNs will likely become less complete, because more are being submitted. EPA estimates that 800 PMNs, almost twice the number in fiscal year 1981, will be submitted in fiscal year 1982.

The premanufacturing review program is designed to screen out risky substances before they enter commerce. Making decisions at that point is more protective of public health, and has the additional advantage of identifying hazards before industry had tied up large amounts of money in manufacture and distribution. Realization of these objectives apparently will require more people as the burden to review PMNs increases at EPA.

Other sections of TSCA specify that EPA can require that industry test substances already present in commerce that "may present an unreasonable risk." Congress, through TSCA, established the Interagency Testing Committee (ITC) to recommend chemicals for testing, and to date EPA has considered only ITC-recommended substances for testing requirements. Even so, EPA has fallen behind schedule in meeting its requirements to develop test rules.

One criticism leveled at EPA's process of developing a test rule is that it spends more effort than necessary to make the case that a substance "may present an unreasonable risk." If the criticism is correct, EPA may be able to improve its procedures and reduce the time and effort necessary to produce test rules. However, even if that is possible, the same EPA program which is overburdened by the PMN process is also responsible for developing test rules.

A critical problem in implementing TSCA has been understaffing. Additional resources should improve EPA's performance in meeting the requirements of TSCA.

OPTION 9

Amend TSCA to require industry to submit to EPA at least a minimal amount of information about each new chemical in PMNs.

Implementation of this option would allow EPA to assess more effectively the potential hazards of new chemical substances. It would require manufacturers or processors to provide a "base set" of information including some information about toxicity. Such important information is not required and is often lacking in PMNs that are submitted under the current law. Its inclusion would allow EPA to assess hazards more completely and efficiently. Information requirements could remain flexible to meet varied needs, and EPA might be granted authority to exclude from this requirement those chemical categories not considered to pose a risk.

Requiring industry to generate a base set of information is viewed by some as costly and burdensome. There is also the additional issue of whether the increased costs would retard innovation and keep potentially useful chemicals off the market. However, the system is deemed feasible by other organizations. The Organization for Economic Cooperation and Development, in which the United States participates, has recommended that its member nations adopt a similar system.

OPTION 10

Amend TSCA to shift from Government to industry the burden of proof for demonstrating that additional testing is unnecessary for existing chemical substances suspected of being toxic.

EPA is slow in requiring industry to generate toxicity information about chemicals suspected of presenting an unreasonable risk. An amendment to TSCA that shifts much of the burden of proof for demonstrating an "unreasonable risk" from the Federal Government to manufacturers and processors of chemical substances might improve EPA's capability to reach the goals established by TSCA.

To decide about risks associated with pesticides, EPA established the "rebuttable presumption against registration" (RPAR) process which places much of the burden of proof on industry. Under the RPAR process, once a preliminary finding is made that a substance "may present an unreasonable risk" and that available information is insufficient to perform a reasoned evaluation, industry has to produce evidence that the pesticide does not present such a risk or the pesticide is no longer allowed in commerce. TSCA could be amended to permit a similar approach to other substances.

The strength of the RPAR process is that if EPA determines that a pesticide reaches or exceeds specific risk criteria, it is the responsibility of registrants and other interested parties to offer rebuttal evidence within a given time period. A system patterned in concept after RPAR could be incorporated into TSCA to alleviate much of the burden on EPA and speed the process along. The term "concept" is emphasized because the RPAR approach has not so far resulted in an expeditious review of pesticides. Congress may want to examine carefully EPA's current efforts in regard to pesticides and consider the National Academy of Science's recommendations for improving the RPAR process.

A major disadvantage of this option stems from differences between the universe of substances covered under TSCA and the narrower range of substances covered by the Federal Insecticide, Fungicide, and Rodenticide Act. All pesticides are biologically active and, as a class, they are expected to more frequently be toxic than chemicals in general. An RPAR-like process, which requires EPA to develop only a minimal amount of information about hazards posed by substances which are already suspect, may be more appropriate to pesticides than the wide spectrum of substances regulated under TSCA.

An option concerning the mechanism by which technical decisions are made about hazard and risk for regulatory purposes.

OPTION 11

Consider establishment of a central panel for making technical decisions for regulatory purposes.

A number of organizations, including the Office of Science and Technology Policy, the American Industrial Health Council (a trade association), and some members of Congress have proposed the establishment of a panel either to make decisions about carcinogenicity for all regulatory agencies or to review all contested decisions. Consumer, environmental, and labor groups, and the Federal regulatory agencies oppose these suggestions and favor that the regulatory agencies continue to make their own decisions about which substances pose risks. The arguments advanced pro and con about the panel are discussed above and in other parts of the assessment. In brief, proponents hold that scientific decisions about toxicity and risk can be made separately from policy decisions about regulation and find merit in a single panel making scientific decisions for all agencies. The opponents see the division between science and policy as illusionary when making decisions about cancer and see each agency as capable of making its own technical decisions. Furthermore, they view a panel as a layer of unnecessary bureaucracy.

Congress is aware of this controversy and has mandated a study of the feasibility of a panel. The study is to be completed in June 1982, and

should produce a great deal of information about the pros and cons of a panel. Congress could require that the study investigate past controversial decisions to see if scientific errors would have been prevented by a science panel.

The objectives of the congressionally mandated study are to:

- assess the merits of an institutional separation of the scientific functions of developing objective risk assessment from the regulatory process of making public and social policy decisions;
- consider the feasibility of unifying risk assessment functions;
- consider the feasibility of developing coherent risk assessment guidelines for use by all regulatory agencies with decisionmaking responsibility; and
- address relevant procedural and institutional issues that may arise in the interaction between the suggested programs of risk assessment and the regulatory process.

In addition to those important subjects, an examination of controversial decisions to determine if scientific or technical mistakes have been made in the past would shed light on the necessity for such a panel.

It may be that Congress is satisfied that hearings and expert opinions have already produced sufficient information to consider the merits of a central technical panel before this study is completed. If a panel were established, it would initiate a new system that will be seen as a turn away from the procedures of the past. In some people's view, those procedures have produced unnecessary regulations, and a panel would be seen as a mechanism to improve regulatory decisionmaking and, perhaps, reduce the regulatory burden. Others would see the panel as a further obstacle in the path of producing regulations to protect the public health.

2.
Cancer Incidence and Mortality

Contents

Cancer Incidence and Mortality

INTRODUCTION

In 1979, cancer killed more than 400,000 Americans (254) and 765,000 new serious cancers* were diagnosed (6) (see table 3). Over 3 million Americans alive today have had a diagnosed cancer. Cancer accounts for about 20 percent of total U.S. mortality, second only to heart diseases, which are responsible for about 38 percent of deaths. Moreover, cancer is the number one killer of adult Americans, ages 25 to 44 (see table 4).

Of equal or greater importance than knowing the number of cancers and cancer deaths is the matter of whether age-specific cancer *rates* are increasing, decreasing, or remaining constant. Are people of a given age at greater risk of developing cancer today than were people of that age in the past? This question of changing rates bears on whether aspects of the modern en-

*Not including nonmelanoma skin cancers, estimated at 400,000 per year.

vironment, largely introduced within the last two to four decades, might be causing today's cancers. If so, preventive efforts should start by identifying these elements in the environment and modifying them. If most of the now common cancers have been common for a long time, it might suggest that the causes of cancer have not changed greatly. In that case, prevention might require changes in long-established aspects of the American lifestyle.

When seeking means to prevent cancer, special attention must be given to increases in cancers at particular sites. This attention is warranted because the increase indicates that the cause (or causes) might have been introduced recently and can presumably be identified and eliminated. However, to concentrate on a search for new agents to the exclusion of other causes may ignore the possibility of preventing pres-

Table 3.—Estimated New Cancer Cases and Deaths by Sex for Major Sites, 1981

| | Total cases | | Total deaths | | Females | | | | Males | | | |
| | | | | | Cases | | Deaths | | Cases | | Deaths | |
Site	Number	Percent of total	Number	Percent of total	Number	Percent of total	Number	Percent of total	Number	Percent of total	Number	Percent of total
Lung	122,000	15.0	105,000	25.0	34,000	8.3	28,000	14.5	88,000	21.8	77,000	33.8
Colon-rectum ..	120,000	14.7	54,900	13.1	62,000	15.0	28,700	14.9	58,000	14.4	26,200	11.5
Breast	110,900	13.6	37,100	8.8	110,000	26.7	36,800	19.1	900	0.2	300	0.1
Prostate	70,000	8.6	22,700	5.4	—	—	—	—	70,000	17.4	22,700	10.0
Uterus	54,000[a]	6.6	10,300	2.5	54,000	13.1	10,300	5.4	—	—	—	—
Urinary	54,600	6.7	18,700	4.5	16,600	4.0	6,500	3.4	38,000	9.4	12,200	5.4
Oral (Buccal cavity and pharynx)	26,600	3.3	9,150	2.2	8,200	2.0	2,850	1.5	18,400	4.6	6,300	2.8
Pancreas......	24,200	3.0	22,000	5.2	11,500	2.8	10,500	5.5	12,700	3.2	11,500	5.1
Leukemia	23,400	2.9	15,900	3.8	10,400	2.5	7,000	3.6	13,000	3.2	8,900	3.9
Ovary.........	18,000	2.2	11,400	2.7	18,000	4.4	11,400	5.9	—	—	—	—
Skin	14,300[b]	1.8	6,700	1.6	7,300	1.8	2,700	1.4	7,000	1.7	4,000	1.8
All others	177,000	21.7	106,150	25.3	80,000	19.4	47,750	24.8	97,000	24.1	58,400	25.7
Total	815,000		420,000		412,000		192,500		403,000		227,500	

[a]Invasive cancer only.
[b]Melanoma only.

NOTE: Estimates of new cancer cases and deaths are offered as a rough guide and should not be regarded as definitive.

SOURCE: American Cancer Society, 1980.

Table 4.—Ranked Causes of Death by Life Stages, United States, 1977
(based on age-specific death rates)

Cause of death	Total population (all ages)	Infants (under 1)	Children (1-14)	Adolescents/ young adults (15-24)	Adults (25-44)	Adults (45-64)	Older adults (over 65)
Chronic diseases							
Cancer	2	—	3	5	1	2	2
Heart disease	1	—	7	6	2	1	1
Stroke	3	—	8[b]	9	8	3	3
Arteriosclerosis	9[a]	—	—	—	—	—	5
Bronchitis, emphysema and asthma	—	—	—	—	—	10	8
Diabetes mellitus	7	—	—	10	10	8	6
Cirrhosis of the liver	8	—	—	—	7	4	9
Infectious diseases							
Influenza and pneumonia	5	2	6	8	9	9	4
Meningitis	—	—	8[b]	—	—	—	—
Septicemia	—	3	—	—	—	—	—
Trauma							
Accidents:							
Motor vehicle	6	—	2	1	3	7	10
All other	4	4	1	2	4	5	7
Suicide	9[a]	—	10	3	5	6	—
Homicide	—	—	5	4	6	—	—
Developmental problems	—	1	4	7	—	—	—

[a]Rates for arteriosclerosis and suicide are at about the same level in the total population.
[b]Rates for meningitis and stroke are at about the same level among children aged 1 to 14.

SOURCE: Public Health Service (299).

ent-day cancers which are due to factors prevalent in the Western World since the last century or before.

Apart from whether or not cancer rates are changing, many variables contribute to the greater prominence accorded the disease today as compared to even a few decades ago. A major factor in its emergence is the sharp decrease in deaths from infectious diseases such as tuberculosis, dysentery, and diphtheria over the past 150 years. Before the mid-19th century, these diseases killed far more people than did chronic diseases. General improvements in living conditions, public sanitation, and nutrition began to reduce the rates of infectious diseases, and the decline was hastened by advances in biology and medicine early in the 20th century.

As the decades passed, these improvements have shifted the age structure of the population upward. As a result, there is a larger proportion of people over 65, and cancer risks have always been 10 or 100 times greater among them than among younger people. This increases the actual number of cases and deaths (crude incidence and crude mortality) but not necessarily the age-standardized cancer rates.

Second, cancer has become *relatively* more common as a cause of death because of the prevention or cure of other diseases. This phenomenon is illustrated by the mortality data for females in 1935 and 1975 (see table 5). Nonrespiratory cancer death rates decreased substantially, but the death rates from all other causes decreased even more. Therefore, the *percentage* of female deaths attributable to nonrespiratory cancer was greater in 1975 than 40 years earlier, even though female cancer risks had declined during that period.

Third, many cancers, which might previously have gone unnoticed, are now diagnosed both during medical treatment and in subsequent death certification. This change is especially pronounced among the elderly who today receive more medical attention than in premedicare years.

Table 5.—Death Rates per 1,000 Females, 1935 and 1975

Year	All causes except cancer	All nonrespiratory cancers	Respiratory tract cancers	All causes
1935 (1933–37)	11.92[a] (87.6%)[b]	1.65 (12.1%)	0.03 (0.2%)	13.60 (100%)
1975 (1973–77)	4.96 (78.8%)	1.17 (18.6%)	0.16 (2.5%)	6.29 (100%)

[a]All ages, age-standardized to the U.S. 1970 census population.
[b]Percentage of rate for all causes.

SOURCE: Doll and Peto (93).

Finally, cancer is discussed more openly in the media and among friends and relatives of cancer patients; public figures no longer try to conceal their diseases. Previously, such matters were often hushed up and the diagnosis perhaps withheld even from the victim. The jump in the reported incidence of breast cancer in 1974 and 1975 is attributed to the publicity surrounding Happy Rockefeller's and Betty Ford's breast cancer surgery. Greater public awareness led to more women being examined and the detection of more cancers, but the reported increase in those years is not considered to reflect a real increase in incidence.

Cancer has a major impact on the Nation's economy, both from the personal costs of treatment and lost income, and from public expenditures for screening programs, public education, and cancer research. In 1977, the most recent year for which information is available, direct costs for all cancers, including hospital care and physicians' services, amounted to about 7 percent of these costs for all illness (168). Indirect costs, based on a lost earnings approach (discounted at 6 percent), amounted to approximately 19 percent of total indirect costs (preliminary estimate; 168). The costs of cancer are not exclusively economic, though these are enormous. Social costs have taken on increasing prominence in recent years, and include more than the obvious pain and suffering of the victim. Relatives and friends of victims and care givers may suffer direct consequences of the victim's morbidity and mortality. Social isolation, economic dependence, lost personal and business opportunities, and many undesirable alterations in lifestyle are inevitable. Serious emotional and psychological problems requir-

ing professional attention are not uncommon among victims and their family members, often producing irreversible changes in family structure and relationships.

A common measure of disease impact is the number of years of life lost due to premature mortality. This index takes into account both the number of deaths and the age at which people die. Therefore, the death of a younger person will contribute more person-years lost than will the death of a person who is closer to having lived to full life expectancy. Cancer accounted for approximately 19 percent of all deaths in 1975, and about 16 percent of all years of life lost (308), indicating that the average age of those who die from cancer is greater than the average age of those who die from the aggregate of all other causes of death.

Cancer Biology

The 200 or so human cancers are diseases in which some cells replicate out of control of normal growth processes. Such cells produce millions of similar self-replicating descendent cells. The cancerous state is reached when parts of this cell mass cross the boundaries of their "normal territory" and invade neighboring tissue directly, or travel to distant sites through the circulatory system. This event is called metastasis. The ability to invade or to metastasize characterizes these tumors as malignant, or cancerous, in contrast to benign tumors which remain confined to the tissues in which they arise. The possibility of complete surgical removal and cure is very high for benign tumors, with some notable exceptions, but declines precipitously with metastasis.

Over the past several years, a preponderance of evidence has accumulated supporting the view that cancers may arise from single cells, a conclusion reached after long debate. This evidence means that changes occurring in only 1 of the 10 trillion cells in the body can initiate a tumor. However, not all cells are at equal risk, which is obvious from the orders of magnitude differences in the occurrence of cancer at different sites (see table 3).

Certain characteristics of cells have been identified as contributing to the observed differences. The rates of cell growth and division in adults vary from organ to organ, from constant and fairly rapid multiplication, to none at all. Some common cancer sites, particularly the gastrointestinal tract, skin, and bone marrow, are those at which regular cell division occurs throughout life. The cells of other organs, for example those of the liver, and cells of the thyroid and other glands seldom multiply but retain that capability to repair tissue damage. They are important, but somewhat less common, cancer sites. At the other extreme, nerve cells have no capacity for multiplication at maturity, and cancers of these cells are not found in adults. This distinction is not a rigid one, but the rate of cell division contributes in some way, at least in many sites, to the total probability of cancer development.

Another determinant of the frequency of cancer at different sites seems to be the degree of exposure of the cells to outside influences. More than half of all cancers arise in external epithelial cells which are in direct contact with the outside environment. The sites affected are mainly the skin and the linings of the gastrointestinal tract, lung, and cervix. This observation supports the view that most cancers are caused by the environment and are not simply inevitable consequences of the aging process. (For a general discussion of cancer biology, see Cairns (42).)

Cancer causation is thought to involve several steps. The simplest multistage process consists of two parts: initiation and promotion. Initiation is seen as occurring in response to an external stimulus and produces a cell that is "latently premalignant" (302). The initiation event may be a mutational change in the cell's genetic material, but the change is unexpressed, i.e., it causes no detectable change in the cell's growth pattern. "Initiated cells can remain as such for at least a large segment of the animal's life without being removed, destroyed, or otherwise harmed in any measurable way" (116).

In laboratory experiments, exposure of an initiated cell to another substance, a promoter, converts the cell to an "irreversible malignancy" (302). Promoters convert only initiated cells to tumor cells and have no lasting effect on noninitiated cells. (A review and discussion of current research about initiation and promotion can be found in 240.)

Many different agents may be initiators or promoters or both, and depending on an individual's exposures, years may elapse between initiation and promotion. The introduction of a potent initiator into society this year might cause no detectable increase in cancer for several years because of the rarity of the required subsequent promotion stage. Alternatively, a potent promoter that interacts with previously initiated cells might result in an increase being seen in a shorter time.

Classification of Neoplasms

There are three main classes of malignant neoplasms. Cancers of the epithelia, including the external epithelia and the internal epithelia which line various glands, are called *carcinomas*. These afflictions account for over 90 percent of all cancers, excluding the common, but not usually fatal, nonmelanoma skin cancers. The remaining cancers are either *sarcomas* (cancers of supportive tissues, e.g., bone, muscle, tendon, cartillage), or *leukemias* and *lymphomas* (cancers of circulating cells).

Cancers in these broad categories are conventionally recognized and recorded by the site at which they occur and by the cell type of the malignancy, and are regarded, for the most part, as separate disease entities. As knowledge of causation of specific cancers has improved, and definite associations elucidated between exposures and the development of cancers, it has become clear that sites are selectively affected by particular exposures and behaviors, and the classification system has some validity for considering preventive strategies.

Reducing Cancer's Impact

There are three approaches to reduce cancer's impact: prevention, the ultimate goal; earlier detection; and improved treatment. The general consensus that most cancers are caused by extrinsic forces has led to the view that many cancers are preventable. Estimates of theoretically preventable cancers have reached as high as 90 percent of the total, though the practical limits undoubtedly will be lower.

Once identified, exposures to carcinogens may be reduced either through voluntary or regulatory methods. There has been one notable success among efforts to influence personal behavior—reduction in cigarette smoking among adults. The decrease is most notable among adult males, and can confidently be attributed to the publicity and attention given to adverse health effects of tobacco. Between 1965 and 1979, the proportion of adult male smokers dropped from 51 to 37 percent. The decline among women over the same period was much smaller, from 33 to 28 percent (287).

It is generally believed that American eating habits are healthier than they were early in this century and that some of the changes, though not specifically identified, may have spurred the decrease in stomach cancer rates. Future cancer-reducing changes in dietary habits may result from research into mechanisms by which dietary components cause or prevent cancers, or from epidemiologic observations of associations between dietary components and cancers.

About two dozen laws provide for the regulation of carcinogenic agents to protect public health. Through them, exposures to some 100 chemicals are controlled. (Ch. 6 describes laws and regulation.)

Early detection of cancers may improve overall survival rates when efficacious treatment is available. Localized cancers detected before they metastasize can be excised completely, leaving the patient with an excellent chance for survival. Between the early 1950's and the late 1960's, the proportion of prostate cancers diagnosed as "localized" increased from 48 to 63 percent. Over that period, the 5-year relative survival for prostatic cancer climbed from 43 to 57 percent. The overall relative survival rate is the ratio of the observed survival rate of the treated group to the expected survival rate for persons of the same age, sex, and race in the general population. Three elements may contribute to the apparent improvement. Part may be artifactual and result from detecting less serious tumors in the late 1960's, that, had they occurred in the early 1950's, would not have come to clinical attention. Some of the improvement probably resulted from better treatment. However, a major component of the gain resulted from detection of tumors at earlier stages when they could be more successfully treated (247).

Surgery, radiation therapy, and chemotherapy are the mainstays of cancer treatment. Vincent DeVita, Director of the National Cancer Institute (NCI), asserted that "approximately 41 percent of patients with the more serious forms of cancer are curable using therapies now available . . . . By cure we mean that a patient remains free of disease and has the same life expectancy as a person who never had cancer" (85). Attaining a 41-percent cure rate is dependent, however, on every patient receiving optimal treatment.

Advances have occurred in all three areas: Surgical techniques have been refined, radiotherapy is more widely available, and aggressive chemotherapy is developing and appears to hold the greatest potential. To date, the number of people actually helped by chemotherapy is modest, but dramatic advances have been made against many of the leukemias and lymphomas. Chemotherapy, used along with surgery and radiotherapy, has proven successful for a significant, but small, fraction of patients with some cancers. These represent promising medical advances, but because most people who receive the drugs, which are often accompanied by undesirable side effects, experience no gain in life expectancy, a backlash against chemotherapy has developed (86).

CANCER RATES

The examination of cancer rates focuses on each body site individually, since some are increasing, some decreasing, and some remaining more or less stable. Trends for the aggregate of all cancers obscure these individual trends.

The trend that dominates all others is the increase in lung cancer, largely a result of the widespread adoption of cigarette smoking earlier in this century. Male lung cancer rates have been rising steadily for at least half a century. Female lung cancer rates started to rise about 25 years ago and are now increasing rapidly. All other changes are small in comparison with the large increases in smoking-related cancers, although the decreases in cancer of the stomach and uterus are also important.

Currently, there is a general tendency for the rates of change at each cancer site to be slightly more favorable for people under 65 than for those over 65: If the site-specific rate for all ages is increasing, it is increasing at a slower pace among the younger group. If the rate is decreasing, the decrease is more pronounced in those under 65. Two clear exceptions stand out. First, skin cancer in males is increasing much more rapidly among people under 65 than among those over 65. Second, mortality rates of brain tumors appear to be moving in opposite directions. Despite falling death rates in middle age, there are large increases in old age, perhaps because diagnosis has improved for older people.

If attention is restricted to those younger than 65, for almost all types of cancer except those strongly affected by smoking (cancers of the respiratory and upper digestive tracts), the most recent trends in mortality are downward. The chief exceptions are pancreatic cancer in women, and melanoma in whites of both sexes.

Incidence and mortality rates differ because not all people who contract cancer die of it. Rates are calculated by relating the number of cases or deaths to the "population at risk" of either contracting cancer or dying from the disease. "Crude rates" are the total number of cases or deaths divided by the total population. These rates are affected by changes in the age structure of the population, that is, the fact that there are more older people in the population today, and hence more people contracting and dying of cancer means that the crude rates will increase. All of the overall comparisons in this report are based on rates "age-standardized" to the composition of the population determined in the 1970 census. Changes in these rates occur because of changes in the risk of cancer among people of a given age; increases or decreases in the proportion of old people in the population do not affect age-standardized rates. When a figure or comparison refers to a specific age class, the rates are based on the cases or deaths as a proportion of the total number of people in that class.

The remainder of this chapter deals with the data used in computing cancer rates and in analyzing trends, and some of the problems associated with those processes. A discussion of cancer at body sites of major importance follows.

Population Estimates

To evaluate changes in either incidence or mortality over time, it is necessary to know the population at risk, i.e., the number of people in the United States who might contract or die from the disease. Ideally, one would like this information cross-classified by such characteristics as age, race, and sex. More detailed information, such as the socioeconomic characteristics of the population, is also desirable.

The principal source of population data is the Census of Population, which is carried out once every 10 years. For each year after the census, all years ending with 1 through 9, "postcensal estimates" are prepared, using statistical techniques which use the data from the last census and possibly earlier censuses, along with vital statistics data, immigration data, and other data relating to population change. When the next decennial enumeration is completed, these estimates are replaced by "intercensal estimates," prepared by interpolation between the two censuses. However, the intercensal estimates are not available until several years after the latest census is completed. Thus, there may be large discontinuities between the later postcensal population estimates and the actual census count— the adjusted estimate for the number of males age 85 or older between 1959 (*postcensal* estimate based on the 1950 census) and 1960 (census enumeration) shows a 50-percent increase. These discrepancies are not present when *intercensal* estimates for 1959 are compared to 1960 figures.

The censuses have been characterized by underenumerations which vary from census to census. The undercounts are thought to be small, near zero, for some demographic groups, such as white females 40 to 45 years old (in 1970), but are considerably greater for other groups, such as black males 25 to 45 years old, for whom the estimated undercounts are on the order of 10 percent or more (see fig. 1) (349). A number of studies have shown that serious undercount of the population exists for the very elderly, those age 85 years and over (350).

Mortality Data

Information on deaths has been collected through the national vital registration system since the beginning of this century and is the most reliable basis for calculating U.S. cancer rates. Since 1933, data have been collected continuously for the entire United States. National vital statistics functions are centered in the Division of Vital Statistics of the National Center for Health Statistics (NCHS). U.S. mortality statistics are based on information obtained directly from copies of original death certificates received from the registration offices and from data provided to NCHS through the Cooperative Health Statistics System. A number of States now provide their data—medical and demographic—entirely on computer tapes.

NCHS is not a repository of original certificates. Those are available only from the States. U.S. mortality statistics for all years except 1972 are based on information for all deaths. In 1972, they were based on a 50-percent sample, because of unusual budgetary and personnel constraints.

The mortality figures used in this report are based on vital statistics information from NCHS, which (except for the most recent years) have been published in the annual volumes of *Vital Statistics of the United States, Volume II, Mortality.* The data refer to the aggregate population of the 50 States and the District of Columbia.

Incidence Data

While mortality data are extremely useful for studying cancer, incidence data are necessary to advance the state of knowledge about when and where cancers occur, irrespective of outcome. Population-based cancer registries are attempts to identify all incident cases in a defined population. In practical terms, registries cover discrete political or geographic areas. There are a number of countrywide cancer registries (e.g., Canada, Norway, and Sweden). These registries have generally taken advantage of preexisting, centralized data-collection mechanisms. There is no nationwide cancer registry in the United States. By law, cancer is a reportable disease in about 30 States and the District of Columbia (58), but most States have not put in place the mechanisms necessary to handle reported data. The most prominent efforts by States are Connecticut's statewide registry, operating since 1935, and the New York State registry, in operation since 1940 (New York City was not included until 1973).

The first major cancer incidence surveys in the United States were the Ten Cities Surveys of 1937 and 1947, (now referred to as the First and Second National Cancer Surveys, FNCS and SNCS, respectively; see table 6), and the Iowa study of 1950. Metropolitan areas were chosen for FNCS and SNCS to assure a high percentage of correctly diagnosed cases. The areas surveyed were selected to provide reliable data and included about 10 percent of the U.S. population. The sample population was representative of the geographic distribution of Northern, Southern, and Western cities with populations greater than 100,000, but was not entirely demographically representative of the U.S. population.

Figure 1.—Comparison by Race and Sex of Percent Net Census Undercounts, by Age, 1960 and 1970

Percent Net Undercounts, by Age, Race, and Sex, 1960

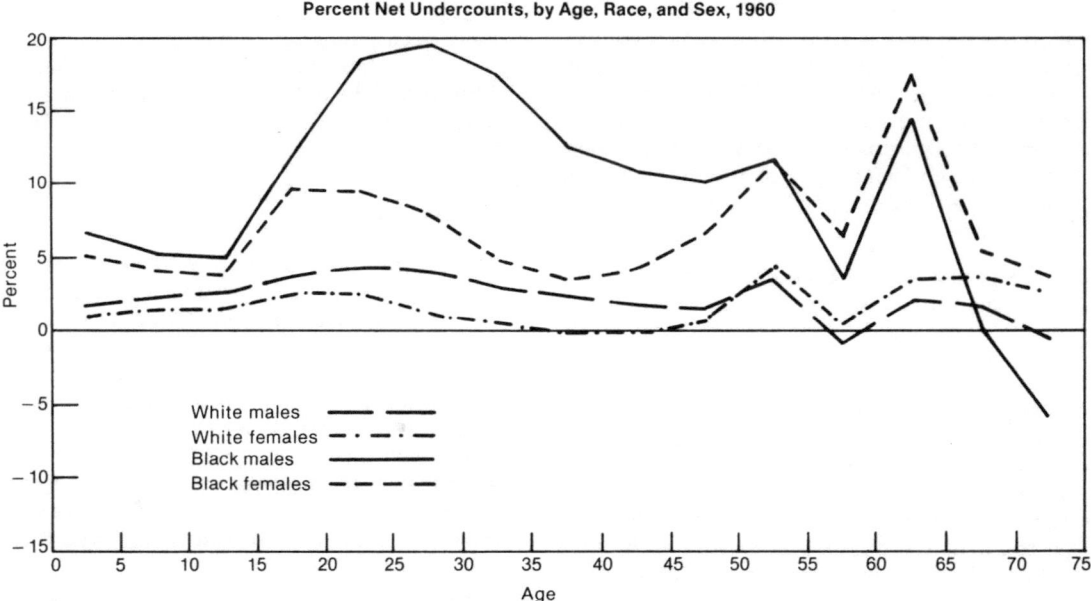

Percent Net Undercounts, by Age, Race, and Sex, 1970

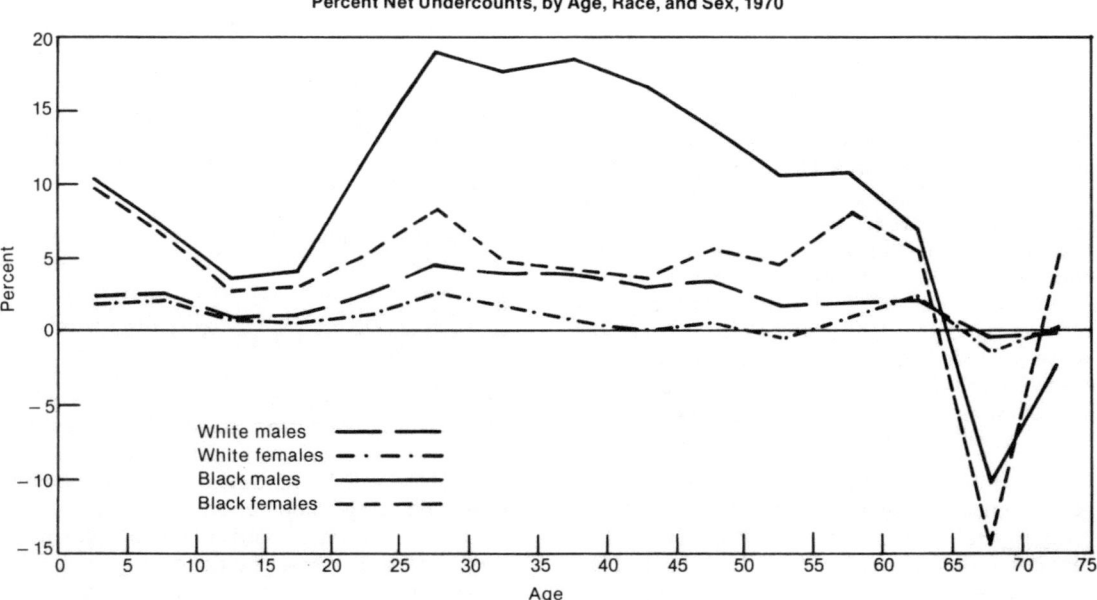

Note: Estimates for 1970 are based on adjusted census data. A negative sign denotes a net census overcount.

SOURCE: U.S. Bureau of the Census (349).

Table 6.—Areas Covered by the Three National Cancer Surveys and the Surveillance, Epidemiology, and End Results Program of NCI

Area	FNCS (1937–39)	SNCS (1947–48)	TNCS (1969–71)	SEER 1973-present	SEER + 1–3 NCS[a]	SEER + TNCS[b]
Atlanta	Cherokee, Clayton, Cobb, DeKalb, Douglas, Fayette, Forsythe, Fulton, Gwinnett	Cherokee, Clayton, Cobb, DeKalb, Douglas, Fayette, Forsythe, Fulton, Gwinnett	Clayton, Cobb, DeKalb, Fulton, Gwinnett	X	X	X
Birmingham	Jefferson	Jefferson	Jefferson, Shelby, Walker			
Dallas	Dallas	Dallas	Collin, Dallas, Denton, Ellis, Kaufman, Rockwell			
Denver	Denver	Adams, Arapahoe, Denver, Jefferson	Adams, Arapahoe, Denver, Jefferson, Boulder			
Detroit	Wayne	Wayne	Macomb, Oakland, Wayne	X	X	X
Pittsburgh	Allegheny	Allegheny	Allegheny, Beaver, Washington, Westmoreland			
San Francisco-Oakland	Alameda, San Francisco	Alameda, San Francisco	Alameda, Contra Costa, Marin, San Francisco, San Mateo	X	X	X
Chicago	Cook	Cook				
New Orleans	Orleans	Orleans		X[c]		
Philadelphia	Philadelphia	Philadelphia				
Fort Worth	Tarrant		Johnson, Tarrant			
Colorado			Entire State			
Iowa			Entire State	X		X
Minneapolis-St. Paul			Anoka, Dakota, Hennepin, Ramsey, Washington			
Seattle - Puget Sound Area (13 counties)				X		
Connecticut (entire State)				X		
Hawaii (entire State)				X		
Utah (entire State)				X		
Puerto Rico				X		
New Mexico (entire State)				X		

Abbreviations: FNCS — First National Cancer Survey.
SNCS — Second National Cancer Survey.
TNCS — Third National Cancer Survey.
SEER — Surveillance, Epidemiology and End Results.
NCS — National Cancer Survey.

[a]"X" indicates area was covered by all 3 NCSs and SEER.
[b]"X" indicates area was covered by TNCS and SEER.
[c]New Orleans is being dropped from the SEER program in 1981.

SOURCE: Devesa and Silverman (84) and Office of Technology Assessment.

Several changes took place in the next major effort, the Third National Cancer Survey (TNCS) of 1969 through 1971 (84). The reporting period was 3 years instead of 1. The timeframe was used to improve data for rare cancers and for smaller population groups. Working under contract to NCI, local, non-profit medical organizations (e.g., schools of public health, medical schools, health department offices) conducted the project at each site. Ten percent of the cancer patients were included in a more intensive survey to determine methods of treatment used, duration of hospitaliza-

tion, cost of medical care, and economic impact on the family. There was considerable geographical overlap between FNCS, SNCS, and TNCS. Seven of the original 10 cities were included in TNCS, although coverage was expanded from only central city areas to their Standard Metropolitan Statistical Areas. The entire state of Iowa was added. The Commonwealth of Puerto Rico cancer registry also supplied data (see table 6).

The first nationally coordinated, continuous-registration system, the Surveillance, Epidemiology, and End Results (SEER) program, was begun in 1973 by NCI. NCI derives the SEER program mandate from the National Cancer Act of 1971 which directs that the Director of NCI:

> Collect, analyze, and disseminate all data useful in the prevention, diagnosis, and treatment of cancer . . . . (sec. 407(b)(4)).

In SEER areas, attempts are made to ascertain every primary cancer, excluding nonmelanoma skin cancer. All information pertaining to a case is consolidated into one record, to facilitate followup and to correlate survival data with treatment, age, and other variables.

Eight geographical locations, four in common with TNCS were chosen originally, and three were added subsequently (see table 6). Recently, one area, New Orleans, was dropped from the program. Approximately 10 percent of the U.S. population resides in SEER areas. A SEER report for the first 4 years of operation compared the demographic characteristics of the population with the total U.S. population (248):

> . . . the participants . . . are fairly representative with respect to age. Blacks are somewhat underrepresented while other nonwhite populations (Chinese, Japanese, Hawaiians, and American Indians) are somewhat overrepresented. Rural populations (especially rural blacks) are also underrepresented.

The SEER program has considered adding registration areas toward the goal of improving the reliability of data for all segments of society. Exact proportional representation is not, however, the ideal situation, since for small demographic groups overrepresentation may be necessary to produce reliable data.

As of September 1980, data were available from the first 6 years of SEER operation. NCI plans to publish complete incidence and mortality data every 5 years, and to make available data for interim years. A small amount of treatment and survival data have been published as the "Cancer Patient Survival" reports (247,251) following the earlier "End Results in Cancer" series. As more years of followup data are accumulated, NCI survival analyses will increasingly draw on SEER program information.

Error and Bias in Mortality and Incidence Data

There are various sources of error and bias in both mortality and incidence data. Reasoned interpretation of trends depends on understanding the forces, other than true changes in incidence and mortality, which impact on certified mortality (cause of death as reported on death certificates) and registered incidence. The important impacts are outlined below:

1. *Improper diagnosis.*—Individuals may contract cancer and die but the correct diagnosis may never be made, affecting both incidence and mortality rates. It is possible, for reasons of inadequate medical care or simple oversight, for lung cancer to be diagnosed as pneumonia; brain cancer as stroke or senility, and leukemias or lymphomas as infectious diseases. Conversely, cancer may be reported as the cause of death for people dying of other causes. For instance, in a 1970 autopsy series in Atlanta, Engel et al. (99) found that 86 percent of cancers found at autopsy were listed as the underlying cause of death on the death certificate. A missed diagnosis of cancer in a dying patient is presumably more likely to occur among old than among young cancer patients, if only because the old are less likely to be hospitalized. These errors are likely to have become less numerous over the past few decades, particularly in older people after the introduction of medicare in 1966.

2. *Improvements in ascertainment.*—It is likely that fewer cancers are missed today than in the past, affecting both incidence and mortality rates, probably to a greater degree in the older age groups. In addition, incidence rates may be influenced by a progressive improvement in the readiness of physicians to collaborate with a cancer registry. Data from the Connecticut cancer registry suggest that since its inception in 1935, the completeness of coverage may have improved so as to in-

troduce substantial upward biases into the rates. Better ascertainment of incident cases is also seen in comparing SNCS to TNCS. The proportions of cases that were ascertained by death certificate only, and for which no clinical record was ever found, were 11.8 and 2.2 percent, respectively (84). This suggests that the earlier survey may have underestimated total incidence rates. Overall, there is a tendency for better recording of cases over time, which causes an apparent increase in incidence.

3. *Primary site not specified.*—The site of the primary cancer in patients with metastatic disease may never be determined. Six to eight percent of American cancer death certificates are for cancer of an unspecified primary site (255). This percentage is a little lower among whites than among nonwhites, and among middle-aged than among older people, but it has not materially changed for decades, and may not seriously bias the assessment of trends in cancers at specified sites. However, the more than 20,000 cancer deaths per year now classified as unspecified represent an uncomfortably large amount of missing information.

4. *Incorrect primary site or cell type.*— Misdiagnosis of the primary site or cell type of fatal cancer is probably the most important bias affecting cancer death certification rates. Patients with cancer of one primary site (e.g., lung) may be misdiagnosed as having a cancer originating from another site (e.g., pancreas or brain), if the cancer has either extended itself to other nearby organs, or metastasized to distant organs. Boyd et al. (93), concluded that at ages over 65 most bone tumor deaths were in fact misdiagnosed secondaries from other sites. This may also have been true in the past for liver cancer, since bone and liver are not sites where cancers commonly arise but, along with brain and lung, are sites to which cancers commonly spread. Likewise, cancers of one particular cell type may be misdiagnosed as cancers of another cell type. This problem can sometimes be circumvented by grouping together particular types of cancers which are often misdiagnosed as each other, e.g., all benign and malignant brain tumors or all colon and rectal cancers. Colon and rectum cancers, which together account for 18 percent of cancer deaths, are often lumped together to improve the reliability of the statistic. However, they are different diseases and their individual characteristics are obliterated by this procedure.

5. *Incomplete transfer of information to death certificates.*—Even if the cancer is correctly diagnosed while the patient is alive, the correct information may never reach the death certificates. Percy, Stanek, and Gloeckler (291) tabulated correspondence between the primary site of cancer, as diagnosed in the hospital, and the primary site as it eventually appeared on the death certificate for 48,826 patients in TNCS. Many discrepancies emerged. Cancers of the colon were overreported while cancers of the rectum were underreported on death certificates as compared to hospital records. In addition, in over 50 percent of all cases where a more specific cancer site (cecum, ascending colon and appendix, transverse colon, etc.) appears in hospital records, it was recorded differently—most often as "colon, not otherwise specified"—on the death certificate. Cancers of specific uterine sites (cervix and corpus) suffer from the same problem. Cancers of the buccal cavity are underreported on death certificates, while bone cancer is overreported, and other sites are misreported to varying degrees.

6. *Inclusion of prevalent cases.*—This bias is limited to incidence data. In a study which runs for a relatively short period, "prevalent" cases, which were actually diagnosed before the start of the study period, may inadvertently be included. This was more likely a problem in FNCS and SNCS, somewhat less so in TNCS, and less still in the ongoing SEER program.

7. *Changes in the definitions for some cancers.*—The definition of what constitutes a

cancer changes with increasing knowledge. For instance, all salivary gland tumors, whether malignant or of mixed cellularity, were classified as cancer up to 1967, but the mixed tumors were dropped thereafter. Likewise, all brain tumors were counted in SNCS, while only those specified as malignant were included in TNCS, causing a substantial artifactual decrease in brain tumor incidence between the two surveys (84).

8. *Increased access to medical care and changes in diagnosis.*—An even more serious bias stems not from classification changes but from the more vigorous search for lumps, and improvements in diagnostic procedures which affect mainly incidence rates. By old age the human body may contain various lumps which, if examined histologically, would be classified as cancer, yet many are biologically benign and cause no reductions in lifespan. For instance, by age 70, 2.5 percent of males in the areas covered by TNCS were diagnosed as having prostatic cancer, while at autopsy 25 percent of males aged 70 or over who died of unrelated causes were found to have cancerous prostates (33). Similarly, among women undergoing mastectomy for cancer of one breast, and in whom cancer is not clinically evident in the opposite breast, biopsy and histological examination of the opposite breast finds 15 to 20 percent of them cancerous (93). Normally only 0.5 percent of these women will develop clinical evidence of cancer in the opposite breast. The scope for biased trends in incidence which are due to either more complete registration or the identification of cancer which would not cause a serious disease is probably large but unknowable with current procedures.

INCIDENCE AND MORTALITY TREND ANALYSIS

The magnitude and rate of change in incidence and mortality at any particular cancer site are seldom equal. Highly fatal cancers are the exception. In fact, comparable incidence and mortality rates are seen for pancreatic and lung cancers which have the poorest survival rates of the leading cancer sites. The same does not hold true for cancers of the endometrium, breast, or bladder, for which survival rates are much higher and improved over the recent past.

Major problems confront analysis of existing U.S. cancer incidence data, while such problems are less severe for mortality data. Incidence data representative of the U.S. population were collected at only three points in time over a period of more than 30 years before 1973. During that time there were changes in survey methods, definitions of disease, diagnostic patterns, classification of disease, and in the rules for assigning cause of death, as well as improvements in access to medical care. All of these factors may have affected registered incidence. The more recent SEER data, while collected according to the same basic procedures since the program's inception, may reflect different degrees of ascertainment in startup years as compared with subsequent years. More importantly, the program has been operating for too short a time for trends which are real but small in magnitude to emerge. Comparing SEER data with information from one or more of the earlier surveys raises questions about whether data from such different sources can be analyzed together with sufficient validity. Despite these drawbacks, data from the national cancer surveys and SEER have been analyzed for trends, and provide some useful indicators, though authors of the analyses acknowledge inherent problems.

Devesa and Silverman (84) analyzed incidence data from the national cancer surveys when TNCS was completed, along with mortality data for corresponding years. They reported that between the two survey points, 1947 and 1970, the "overall age-adjusted incidence rate for all sites combined decreased 3.9 percent." This summary figure is the result of ups and downs in race-sex-site groups, including an overall striking decrease for women and an overall increase for men. Lung cancer was by far the most active site, increasing more than 350 percent between FNCS, when it ranked eighth in incidence as a primary site, and TNCS, when it took first place. Uterine cancer, which had the highest incidence rate in FNCS, had decreased 40 percent. Even more dramatic was the overall 72 percent decrease in stomach cancer by the time of TNCS. Incidence trends for the most frequent sites and for all sites combined, as reported by Devesa and Silverman are displayed in figures 2 and 3.

Devesa and Silverman believe that some of the apparent changes may be artifactual, notably part of the dramatic increase in cancers of the lung and prostate in nonwhite males. In addition, the lower rates for nonwhites in the earlier periods may reflect underdiagnosis. However, they conclude (84):

> Changes are likely to have occurred in the prevalence of carcinogenic agents either in the general or personal environment, since the shifts in trends, especially when considered by race and sex, are greater than those that could be explained by the problems discussed earlier.

Doll and Peto (93) conclude that the most reliable estimates of trends in cancer incidence are probably those derived by direct comparison of SNCS and TNCS, though even in this comparison substantial artifacts are possible. Figures 4 and 5 display the age-standardized male and female incidence data from SNCS and TNCS, respectively. Figures 6 and 7 display age-standardized mortality for the period 1955 through 1975. The important changes are increases in lung cancers and melanomas, a decrease in stomach cancers for both sexes, increasing rates of prostate, bladder, and kidney cancers in males, and a sharp decrease in cervical cancer in women.

Pollack and Horm (296) presented the first analysis of cancer incidence rates from SEER data. The paper, according to the authors, had three objectives:

1. to assess the comparability of the cancer incidence rates across the total SEER program over the period 1973-76;

2. to assess the validity of use of TNCS incidence rates for 1969-71 and SEER rates for 1973-76 to analyze incidence trends over the period 1969-76; and

3. to present trends in cancer incidence and mortality for 1969-76, where data are sufficiently comparable, for some of the major forms of cancer and to summarize these trends by use of a convenient set of measures.

For whites, rates for all SEER areas combined, for individual cancer sites and all cancer sites combined were found to be "reasonably comparable." However, rates for blacks over the 4-year period are not comparable, and therefore analysis of incidence data was carried out for whites only; mortality data were analyzed for whites and blacks. The authors concluded, regarding the second stated purpose, that "the use of incidence rates for TNCS areas for 1969-71 and for SEER areas for 1973-76 appears to provide a good approximation to trends over that total time period for the white population" (296). Pollack (295) reached the same conclusion after comparing Connecticut tumor registry data, the data from the three national cancer surveys and the SEER program.

The authors (296) calculated the average annual percent change in incidence at each site and all sites combined for each sex (see table 7). However, they caution that "it can be misleading to focus on the picture for all sites" because these overall figures are affected by many dynamic rates for different sites. For all sites combined, the incidence rate increased an average of 1.3 percent/yr for white males, and 2.0 percent/yr for white females. Mortality rates for all sites combined increased an average of 0.9 and 0.2 percent/yr for white males and white females, respectively. Mortality rates for blacks increased an average of 2.1 and 0.6 percent/yr for males and females, respectively.

Figure 2.—Age-Adjusted Cancer Incidence Trends Among Males for All Sites
Combined Showing the Most Frequent Sites

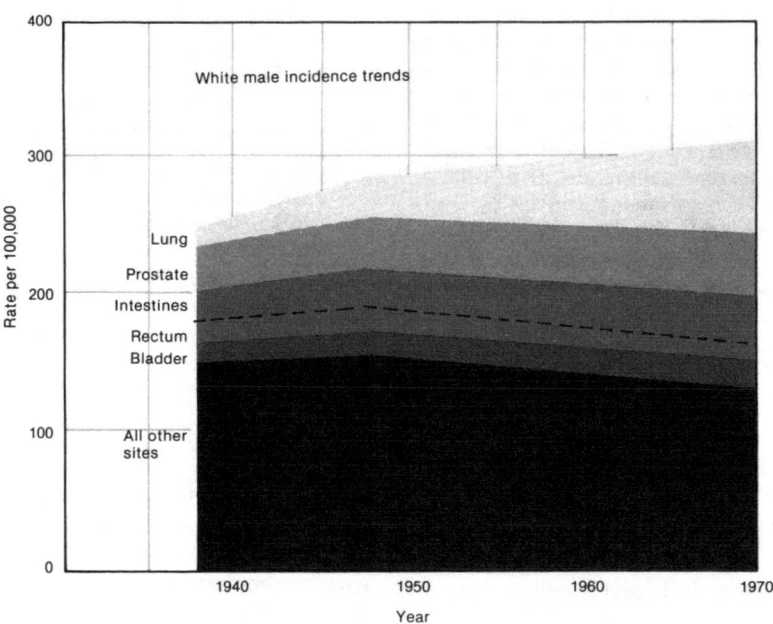

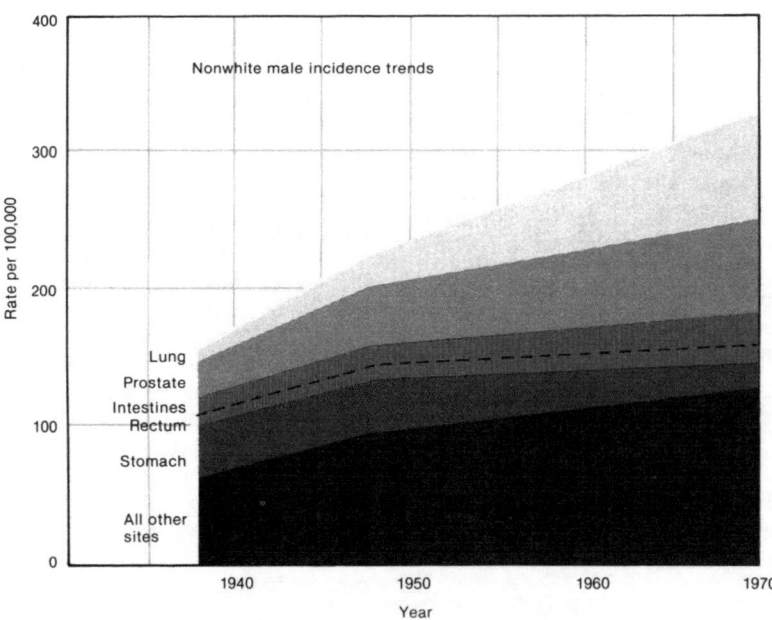

SOURCE: From Devesa and Silverman (84).

Figure 3.—Age-Adjusted Cancer Incidence Trends Among Females for All Sites Combined Showing the Most Frequent Sites

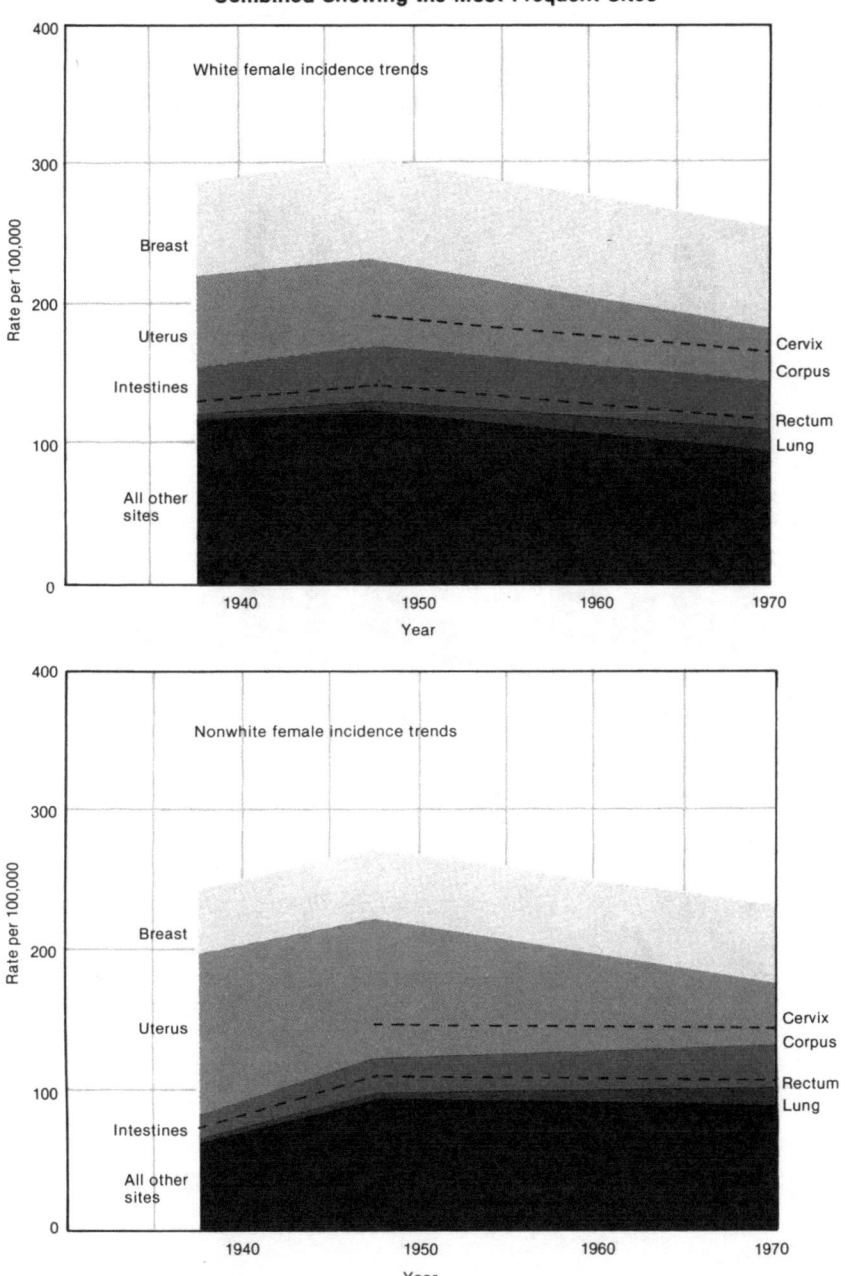

SOURCE: From Devesa and Silverman (84).

Figure 4.—Site-Specific Cancer Incidence Rates per Million Males, All Ages[a]

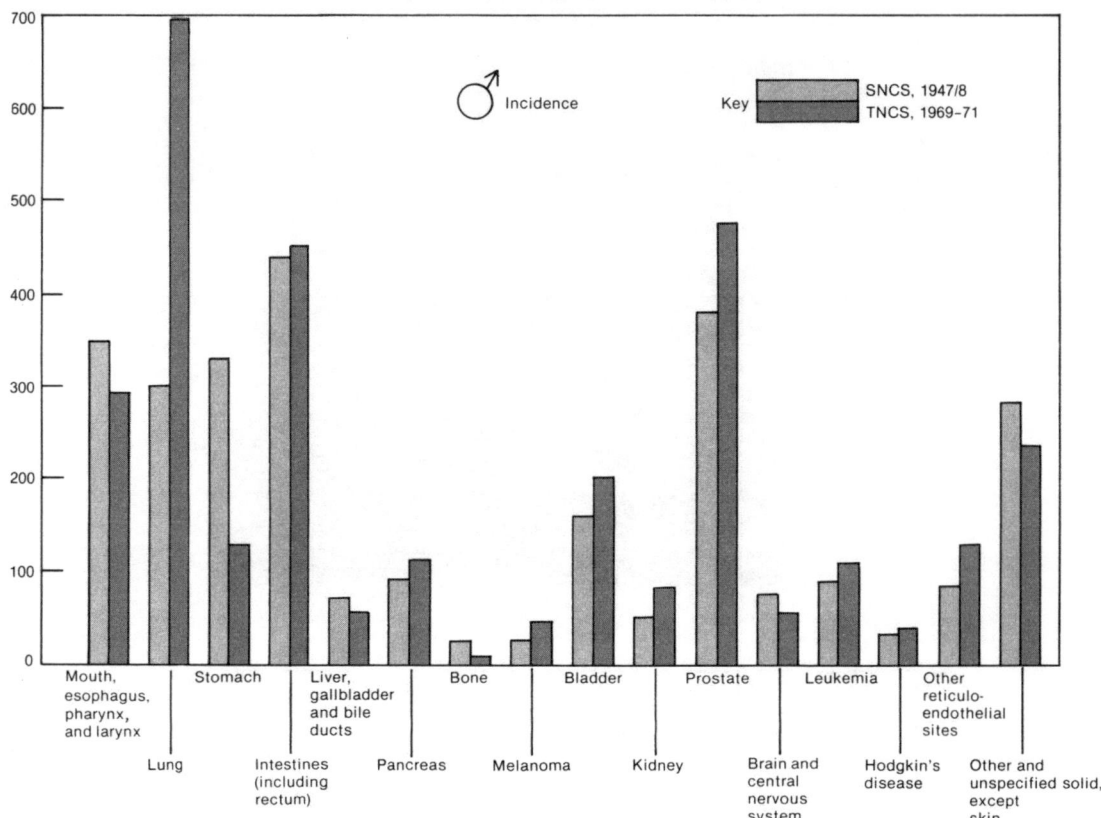

[a] Age-standardized to 1950 U.S. Census population, assuming 90 percent of the population is white.

SOURCE: Doll and Peto (93).

Figure 5.—Site-Specific Cancer Incidence Rates per Million Females, All Ages[a]

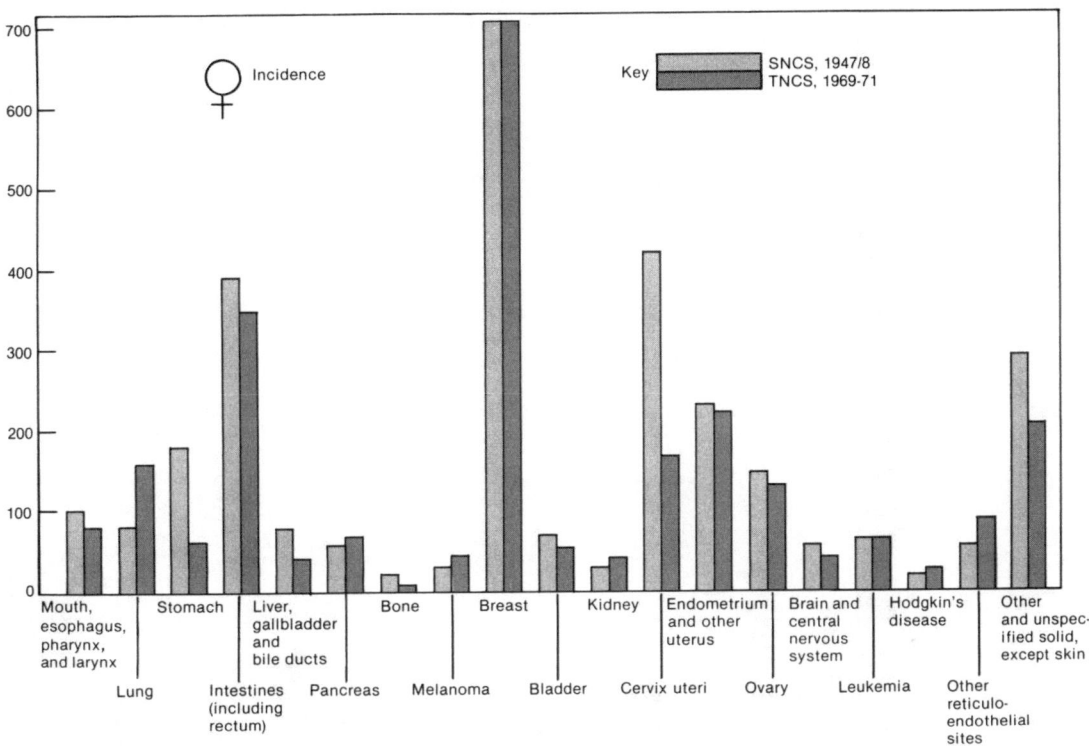

[a] Age-standardized to 1950 U.S. Census population, assuming 90 percent of the population is white.

SOURCE: Doll and Peto (93).

Figure 6.—Site-Specific Cancer Mortality Rates per 100 Million Males at Ages[a] 0-64 Years: 1953-57; 1963-67; and 1973-77

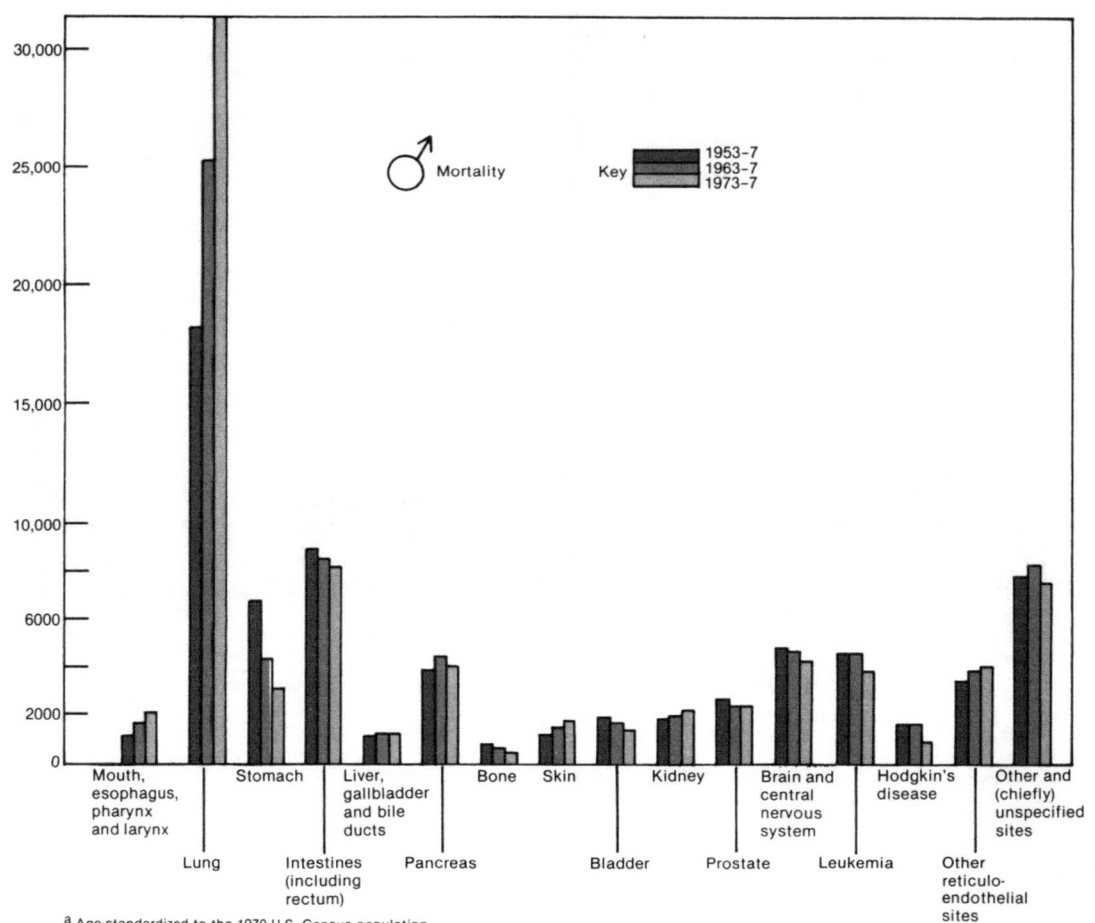

[a] Age-standardized to the 1970 U.S. Census population.

SOURCE: Doll and Peto (93).

Figure 7.—Site-Specific Cancer Mortality Rates per 100 Million Females at Ages 0-64 Years: 1953-57; 1963-67; and 1973-77

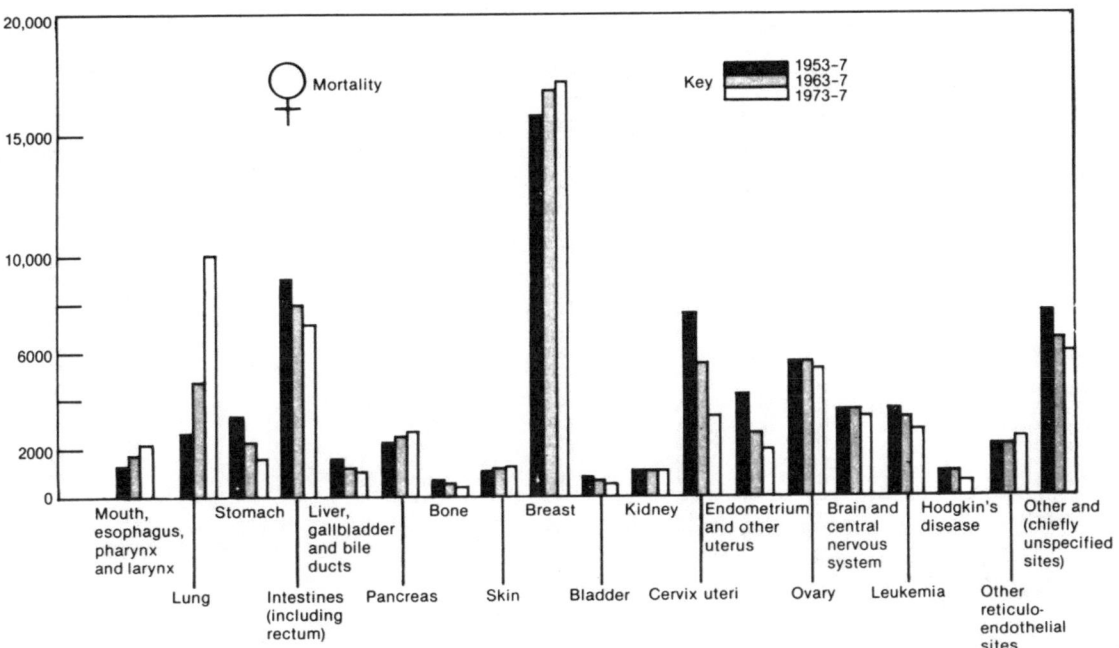

a Age-standardized to the 1970 U.S. Census population.

SOURCE: Doll and Peto (93).

Table 7.—Age-Adjusted[a] Cancer Incidence Rates per 100,000 Population for Selected Sites by Sex and Year, and Average Annual Percent Change, TNCS Areas 1969-71 and SEER Areas 1973-76: Whites

Site	Sex	Incidence rate/100,000 population							Average annual percent change	95% confidence interval	
		1969	1970	1971	1973	1974	1975	1976			
All sites	M	346.6	343.7	337.2	355.5	365.3	365.8	374.0	1.3	0.74	1.86
	F	271.5	268.6	270.9	287.3	305.2	301.8	301.2	2.0	1.28	2.72
Stomach	M	15.4	14.1	13.4	13.8	13.1	12.7	12.6	−2.3	−3.34	−1.26
	F	7.1	7.0	6.3	6.1	5.9	5.4	5.6	−3.7	−4.70	−2.70
Colon excluding rectum......	M	34.5	33.2	32.4	34.2	37.3	35.5	36.9	1.5	0.29	2.71
	F	30.6	28.9	28.6	29.7	30.1	30.6	31.4	0.7	−0.22	1.62
Rectum	M	17.5	17.8	18.1	18.8	19.3	18.3	19.4	1.3	0.60	2.00
	F	11.1	10.6	10.6	11.3	11.2	12.0	11.4	1.2	0.18	2.22
Pancreas	M	12.1	12.1	12.3	12.7	11.2	12.5	11.5	−0.5	−1.96	0.96
	F	7.5	7.3	7.0	7.5	8.0	7.2	8.0	0.9	−0.61	2.41
Lung......................	M	70.6	71.5	70.0	72.3	74.5	76.4	77.8	1.4	0.87	1.93
	F	13.3	14.4	15.5	17.7	20.0	21.8	23.7	8.6	8.06	9.14
Melanoma	M	4.4	4.7	4.7	5.8	6.3	6.4	6.8	6.8	5.75	7.85
	F	4.1	4.2	4.8	5.1	5.5	6.0	6.1	6.2	5.32	7.08
Breast[b]	F	73.9	76.1	75.1	81.0	92.5	86.2	83.5	1.8	1.17	2.43
Cervix....................	F	16.0	14.5	14.3	12.6	11.5	10.7	10.6	−5.9	−6.67	−5.13
Corpus—uterus NOS[c]	F	22.6	22.7	24.6	29.0	31.1	32.4	31.2	5.9	4.48	7.32
Ovary	F	14.9	14.2	13.6	14.2	14.9	14.2	13.6	−0.4	−1.61	0.81
Prostate gland	M	59.0	57.4	56.7	61.0	62.1	64.8	68.6	2.3	1.27	3.33
Bladder	M	23.8	23.3	23.4	25.5	27.1	25.8	26.4	2.3	1.31	3.29
	F	6.3	5.9	6.3	6.1	6.9	6.9	7.3	2.5	1.01	3.99
Kidney	M	9.0	8.7	8.2	9.4	9.1	9.0	9.6	1.2	−0.20	2.60
	F	4.3	4.0	3.8	4.4	4.1	4.0	4.8	1.3	−1.09	3.69
Leukemia..................	M	13.2	13.6	12.2	13.2	13.4	12.5	13.1	−0.2	−1.51	1.11
	F	8.0	7.6	7.2	7.8	7.5	7.3	7.1	−1.0	−2.14	0.14

[a]1970 U.S. population was used as standard.
[b]1974 and 1975 were not included in the computation of trend for breast cancer.
[c]Not otherwise specified.

SOURCE: Pollack and Horm, 1980.

Schneiderman (320) also reported incidence trends from TNCS/SEER data, and his estimates of site-specific and overall change are similar to those of Pollack and Horm. The Toxic Substances Strategy Committee (TSSC) (345) stated that "even after correcting for age, both mortality (death) rates and incidence (new cases) of cancer are increasing," based on Schneiderman's analysis. However, TSSC was cautious about drawing firm conclusions about the magnitude of any increase because of the problems and uncertainties inherent in the data and the comparison of data sets.

Doll and Peto (93) consider the TNCS/SEER comparison "completely unreliable." These authors compared incidence from the SNCS/TNCS/SEER series with registered incidence from Connecticut and upstate New York. They also looked at U.S. mortality for the concurrent period, and found that the TNCS/SEER portion yielded "fantastic and irregular variations in incidence . . . ten times greater than could plausibly be attributed to chance, and a hundred times greater than the corresponding annual changes in mortality over the past few decades." Morgan (242) and Rothman (314) also have challenged the validity of analyzing incidence trends using a TNCS/SEER comparison. Further, they do not feel there is adequate evidence to support claims that incidence is rising. Resolving the differences of opinion concerning trends is not possible at this time.

TRENDS IN SITE-SPECIFIC CANCER RATES

After allowing for all the biases and difficulties in interpretation, it is refreshing that some conclusions can be drawn about trends in cancer rates at specific body sites. As discussed earlier in this chapter, mortality rates in this country are more reliable than the available incidence rates, thus this discussion of site-specific trends relies more heavily on mortality than incidence rates.

Although it is uncertain how far back cancer death certification rates can be considered reliable, 1950 is a sensible starting point for discussing modern trends. In 1950, there were new rules for coding death certificates and a new census. The classification of cancers had just begun to be based on a reasonably modern International Classification of Diseases (the sixth ICD). For example, Hodgkins' disease was classified as a neoplasm rather than an infectious disease, the lymphomas were listed separately, and the important distinction between cancer of the cervix and other uterine cancers had recently begun. Moreover, by 1950, fairly modern standards of diagnostic radiology already existed, and nontoxic anesthesia and the chemotherapy of infectious diseases had just developed, allowing for successful operations against cancer (93).

Trends in mortality rates from all malignancies are depicted in figure 8. Mortality rates and rate of charge differ between whites and nonwhites and between males and females. Consideration of such overall rates are not so informative as consideration of rates at particular sites, which follows. The discussions draw on data presented in tables 8 and 9 which display cancer mortality rates for people under 65 and over 65, respectively and figures 9 through 17 which present age-standardized cancer mortality trends for the years 1950-78.

Figure 8.—Mortality Rates for All Malignancies (ICD 8: 140-209) per 100,000, Age-Standardized to U.S. 1970 Population: 1950-77

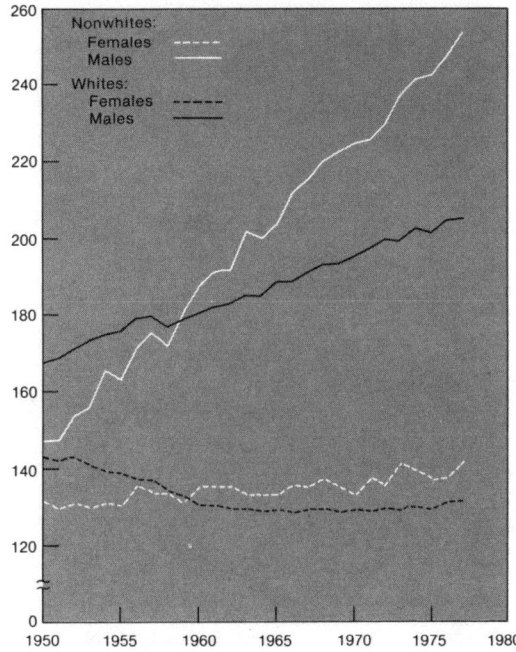

SOURCE: Office of Technology Assessment.

Respiratory cancer sites, dominated by lung cancer, shows the most dramatic increases (see fig. 9). Male respiratory cancer rates appear to have been rising for at least half a century. Female respiratory cancer death certification rates started to rise 25 years ago and are now increasing rapidly. Before 1950, almost the whole of the apparent increase in female lung cancer and some of the apparent increase in male lung cancer may be artifactual, due to increasingly accurate detection during the period 1933 to

**Table 8.—U.S. Age-Standardized Cancer Death Rates for Males and Females Under 65
1953–78**

Site	Sex	Average annual rates/100 million aged under 65[a]					
		1953–57	1958–62	1963–67	1968–72	1973–77	Only 1978
Mouth, pharynx, larynx, or esophagus[b]	M	5,936	6,485	6,858	7,059	7,123	7,200
	F	1,213	1,478	1,700	2,000	2,143	2,111
Remaining respiratory:							
Trachea, bronchus, or lung[c]	M				28,799	30,911	32,080
	F				7,133	9,803	11,598
Pleura, nasal sinuses, and all other	M				475	447	408
	F				215	192	178
Both	M	18,275	21,290	25,390	29,274	31,358	32,488
	F	2,714	3,378	4,734	7,348	9,995	11,776
Stomach	M	6,808	5,539	4,478	3,753	3,270	2,983
	F	3,293	2,717	2,216	1,815	1,551	1,403
Intestines (chiefly large intestine, i.e., colon and rectum[d])	M	8,954	8,739	8,624	8,521	8,298	8,276
	F	9,014	8,576	7,977	7,486	7,130	6,807
Liver[e]	M				807	795	789
	F				354	347	383
Gallbladder and ducts[f]	M				535	488	487
	F				712	644	625
Both	M	1,203	1,396	1,362	1,342	1,283	1,277
	F	1,520	1,425	1,219	1,066	991	1,008
Pancreas	M	3,984	4,336	4,536	4,464	4,267	4,148
	F	2,210	2,363	2,459	2,482	2,598	2,618
Remaining digestive (chiefly peritoneum[g]	M	465	427	404	351	283	256
	F	414	370	330	265	212	193
Bone	M	936	795	747	680	600	575
	F	656	552	483	444	380	360
Connective and soft tissue sarcomas	M	355	419	492	516	464	473
	F	276	338	373	421	414	426
Skin (chiefly melanoma[h])	M	1,325	1,410	1,659	1,547	1,828	1,996
	F	916	935	1,040	1,022	1,086	1,161
Breast	M	138	127	121	130	123	110
	F	15,880	16,158	17,053	17,358	17,260	17,229
Bladder[i]	M	2,066	1,919	1,810	1,658	1,538	1,386
	F	760	676	655	547	500	455
Kidney[i]	M	2,012	2,051	2,134	2,206	2,236	2,300
	F	1,008	1,006	991	1,018	1,016	1,011
Cervix uteri	F	7,550	6,651	5,673	4,423	3,365	2,911
Endometrium[j]	F	4,218	3,282	2,650	2,193	1,966	1,815
Ovary	F	5,692	5,736	5,680	5,621	5,304	5,042
Prostate	M	2,785	2,602	2,549	2,555	2,612	2,590
Other genital:							
Malignant	M	854	852	837	811	729	540
Malignant	F	356	326	291	274	246	224
Benign and unspecified	F	835	444	302	173	95	53
Brain or nerves, malignant, or benign[k]	M	4,908	4,822	4,831	4,693	4,475	4,293
	F	3,675	3,663	3,653	3,520	3,364	3,246
Eye	M	127	120	102	92	77	70
	F	116	106	100	82	66	58
Thyroid	M	236	207	186	182	153	146
	F	340	304	255	210	177	181
Leukemia	M	4,754	4,843	4,705	4,344	4,036	3,845
	F	3,562	3,477	3,338	3,049	2,753	2,622

Table 8.—U.S. Age-Standardized Cancer Death Rates for Males and Females Under 65, 1953-78 (Continued)

Site	Sex	Average annual rates/100 million aged under 65[a]					
		1953-57	1958-62	1963-67	1968-72	1973-77	Only 1978
Hodgkin's disease	M	1,775	1,770	1,770	1,573	1,065	830
	F	992	999	1,025	918	620	486
All other lymphomas[l]	M	3,603	3,862	4,070	4,429	4,254	4,267
	F	2,260	2,543	2,720	2,884	2,875	2,876
Remainder (chiefly[m] deaths where the anatomic site or origin of the cancerous cells was not recorded)	M	5,935	5,775	6,490	5,805	6,029	6,304
	F	5,244	4,800	4,868	4,669	4,734	4,613

a There are currently about 100 million people of each sex aged under 65, so the cited rates are roughly similar to the actual numbers of such deaths.
b These are the cancers which are strongly affected both by alcohol and by all forms of tobacco.
c Lung (including trachea and bronchus) cancer rates are affected more strongly by cigarette than by pipe smoking, and the increases in respiratory cancer among people aged under 65 during the past quarter century can be chiefly ascribed to prior widespread adoption of cigarette smoking.
d Cancer of the intestines may arise in the small intestine, in the ascending, transverse, descending or sigmoid colon, or in the rectum. U.S. mortality data do not seem to be sufficiently precise to allow unbiased examination of the trends in *any* of these separate parts, not even merely "colon" and "rectum".
e Liver specified as primary, including the bile ducts inside the liver.
f Gallbladder, including the bile ducts outside the liver.
g Mesentery, peritoneum and unspecified digestive sites (the latter comprising the minority in 1948, when separate totals were last published).
h In middle age there are now so few deaths from nonmelanoma skin cancers that the data for "total skin" represent the melanoma death rates reasonably accurately, but in old age the continuing decrease in the death rates from nonmelanoma skin cancers still dilutes the progressive increase in melanoma death rates.
i "Other urinary organs" (ureter and urethra, where cancers are rare) were included with "bladder" up to 1967, and were then transferred to "kidney" from 1968 onwards.
j Endometrium, including all cancers of unspecified parts of the uterus.
k The distinction between "malignant" and "benign" is less clear-cut for brain tumors than for most other neoplasms, and so the most meaningful analysis seems to be of all fatal tumors of the central nervous system, irrespective of histology. However, even here, large biases are possible, for in old age symptoms due to brain tumors may be misdiagnosed as due to senility or vascular disease. Such errors are, of course, less likely in middle age, which may account for the marked upward trend in brain tumor death *certification* rates in old age being entirely absent in middle age.
l There is considerable diagnostic uncertainty between lymphosarcoma, reticulum cell sarcoma and various other lymphomas, so we have not attempted to examine them separately. Myeloma is also included since data on myeloma were published separately only from 1968.
m In years when any distinction between them can be made from the U.S. Government publications, the "unspecified site" death certificates greatly outnumber the "specified sites" among those remaining cancers, although the distinction between them seems surprisingly erratic (e.g., comparing 1957 with 1958).

SOURCE: Doll and Peto (93).

1950, but some of the pre-1950 male increase and virtually all of the more recent increases in both sexes are real and largely or wholly caused by the delayed effects of the adoption of the habit of cigarette smoking decades ago.

The long delay between cause and full effect arises because the exact age at which smoking began during the late teens or early twenties is a surprisingly important determinant of lung cancer risks in middle or old age. The dependence of lung cancer risks in old age on cigarette smoking habits in early adult life means that lung cancer rates among people in their sixties during the 1970's are strongly influenced by the smoking habits of teenagers and people in their early twenties back about 1930 (93).

An encouraging sign is the decrease in lung cancer mortality rates among white men in all age groups under age 50 (fig. 10). This decrease is associated with both decreased smoking rates among men and decreased tar yield of new ciga-

rettes. Smoking rates among women rose at least throughout the 1960's. (Trends during the 1970's are not clear.) As a result, all age-specific female rates are still rising, except those at ages 30 through 39, which apparently have stopped rising. These increasing rates suggest that by the turn of the century, lung cancer rates among middle-aged women may no longer be rising, but rates among older women will probably continue increasing because of higher smoking rates during their early adult lives (93).

Mouth, pharynx, larynx, and esophagus (figure 11) are the sites at which cancers can be caused by alcohol and by tobacco, including the pipe tobacco which men have used since the last century. The combination of both alcohol and tobacco exposure seems to cause an increase in the risk of these cancers which greatly exceeds the sum of the two separate risks. Mortality rates at these sites have remained relatively constant since 1950 for whites, but nonwhite males

Table 9.—U.S. Age-Standardized Cancer Death Rates for Males and Females Over 65, 1953-78

Site	Sex	Average annual rates/10 million aged 65 or over[a]					Only 1978
		1953–57	1958–62	1963–67	1968–72	1973–77	
Mouth, pharynx, larynx, or esophagus[b]	M	8,027	7,580	7,214	7,324	7,478	7,487
	F	1,786	1,654	1,551	1,643	1,787	1,933
Remaining respiratory:							
Trachea, bronchus or lung[c]	M	—	—	—	31,539	37,424	40,888
	F	—	—	—	4,692	6,550	8,296
Pleura, nasal sinuses, and all other	M	—	—	—	483	492	468
	F	—	—	—	205	195	203
Both	M	14,277	19,016	24,823	32,022	37,916	41,356
	F	2,937	2,981	3,442	4,897	6,745	8,499
Stomach	M	14,368	11,827	9,552	7,708	6,519	5,892
	F	7,547	5,930	4,635	3,667	3,047	2,870
Intestines (chiefly large intestine, i.e. colon and rectum[d]):	M	17,916	17,749	17,761	17,958	18,265	18,839
	F	15,502	14,672	14,024	13,497	13,256	13,437
Liver[e]	M	—	—	—	926	957	1,067
	F	—	—	—	364	376	395
Gallbladder and ducts[f]	M	—	—	—	1,267	1,193	1,192
	F	—	—	—	1,749	1,479	1,459
Both	M	1,921	2,106	2,208	2,193	2,150	2,259
	F	2,651	2,561	2,357	2,113	1,855	1,854
Pancreas	M	5,816	6,426	6,899	7,090	7,169	7,247
	F	3,842	4,074	4,226	4,390	4,463	4,637
Remaining digestive (chiefly peritoneum[g]	M	729	668	628	500	483	417
	F	649	610	540	431	365	317
Bone	M	837	617	521	502	465	436
	F	468	359	308	286	261	244
Connective and soft tissue sarcomas	M	228	273	323	357	353	355
	F	156	184	209	243	244	273
Skin (chiefly melanoma[h])	M	1,867	1,739	1,679	1,448	1,527	1,608
	F	1,118	961	863	780	789	840
Breast	M	201	166	175	192	188	181
	F	11,356	10,633	10,351	10,603	11,087	11,070
Bladder[j]	M	5,416	5,496	5,501	5,626	5,781	5,732
	F	2,258	2,042	1,876	1,673	1,615	1,623
Kidney[j]	M	1,735	1,969	2,166	2,488	2,543	2,670
	F	1,047	1,066	1,105	1,160	1,222	1,252
Cervix uteri[j]	F	3,127	2,884	2,513	2,021	1,642	1,403
Endometrium[j]	F	4,068	3,512	3,175	2,861	2,662	2,593
Ovary	F	3,195	3,344	3,460	3,680	3,743	3,796
Prostate	M	19,300	18,584	18,488	18,591	19,465	20,392
Other genital:							
Malignant	M	435	359	320	295	252	224
Malignant	F	645	604	545	514	495	470
Benign and unspecified	F	240	147	115	72	51	39
Brain or nerves, malignant or benign[k]	M	935	1,068	1,375	1,731	2,163	2,581
	F	596	692	857	1,187	1,522	1,862
Eye	M	131	123	106	112	99	102
	F	106	91	79	79	70	64
Thyroid	M	276	251	234	232	210	217
	F	524	450	417	372	338	310
Leukemia	M	3,924	4,512	4,855	5,015	5,053	5,142
	F	2,273	2,474	2,612	2,704	2,609	2.627

Table 9.—U.S. Age-Standardized Cancer Death Rates for Males and Females Over 65, 1953-78 (Continued)

Site	Sex	Average annual rates/10 million aged 65 or over[a]					
		1953–57	1958–62	1963–67	1968–72	1973–77	Only 1978
Hodgkin's disease	M	626	600	626	592	468	384
	F	388	374	397	385	296	261
All other lymphomas[l]	M	2,701	3,303	3,900	5,126	5,787	6,266
	F	1,849	2,227	2,634	3,470	3,894	4,184
Remainder (chiefly[m] deaths where the anatomic site or origin of the cancerous cells was not recorded)	M	8,637	7,945	8,650	8,198	9,248	9,666
	F	7,324	6,341	6,294	6,038	6,354	6,502

a There are currently about 10 million Americans of each sex aged 65 or over, so the cited values are roughly similar in magnitude to the actual numbers of such deaths.
b These are the cancers which are strongly affected both by alcohol and by all forms of tobacco.
c Lung (including trachea and bronchus) cancer rates are affected more strongly by cigarette than by pipe smoking, and the increases in respiratory cancer among people aged under 65 during the past quarter century can be chiefly ascribed to prior widespread adoption of cigarette smoking.
d Cancer of the intestines may arise in the small intestine, in the ascending, transverse, descending or sigmoid colon, or in the rectum. U.S. mortality data do not seem to be sufficiently precise to allow unbiased examination of the trends in *any* of these separate parts, not even merely "colon" and "rectum".
e Liver specified as primary, including the bile ducts inside the liver.
f Gallbladder, including the bile ducts outside the liver.
g Mesentery, peritoneum and unspecified digestive sites (the latter comprising the minority in 1948, when separate totals were last published).
h In middle age there are now so few deaths from nonmelanoma skin cancers that the data for "total skin" represent the melanoma death rates reasonably accurately, but in old age the continuing decrease in the death rates from nonmelanoma skin cancers still dilutes the progressive increase in melanoma death rates.
i "Other urinary organs" (ureter and urethra, where cancers are rare) were included with "bladder" up to 1967, and were then transferred to "kidney" from 1968 onwards.
j Endometrium, including all cancers of unspecified parts of the uterus.
k The distinction between "malignant" and "benign" is less clear-cut for brain tumors than for most other neoplasms, and so the most meaningful analysis seems to be of all fatal tumors of the central nervous system, irrespective of histology. However, even here, large biases are possible, for in old age symptoms due to brain tumors may be misdiagnosed as due to senility or vascular disease. Such errors are, of course, less likely in middle age, which may account for the marked upward trend in brain tumor death *certification* rates in old age being entirely absent in middle age.
l There is considerable diagnostic uncertainty between lymphosarcoma, reticulum cell sarcoma and various other lymphomas, so we have not attempted to examine them separately. Myeloma is also included since data on myeloma were published separately only from 1968.
m In years when any distinction between them can be made from the U.S. Government publications, the "unspecified site" death certificates greatly outnumber the "specified sites" among those remaining cancers, although the distinction between them seems surprisingly erratic (e.g., comparing 1957 with 1958).

SOURCE: Doll and Peto (93).

experienced a large increase and nonwhite females a smaller, but notable, increase.

Stomach cancer (fig. 12) is now decreasing throughout the developed world. The enormously encouraging feature of the U.S. stomach cancer trends is that they are continuing downwards throughout middle age, which strongly suggests that as those people and subsequent cohorts age, they will have lower rates in old age than do older people today. The United States, which used to have very high stomach cancer rates, now has incidence rates which are among the lowest recorded in any country in the world.

No single explanation adequately explains the decrease, but several factors have been suggested as contributors: modern techniques of food preparation and storage, increased consumption of green vegetables, fruits, and antioxidants (as food preservatives), and increased milk intake (237). These associations are dif-

ficult to study epidemiologically because individuals may alter their diet throughout life and it is difficult to reconstruct past consumption patterns.

Intestinal cancer (fig. 13) may either be of a specified or of an unspecified part of the intestine. In 1958, about two-thirds of male intestinal cancer deaths were certified as being of some specific intestinal site (small intestine, ascending colon, transverse colon, descending colon, sigmoid colon, or rectum), and one-third were of an unspecified intestinal site, while by 1977 the converse was true. Overall there was little change in total male intestinal cancer mortality during this period. Clearly, although the male death certification rates for each specific intestinal site have been approximately halved, these decreases cannot be accepted as real, since the "unspecified site" rates have doubled.

Moreover, it has been traditional to compile separate data for the "rectum," the last foot or

Figure 9.—Respiratory Cancer (ICD 8: 160-163) Mortality Rates per 100,000, Age-Standardized to U.S. 1970 Population: 1950-77

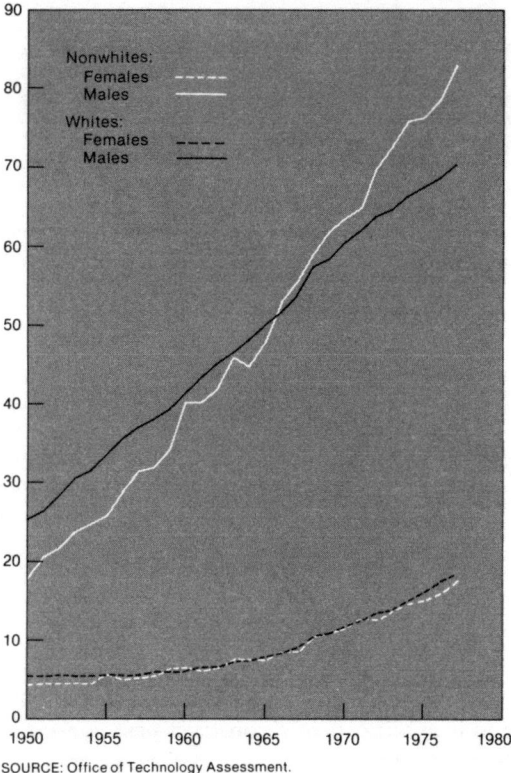

SOURCE: Office of Technology Assessment.

Figure 10.—Trends Since 1950 in U.S. Male Lung Cancer Mortality at Young Ages

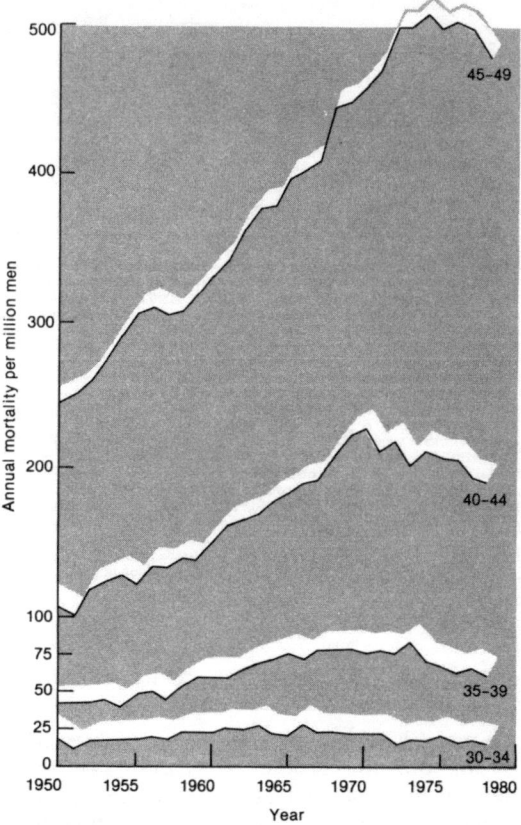

SOURCE: Doll and Peto (93).

so of the large intestine, and to describe the remainder, including unspecified intestinal sites, as "colon." Inspection of the data gives the misleading impression that rectal cancer rates are decreasing and colon cancer rates are increasing, while in fact the decreases in the death certification rates for rectum are if anything slightly less extreme than for other specified parts of the intestines. In view of the fact that half of all fatal cancers diagnosed in hospital as "rectum" in TNCS, were eventually certified as "colon," the most plausible interpretation of the data is that there have been no material trends in either colon or rectal cancer mortality during the past 25 years among males, although both the incidence and mortality data do suggest a slight decrease in onset rates below 65 years of

age (93). Similar difficulties of classification affect data for females, and when all intestinal sites are combined, total female intestinal cancer death rates appear to be decreasing steadily since 1950.

Liver cancer currently accounts for 0.8 percent of cancer deaths among Americans under 65 and no statistically significant trends in liver cancer mortality are evident during the past decade. Incidence trends show a decrease in liver cancer, which is probably artifactual and due to improving differential diagnosis between primary liver cancer and cancers which have metastasized from other sites to the liver. This

Figure 11.—Combined Mouth, Pharynx, Larynx, and Esophagus Cancer (ICD 8: 140-150, 161) Mortality Rates per 100,000, Age-Standardized to U.S. 1970 Population: 1950-77

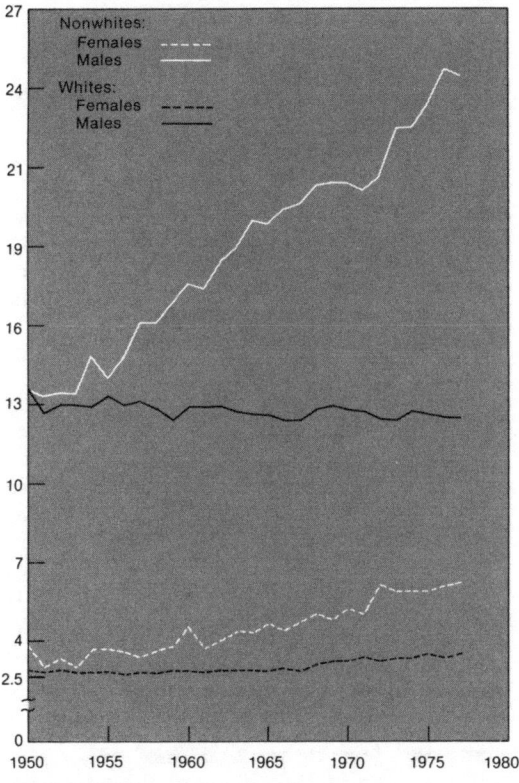

SOURCE: Office of Technology Assessment.

Figure 12.—Stomach Cancer (ICD 8: 151) Mortality Rates per 100,000, Age-Standardized to U.S. 1970 Population: 1950-77

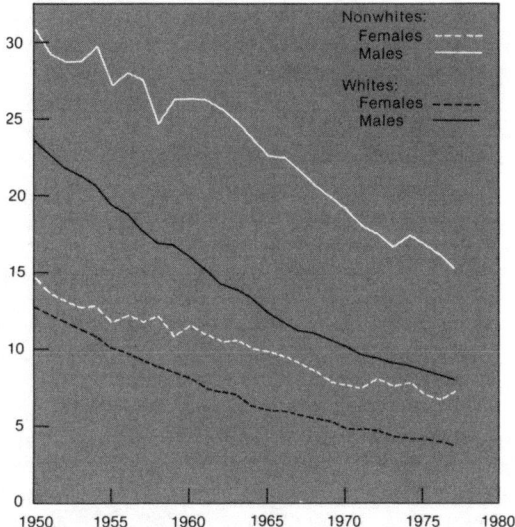

SOURCE: Office of Technology Assessment.

Figure 13.—Combined Small Intestine, Colon, and Rectum Cancer (ICD 8: 152-154) Mortality Rates per 100,000, Age-Standardized to U.S. 1970 Population: 1950-77

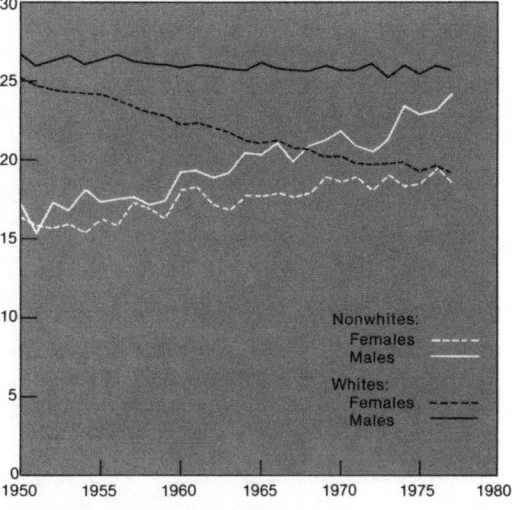

SOURCE: Office of Technology Assessment.

decrease may be somewhat surprising in that the liver is intimately exposed to much of what is ingested, and it is composed of cells which are capable of rapid proliferation when necessary. Moreover, many of the chemicals that have thus far been found to be carcinogenic in animal feeding experiments cause liver cancer in animals.

Gallbladder and *bile duct* cancers are unfortunately not reported separately either in mortality data or in the data from SNCS, though they are in TNCS. Cancers at these sites have different causes, however. Gallstones are a risk factor for gallbladder but not bile duct cancer. According to TNCS data, females develop cancer of the gallbladder more frequently than cancer of the bile ducts, while for males the ratio is the inverse.

Decreases have occurred and are continuing to occur in the aggregate of the two cancers, and these decreases are larger among females than among males. The figures suggest that it is cancer of the gallbladder that is chiefly decreasing, rather than cancer of the bile ducts.

Pancreatic cancer (fig. 14) is now decreasing in males at ages under 65, the decreases in early middle age being particularly rapid. This decrease is especially encouraging because it comes after decades of gradually but steadily increasing rates. Pancreatic cancer is so uniformly fatal that treatment cannot have affected these trends. If the correlation of smoking with pancreatic cancer represents a cause-and-effect relationship, one might expect the ratio of rates among smokers to nonsmokers to be increasing, as has been the case in recent years for lung cancer. If the association is causal, then among middle-aged nonsmokers the trend in pancreatic cancer mortality must be even more steeply downwards than these national data suggest.

Bone cancer death certification (and incidence) have shown apparent decreases, which

Figure 14.—Pancreas Cancer (ICD 8: 157) Mortality Rates per 100,000, Age-Standardized to U.S. 1970 Population: 1950-77

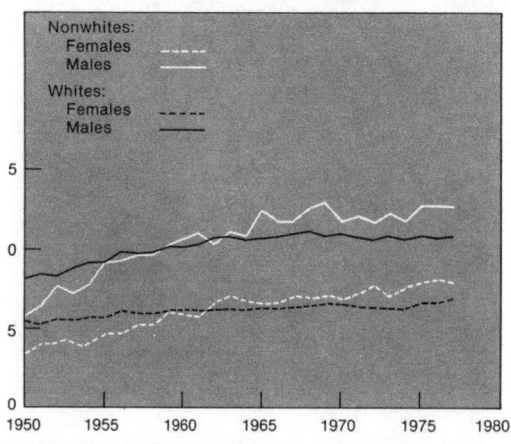

SOURCE: Office of Technology Assessment.

may be due largely to the progressive elimination of misdiagnosed secondaries (93). However, it is now impossible to determine whether or not actual decreases have occurred.

Skin cancer mortality increases from 1950 through 1978 are a result of an increasing death rate from melanomas, offset partially by a decreasing death rate from other skin tumors. The increases are most rapid in middle age, so the rates in old age will probably increase even more rapidly in future decades than is now the case. The causes of melanoma are not well-understood; exposure to sunlight seems to be involved, and people with a genetic deficiency in their ability to repair the damage done to DNA by sunlight are at extraordinarily high risk of melanoma (310). However, people whose work involves regular outdoor exposure seem paradoxically to be at lower risk of melanoma than otherwise similar people who work indoors (93), perhaps because a permanent suntan is protective. This may be at least in part a result of self-selection for outdoor work, or perhaps the conditions that maximize risk are those which involve sudden exposure of untanned skin to sunlight. It is possible that the worldwide increases in melanoma are due merely to some change in the pattern of human exposure to sunlight, e.g., changes in clothing and increases in sunbathing, particularly since the chief increases seem to be in melanoma of the trunk and legs rather than face (93). Alternatively since melanocytes are subject to hormonal influences, it could be that other causes are also important.

Breast cancer (fig. 15) incidence and mortality at ages under 65 show no substantial changes, but that overall rate conceals smaller fluctuations in mortality in particular age groups. Based on the accepted association of age at first childbirth and breast cancer risk (219), Blot (27) has argued that the reproductive patterns of different cohorts of American women can account for some or all of the small fluctuations in breast cancer death rates in particular cohorts of women. Women who were young during the Great Depression of the 1930's somewhat delayed having their children, and their breast cancer mortality now is slightly increased.

Figure 15.—Breast Cancer (ICD 8: 174) Mortality
Rates per 100,000, Age-Standardized to U.S.
1970 Population: 1950-77

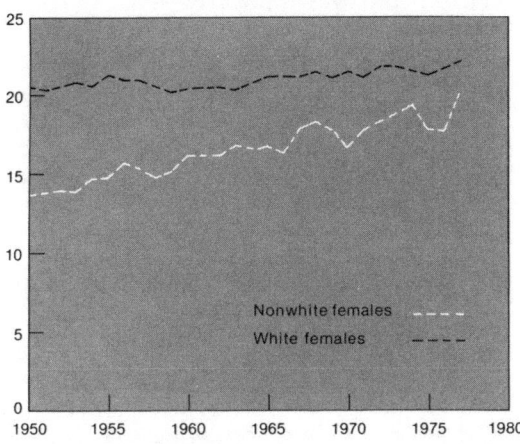

SOURCE: Office of Technology Assessment.

Women bearing children in the postwar baby boom had their babies at earlier ages and have now, in early middle age, substantially decreased breast cancer rates because of their early pregnancies.

Bladder cancer death rates in both sexes are decreasing steadily. The trend is encouraging, since bladder cancer can be caused by occupational exposure to various carcinogens. However, the discrepancy between rising incidence and falling mortality is more marked for bladder than for any other type of cancer except thyroid cancer (see p. 60). These diverging trends may be partly accounted for by improved treatment, but another reason is a shift in the classification of the two types of bladder tumors: papillomas and carcinomas. Lesions that are today considered carcinomas and included in incidence statistics, would formerly have been labeled papillomas, and not counted as such (93).

Kidney cancer death rates have been slowly but continually increasing for 25 years in males under age 65. Rates for females have just recently begun to rise. The mortality increases are accompanied by slight increases in incidence in both sexes. Mutagens have been detected in the urine of male smokers (369), and epidemiologic

studies suggest about a 40 percent excess of kidney cancer among smokers (see ch. 3, "Tobacco"). Additional evidence is needed to confirm or refute an association of kidney cancer and smoking. If confirmed, all or most of the upward trend in mortality from kidney cancer could be attributed to tobacco.

Uterine cancer (fig. 16) mortality has decreased dramatically throughout the past 50 years, the combined effect of large decreases in cervical cancer mortality and smaller decreases in mortality from endometrial cancer. The downward trend in cervical cancer began long before screening for cancer of the cervix became widespread, and is the chief reason for the large, steady decrease in female nonrespiratory death rates over the past 40 years. The causes of this substantial improvement are not fully understood, although effects of improved personal

Figure 16.—Uterus Cancer (ICD 8: 180-182) Mortality
Rates per 100,000, Age-Standardized to U.S.
1970 Population: 1950-77

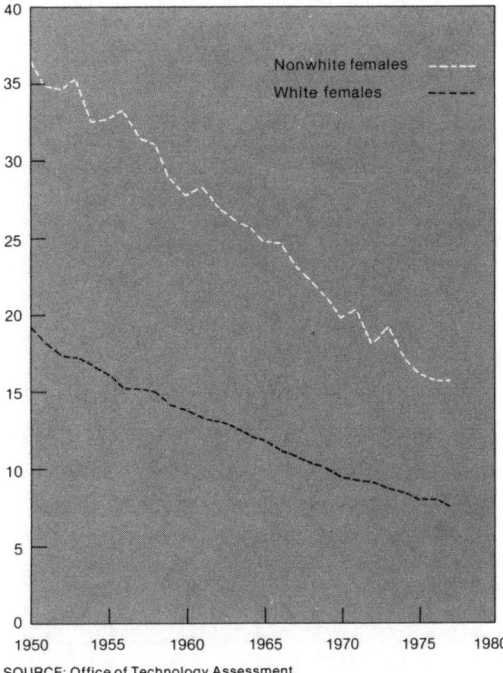

SOURCE: Office of Technology Assessment.

hygiene may be relevant. It is not known what effect cervical cancer screening programs have had on cervical cancer mortality. Also, many cervical deaths between 1933 and 1978 were certified merely as being due to "cancer of the uterus" (with the exact site not otherwise specified). If these deaths could be transferred from *endometrium*, where they now are, to *cervix*, the downward trend in cervical cancer would presumably be much steeper and that from cancer of the endometrium much shallower, which is supported by the trends in incidence. Finally, an increasing percentage of American women in middle and old age, when cancer is most common, have already undergone hysterectomy for various reasons, thereby removing both uterine cervix and endometrium (and, sometimes, both ovaries) from risk. A better statistic for these cancers might be the death rate per uterus or per ovary and not per woman.

Prostate cancer (fig. 17) becomes increasingly common with age, more so than for most other cancers. Incidence rates for prostate cancer probably are not reliable, being influenced by

Figure 17.—Prostate Cancer (ICD 8: 185) Mortality Rates per 100,000, Age-Standardized to U.S. 1970 Population: 1950-77

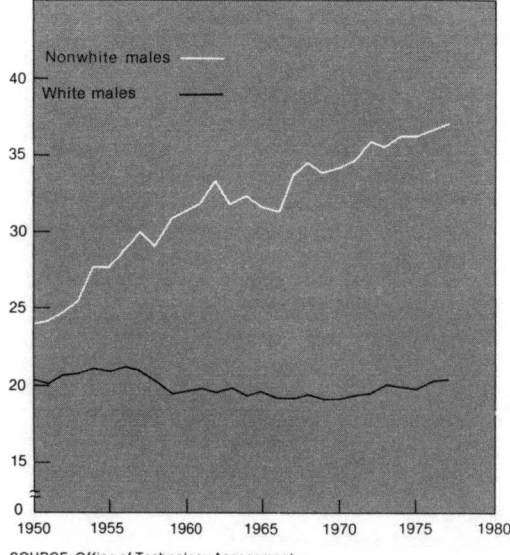

SOURCE: Office of Technology Assessment.

poorer census data for older age groups, and most importantly, the more thorough search for lumps, which would not have come to clinical attention in earlier years.

Mortality data appear to be reliable, however, and indicate a marked divergence of rates for whites and nonwhites. The rate for whites has remained more or less constant since 1950, while the rate for nonwhites has risen steadily, and has not leveled off. The reasons for these patterns are not known.

Brain tumors, whether malignant, benign, or of unspecified types are not reliably distinguishable, therefore the three types are combined to examine trends. Under age 65, a 1-percent per year decrease in brain tumor death rates is seen. Over 65, the opposite is true, and there is a very rapid increase in brain cancer death rates, possibly due to a steady improvement of diagnostic standards.

Thyroid cancer is not common, accounting for less than 1 percent of all cancer deaths. Thyroid cancer death rates have fallen steadily from 1950 to the present, while a large increase in incidence occurred through at least 1970. The discrepancy between incidence and mortality can be at least partly explained by the many cases, mostly nonfatal, induced by medical radiation of the thyroid, head, and neck. These X-ray practices have largely been discontinued. The decrease in mortality may be a result of improved treatment, as well as possible real decreases in the incidence of serious cases.

Hodgkin's disease and certain forms of *leukemia* are much more treatable now than a decade or two ago. This fact alone accounts for the observed substantial downward trends in mortality, especially among younger people. The availability of successful treatments may also have encouraged more thorough efforts at correct diagnosis. Reliable estimation of trends in the various completely different types of leukemia is, unfortunately, not possible from the available data. The lack of any net trend in either direction in leukemia mortality among older people may represent a balance between increasingly thorough diagnosis among elderly patients who are dying of leukemia and slightly better treatment of the disease. The incidence data suggest that some decreases in real onset rates for leukemia are in progress, at least among females (93).

Myelomatosis death rates have been rising steadily from 1968 through 1978, more so for older than for middle-aged people, for unknown reasons. The apparent increase may be real, but may be largely or wholly due merely to be improved case-finding, for improved case-finding

must have occurred during 1968-78 and might be expected to have its greatest effect among the old.

Unspecified sites account for 6 to 8 percent of all cancers at ages below 65. The exact percentage varies irregularly from 1950. Rather surprisingly, given better diagnostic criteria in recent years, slight increases in cancer at unspecified sites have been seen during the past decade.

SUMMARY

The ability to analyze cancer incidence and mortality depends on the available data. Qualifications are attached to the reliability of both kinds of data, more to incidence data because they have been collected over smaller geographical regions for shorter periods of time, but certain conclusions can be drawn.

Respiratory cancer incidence and mortality have increased dramatically in both sexes, but the last few years have seen a decline in lung cancer rates among young men. The increases and the more encouraging decreases are associated with changes in smoking habits. The decrease in cancer death rates for females during the last 50 years is partly explained by dramatic decreases in deaths from cancer of the uterine cervix. Stomach cancer mortality has decreased substantially in both sexes.

When cancer mortality from all nonrespiratory sites are considered together, a decrease is seen in females since 1950 (due to decreased cer-

vical and stomach cancers). Male death rates have remained about level over the same period. While stomach cancer death rates have decreased in men increases at other sites have balanced those decreases.

A controversy is swirling around the interpretation of incidence rates. Data collected in TNCS (1969-71) and NCI's SEER program (1973-78) show that overall cancer incidence increased more than 1 percent per year over that decade. The large changes, major increases in lung cancer and decreases in cervical and stomach cancers, are the same as those observed in mortality trends. However, increases seen at other sites are not universally accepted as reflecting actual change, because of differences in methodology between TNCS and SEER. Continuation of the SEER program may provide data to better answer questions about cancer incidence.

3.
Factors Associated With Cancer

Contents

3.
Factors Associated With Cancer

A select committee of the World Health Organization (WHO) broadly defined environmentally caused cancers as those in which extrinsic factors are responsible (364):

> These include all environmental carcinogens (whether identified or not) as well as "modifying factors" that favor neoplasia of apparently intrinsic origin (e.g., hormonal imbalances, dietary deficiencies, and metabolic defects).

This overarching picture of "environment" contrasts sharply with the more usual use of the word "environment." Common usage is restricted to what is seen as the purview of the Environmental Protection Agency (EPA): air, water, and soil.

The WHO committee expressed its belief that "the majority of cancers are caused by, or their causation modified by extrinsic factors" (364). This view represents a general consensus among cancer researchers, and lays the foundation for the theory that the majority of cancers are preventable. Individuals have gone further than the WHO committee, and have used figures of 60 to 90 percent for the proportion of cancers that are potentially preventable (31,115,164, 165,166,368). These and other estimates have been erroneously cited as if they referred only to man-caused pollution or even more narrowly, only to manmade chemicals, in the "environment." In this report, "environment" is used to describe the gamut of exposures and behaviors that are associated with cancer.

GENETICS AND ENVIRONMENT

Environment, as used in this assessment, excludes genetic factors. Genetic makeup does, however, play a role in determining the probability of an individual developing cancer. Knudson (201) classifies all individuals as falling into four groups, according to the participation of heredity and environment in the possible development of cancer:

1. genetic predisposition to cancer even in the absence of environmental variation;
2. predisposition imposed by environmental variation in the absence of genetic variation;
3. predisposition imposed by both genetic and environmental factors; and
4. neither genetic nor environmental predisposition.

The first category represents individuals with a genetic defect who have an extremely high probability of developing one or more particular cancers, regardless of environmental factors. Retinoblastoma, a malignancy of the retina, is a

childhood cancer which develops in about 95 percent of those with the genetic predisposition. Several other childhood tumors—neuroblastoma and Wilms' tumor of the kidney—fall into this category. In adults, polyposis of the colon, an inherited condition, often leads to colon cancer; another hereditary syndrome is characterized by high susceptibility to cancers of the colon and endometrium, and other inherited conditions are associated with other cancer sites. Fortunately, these conditions are relatively rare and are involved in probably 1 to 2 percent of all cancer. Categories 2 and 4 represent cancers which are not dependent on genetic susceptibility.

A well-understood example of the third category is xeroderma pigmentosum, a genetic condition involving a defect in deoxyribonucleic acid (DNA) repair mechanisms. Affected individuals exposed to ultraviolet light, a component of sunlight, develop skin tumors, as well as other skin abnormalities and some internal tumors. However, if sunlight is avoided entirely, these individuals will not develop tumors. Both environmental and hereditary predisposing factors must be present for clinical manifestation of the disease.

Xeroderma pigmentosum is rare, but the occurrence of many common cancers have a genetic component as well. One of potentially large importance is an apparent relationship between genetically controlled responses to cigarette smoke carcinogens (197) and the probability of developing lung cancer.

Daughters of breast cancer patients have a higher risk of developing breast cancer than women without this family history, though many other factors affect the probability of the cancer occurring. Individuals with deeply pigmented skin have a lower risk of skin cancer induced by sunlight. (The above discussion draws heavily on Knudson (201).)

MULTISTAGE DEVELOPMENT OF CANCER

Cancer epidemiology and experimental carcinogenesis have established that the carcinogenic process is multifactor in its causation and multistage in its development (302).

Multifactored causality means that several agents, environmental and genetic, may be involved in cancer occurrence. The multistep development of cancer is pictured as involving at least two steps which must occur in sequence in the cell that is eventually to develop into a tumor. The two steps are generally called "initiation" and "promotion," and more general terms are "early" and "late" events.

Some substances, "complete carcinogens," function both as initiators and promoters. Other substances are known to behave only as either initiators or promoters.

Initiation is seen as occurring in response to an external stimulus and produces a cell that is "latently premalignant" (302). The initiation event is generally thought to be a mutational change in the cell's genetic material, but the change is unexpressed and causes no detectable change in the cell's growth pattern. Initiated cells can remain as such for at least a large segment of the animal's life without being removed, destroyed, or otherwise harmed in any measurable way (116).

In laboratory experiments, exposure of an initiated cell to another substance, a promoter, converts the cell to an "irreversible malignancy" (302). Promoters convert only initiated cells to tumor cells and have no lasting effect on noninitiated cells. The long latency period between exposure to carcinogens and the manifestation of disease may represent the time necessary for the occurrence of a promotional event.

The importance of initiation and promotion (or early and late events in carcinogenicity) in humans is that interference in either one might reduce cancer's toll. Radman and Kinsella (302) draw attention to the possibility of identifying substances which can inhibit the activities of either initiators or promoters.

SHARED RESPONSIBILITY

Attribution of the risk of cancer to specific, single causes is the exception rather than the rule. Genetic factors affecting individual susceptibility are frequently part of the interaction. Of more relevance to this assessment are environmental agents which interact with each other to produce carcinogenic effects.

There is clear evidence that smoking acts synergistically with some other factors. Synergism in this context means that the number of cancers resulting from exposure to two agents is greater than the sum of cancers that would be expected from the two exposures individually. Smoking interacts with ionizing radiation to produce cancer of the lung; and with alcohol to produce cancer of the esophagus. One of the best known synergisms is the interaction of tobacco and asbestos.

Asbestos and Smoking

In 1979, the Surgeon General stated (286):

Asbestos provides one of the most dramatic examples of adverse health effects resulting from interaction between the smoking of tobacco products and an agent used in the workplace.

Exposure to asbestos is one of the most extensively studied occupational health hazards, and one which continues to attract the efforts of epidemiologists, in part because of its interaction with smoking. Indisputable evidence links asbestos to lung cancers and to rare cancer types, mesotheliomas of the pleura and the peritoneum. Smokers exposed to asbestos, especially those exposed at high levels, have a much greater probability of developing lung cancers than either smokers not exposed to asbestos, or nonsmokers exposed to asbestos. Rates for mesotheliomas, on the other hand, are similar for smokers and nonsmokers exposed to asbestos.

Hammond, Selikoff, and Seidman (156) have analyzed mortality data from a large group of U.S. male asbestos insulation workers. Computations were carried out comparing the insulation workers to a control group of males from a large cohort assembled by the American Cancer Society (ACS). Table 10 presents the results of the analysis, supporting the existence of strong synergism between smoking and exposure to asbestos in the production of lung cancer. As the authors explain, if the two exposures

were acting independently in this cohort, one would predict the following (156):

. . . the lung cancer death rate of asbestos workers with a history of cigarette smoking should be very close to the sum of the following three numbers: 11.3 (the rate for the "no,no" group), 47.1 (the mortality difference for the "yes, no" group), and 111.3 (the mortality difference for the "no, yes" group). The sum comes to 169.7 lung cancer deaths per 100,000 man-years . . . . In contrast, the observed lung cancer death rate of the "yes, yes" group was 601.6 per 100,000 man-years. The difference (601.6 − 169.)7 = 431.9 lung cancer deaths per 100,000 man-years, was presumably due to a synergistic effect in men with both of the two types of exposure . . . .

Another measure, in addition to the mortality difference, is the mortality ratio, which in this case is the lung cancer death rate in each of the four exposure groups, divided by the lung cancer death rate in the group of nonsmokers who were not exposed to asbestos (group 1). The mortality ratio for exposure to both agents, 53.24, is much higher than would be expected from the additive effects of cigarette smoking alone (mortality ratio = 10.85) and asbestos exposure alone (mortality ratio = 5.17). The effects appear to be multiplicative.

Attribution of Risk

In the case of smoking and asbestos, and in other cases where two or a variety of factors interact to produce some cases of cancers, the disease may be prevented by interventions in any of the factors. Shared responsibility, however, complicates the attribution of risk to a

Table 10.—Age-Standardized Lung Cancer Death Rates[a] for Cigarette Smoking and/or Occupational Exposure to Asbestos Dust Compared With No Smoking and No Occupational Exposure to Asbestos Dust

Group	Exposure to asbestos?	History of cigarette smoking	Death rate	Mortality difference	Mortality ratio
Control	No	No	11.3	0.0	1.00
Asbestos workers	Yes	No	58.4	+ 47.1	5.17
Control	No	Yes	122.6	+ 111.3	10.85
Asbestos workers	Yes	Yes	601.6	+ 590.3	53.24

[a]Rate per 100,000 man-years standardized for age on the distribution of the man-years of all the asbestos workers. Number of lung cancer deaths based on death certificate information.

SOURCE: Hammond, Selikoff, and Seidman (156).

particular factor. Adding up the numbers of cases that might be prevented by various individual measures taken separately may produce a total number of "preventable" cancers larger than the number that actually occurs. An example of this concept, presented in table 11, is based on Lloyd's (214) analysis of the asbestos insulation worker mortality data described above. He estimated the percentage reduction in lung cancer mortality that would accrue by eliminating smoking cigarettes alone to be 88.5 percent, and by eliminating exposure to asbestos alone to be 79.6 percent. By eliminating both exposures, the total reduction would be 97.8 percent, and not the sum of the individual reductions, which would amount to a whopping 168.1 percent. The multifactorial nature of

Table 11.—Estimates of Percentage Reduction in Lung Cancer Mortality in Asbestos Workers by Elimination of Exposure to Cigarettes and to Asbestos

Status	Percentage reduction from current rate
Current	0.0
Eliminate smoking only	88.5
Eliminate asbestos only	79.6
Eliminate smoking and asbestos.	97.8

SOURCE: Lloyd (214).

cancer means that it is impossible a present a neat balance sheet adding up to 100 percent that indicates the proportion of all cancers that can be attributed to factors X, Y, and Z.

ESTIMATES OF THE AMOUNTS OF CANCER ASSOCIATED WITH ENVIRONMENTAL FACTORS

Diverse methods have been used to produce estimates of the amounts of cancer associated with various exposures and behaviors. The methods are variously described as ranging from "seat of the pants," to "top of the head," to figures based on more quantified inputs. Evidence for associations between various "factors" and cancer ranges from very strong to very weak. There is no relationship between the strength of the association and the estimated magnitude of the amount of cancer associated with a factor. For instance, the strongest associations include those between smoking tobacco and respiratory cancers, between asbestos and cancer of the lung and other sites, and between ionizing radiation and cancer at many sites. While each of the three associations is strong, the percentage of cancer associated with each is different. Smoking is associated with more than 20 percent of cancer, asbestos with between 3 and 18 percent, and natural background radiation, with less than 1 to 3 percent.

The importance of a factor, as measured by the magnitude of the proportion of cancer with which it is associated, is one starting point for deciding on the development of preventive strat-

egies. However, a large proportion, by itself does not give any indication of the practicality or availability of strategies. If all factors were equally well understood, and preventive strategies equally available, one would choose to go for big reductions. Under real conditions, strategies that can be implemented receive preference.

Most numerical estimates of associations are based on cancers occurring today or in the last few years. Therefore, they are not predictors of carcinogenic activity today, but reflections of carcinogenic activity in the past, possibly 20 to 50 years ago. A few authors have attempted to relate today's carcinogenic risk to future cancers and these are also cited.

All factors discussed here have not been investigated equally in the scientific community, either because of perceived differences in relative importance, or because of difficulty in obtaining meaningful results. Therefore, it has not been possible for "equal" evidence to be presented for each factor in this assessment. Evidence for carcinogenicity in humans from good epidemiologic studies is given more weight than are animal data.

The remainder of this chapter discusses what is known about the contributions of the following factors to cancer incidence and mortality: tobacco, alcohol, diet, occupation, pollution, consumer products, medical drugs and radiation, sexual development, reproductive patterns and sexual practices, natural radiation, infection, and other or unknown associations. Current thinking, with some historical background, is presented for the major elements of each factor, and attempts are made to mention studies giving quantified estimates of the importance of various factors.[1]

---

[1]Discussion of the factors draws heavily on a contract report by Sir Richard Doll and Richard Peto, who were charged with reviewing existing literature about the quantified estimates of cancer causation. They also made their own estimates, which are cited in this assessment. Doll and Peto's report, in its entirety, is published in the *Journal of National Cancer Institute* (93).

The categories used are not necessarily "natural" assemblages, nor are they the only possible groupings of the components. The discussion of each factor includes a description of important inclusions and exclusions. For instance, the "diet" section looks at all "foodstuffs," including naturally occurring and added contaminants. Drinking water, which is discussed under "pollution," and "alcohol," which is treated as a factor unto itself, are excluded from diet.

All of the estimates considered in preparing the following discussion of factors are listed in table 19, at the end of this chapter. Only "best estimates," either point estimates or intervals, as presented by each author are included in the table. The primary references should be consulted for acceptable ranges and/or confidence limits, exact data sources and methods, and caveats.

TOBACCO

Diseases related to the smoking of tobacco include lung cancer and cancer at other sites, coronary heart disease and stroke, chronic bronchitis and emphysema, and many other diseases, including peptic ulcers (157). Tobacco smoking "is the single most important preventable environmental factor contributing to illness, disability, and death in the United States" (286). WHO (365) states:

> Smoking-related diseases are such important causes of disability and premature death in developing countries that the control of cigarette smoking could do more to improve health and prolong life in these countries than any single action in the whole field of preventive medicine.

The harmful effects of tobacco are greater when it is smoked as cigarettes than when consumed in other forms. This may be because acid cigarette smoke is less irritating than the alkaline smoke from pipes and cigars and, therefore, more easily inhaled. However, tobacco consumption in any form appears to be accompanied by adverse effects, most recently demonstrated in a study showing that long-time snuff dippers experience a highly increased risk of oral cancer (363).

Tobacco is known to contribute more heavily to the number of cancer deaths than any other single substance. The relationship of cigarette smoking and cancer was first suggested in the 1920's. During the 1950's, results from many epidemiologic studies confirmed this association (287). Many carcinogens have been identified in cigarette smoke, and the differences consistently observed between rates of lung cancer among regular cigarette smokers and lifetime non-smokers is so extreme that it is not likely to be an artifact of the epidemiologic method (287):

> The 1964 Surgeon General's Report reached the following conclusion: 'Cigarette smoking is causally related to lung cancer in men . . . The data for women, though less extensive, point in the same direction.'

Today, cigarette smoking is regarded as the major cause of lung cancer in both males and females and is largely responsible for the recent rapid rise in female lung cancer rates. The 1980 Surgeon General's report, *The Health Consequences of Smoking For Women*, states (287):

. . . the first signs of an epidemic of smoking-related disease among women are now appearing.

It has been predicted that by the early 1980's, the age-adjusted female lung cancer death rate will surpass the breast cancer rate, which is today's leading cause of cancer death in women. The Surgeon General's 1980 report estimates (287):

> . . . smoking will contribute to 43 percent of the male and 18 percent of the female newly diagnosed cancer cases in the United States in 1980 and to 51 percent of the male and 26 percent of the female cancer deaths.

The principal impact of tobacco smoking is on the incidence of cancer of the lung although cancer at many other body sites, including larynx, oral cavity, esophagus, urinary bladder, kidney, and pancreas are also associated (287). By late middle age, the risk of developing lung cancer is more than 10 to 15 times greater in cigarette smokers than in lifelong nonsmokers (152). Present evidence indicates that the effect of smoking on the development of lung cancer is affected by number of years smoked, age when smoking began, the number of cigarettes smoked per day, the degree of inhalation, and the composition of the cigarette.

Studies have shown that discontinuing smoking decreases the risk of developing lung cancer. Ten to fifteen years following cessation of smoking, an ex-smoker's risk of dying of lung cancer decreases to a level only about two times higher than the risk for lifelong nonsmokers (286). This phenomenon is nicely illustrated by data in table 12 from an epidemiologic study of British doctors (92).

Higginson and Muir (166) attributed 30 percent of male and 7 percent of female cancers from 1968 through 1972 in the Birmingham and West Midland region of England to tobacco. They specifically ascribed 80 to 85 percent of lung cancers to smoking. Wynder and Gori (368) estimated that 28 percent of male and 8 percent of female 1976 cancer deaths in the United States can be attributed to smoking. Their estimate is based on calculating the percent difference between U.S. mortality rates and the lowest reported worldwide mortality rates for each site and by considering specific case-control studies.

Table 12.—Lung Cancer Mortality Ratios in Ex-Cigarette Smokers, by Number of Years Stopped Smoking

Years stopped smoking	Mortality ratio
Still smoking	15.8
1–4	16.0[a]
5–9	5.9
10–14	5.3
15 +	2.0
Nonsmokers	1.0

[a]The higher mortality ratios observed in the 1-4 year category after quitting compared to those continuing smoking is believed to be due to those individuals who quit smoking because of illness.

SOURCE: Doll and Peto (93).

Enstrom (100) reported:

> If all Americans did not smoke, the mortality reduction that would occur has been estimated to be 80,000 lung cancer deaths plus 22,000 other cancer deaths of the 1978 total of 390,000 cancer deaths—a reduction of 26 percent.

Data from a representative sample of non-smokers derived from a 1966–68 National Mortality Survey indicated that this group had a total cancer rate which was 24 percent less than that of all U.S. whites (100).

Numerous estimates have been made of the contribution of tobacco to the overall cancer rate. Most have taken advantage of concurrent epidemiologic cohort studies, in which large numbers of people are queried about their smoking habits at the initiation of the study and then followed to determine their causes of deaths. The largest such study involved 1 million Americans who were self-identified as smokers or nonsmokers in 1959 and whose subsequent mortality was monitored by ACS. The magnitude of the excess risk observed for women in the ACS population was less than for men. The difference is thought to be due to women having smoked fewer cigarettes per day, inhaling less deeply, and being more likely to smoke cigarettes with reduced tar and nicotine (153). In addition, women are less frequently exposed to occupational hazards, including those that may act additively or synergistically with tobacco to cause cancer.

Several researchers have evaluated data from the ACS study population. Doll and Peto (93) computed mortality rates from the ACS study group and estimated that between 25 and 40 percent of 1978 American cancer deaths, with a best estimate of 30 percent (94,782 or 43 percent male; 27,266 or 15 percent female), could be attributed to tobacco smoking. Their computation method assumes that the male and female age-specific cancer death rates observed among the ACS nonsmokers, between 1960 and 1972, would have applied to the entire country had no one smoked.

Hammond and Seidman (155) estimated that from 25 to 35 percent of cancer mortality in the U.S. male population and 5 to 10 percent in the female population are "mainly due to smoking of tobacco products and cigarettes." Enstrom (100) calculated a 38-percent reduction in the total cancer rate in the "never smoked regularly" group as compared with all U.S. whites. These estimates from ACS data do not greatly differ and the reported differences can be explained by the different methodological approaches and assumptions used. Hammond and Seidman (155) assumed that the age-specific distribution of smoking habits in the ACS group was similar to the country as a whole and relied on mortality rates computed for individuals classified as smokers in 1959, many of whom are known to have quit the habit by 1967. In the approach taken by Doll and Peto (93), it was unnecessary to speculate on the smoking habits of the general population and instead of using

mortality rates for smokers, they relied on cancer rates in the nonsmoking group. The specifics of Enstrom's (100) calculations were not given.

Data derived from a unique study cohort such as the ACS population are not free of bias, but the risks estimated from the study are comparable with those found in a study of U.S. veterans. Rogot and Murray (312) reported mortality ratios for cigarette smokers versus nonsmokers and ex-cigarette smokers versus nonsmokers in a cohort of 250,000 American World War I veterans. After a 16-year followup period, lung cancer deaths occurred 11.3 times more frequently among smokers; laryngeal cancer 11.5 times, buccal cavity cancer, 4.2 times; pancreas and bladder cancer, approximately 2 times; and deaths from cancer at all other sites 1.38 times more often (see table 13). Studies from Great Britain (94,192) and other countries (286,287) show similar elevated cancer death rates among smokers.

Many of these estimates have been criticized for overstating the impact of tobacco on cancer. Objections are expressed because the studies measured mortality rather than incidence, and because they did not take into account improvements in survival, changes in smoking habits, and changes in cigarette composition. None of the estimates attempt to account for any effects of "passive smoking" and it is only recently that evidence of a carcinogenic effect

Table 13.—Mortality in a Population of U.S. Veterans Classified as Smokers Compared to Mortality Expected for Nonsmokers

Cause of death (7th Revision International Classification of Disease)	Cigarette smokers			Ex-cigarette smokers[a]		
	Observed deaths	Expected deaths	O ÷ E[b]	Observed deaths	Expected deaths	O ÷ E[b]
All cancers (140–207)	7,608	3,590[c]	2.12	2,816	2,025[c]	1.39
Cancer of buccal cavity (140–144)	110	26	4.22	24	14	1.67
Cancer of pancreas (157)	459	256	1.79	170	145	1.17
Cancer of larynx (161)	94	8	11.49	22	5	4.78
Cancer of lung and bronchus (162.1, 162.8, 163)	2,609	231	11.28	517	130	3.97
Cancer of bladder and other urinary organs (181)	326	151	2.16	126	90	1.41
All other cancers	4,010	2,916	1.38	1,957	1,642	1.19

[a]Only ex-cigarette smokers who stopped smoking cigarettes for reasons other than physicians' orders.
[b]O ÷ E values are based on expected numbers to two decimal places.
[c]Values do not exactly total due to rounding.

SOURCE: Rogot and Murray (312).

from such exposure has been documented. Hirayama (167) reported an approximately two-fold increased risk of developing lung cancer among nonsmoking wives of cigarette smokers. The effects may even be greater; a fourfold excess was estimated by Doll and Peto (93), who considered lifelong exposure, as would be the case with children.

A more precise estimate of the proportion of cancer associated with tobacco smoking requires a more exhaustive study of lung cancer. Such an effort might be desirable because of the importance of lung cancer to overall cancer rates. As American lung cancer death rates continue to rise, the estimate of the percentage of cancer deaths caused by tobacco will likewise increase. The future course of lung cancer rates depends largely on patterns of cigarette consumption and possibly on changes in tar and nicotine yields. The latter point may be particularly important in light of the large numbers of smokers who have switched to lower tar and nicotine cigarettes.

There is some evidence to indicate that low-tar/nicotine cigarettes may have a lesser carcinogenic risk (6,153,157,287). The tar and nicotine yield is believed to be a function both of the tar/nicotine content of the tobacco and the number of puffs taken (202). Therefore, a reduced risk is dependent on the smoker's behavior as well as the cigarette itself. The decreased risk from a "less hazardous" cigarette may be somewhat offset by an increase in the number of cigarettes smoked. Reports indicate that with the increased production of low-tar/nicotine cigarettes, there has been an increase in the number of cigarettes consumed per current smoker (286). It is also unknown whether chemicals newly added to cigarettes and changes in the composition of the gaseous phase will have health consequences.

The extent to which the increase in male and female lung cancer rates over the last few decades can be accounted for by tobacco is debated. Doll and Peto (93) argue that the increase within the last century can almost totally be explained by cigarette smoking, while others,

Schneiderman (321) and the Toxic Substances Strategy Committee (345) included, contend that additional factors are responsible. (For a more complete discussion, see ch. 2.)

Examination of cigarette-consumption patterns in this country leads to speculations about future cancer statistics at tobacco-related sites. The proportion of adult men smoking cigarettes has declined from 51 to 37 percent during the period 1965 to 1978 (287). There has also been a slowdown in the rate of initiation of smoking among adolescent males. The decreases began at the time of release of the first Surgeon General's report in 1964, and the widespread discussion of the dangers of smoking that followed (287). This information demonstrates that worthwhile decreases in cigarette consumption can take place even without radical Government intervention, chiefly by increasing public awareness of the hazards of smoking. The proportion of adult women who smoke remained virtually constant at around 32 percent between 1965 and 1976, and has since started declining slightly. Unfortunately, the rate of smoking initiation among young women has not declined (287).

Changes in smoking habits that should lower risks are believed to have already influenced lung cancer rates. The rate of increase in lung cancer among men under 65 years of age has slowed during the last decade (see table 8 and fig. 10). Recent female mortality statistics are also promising, for they indicate that female lung cancer rates in the 30- to 40-year age group are steady or decreasing. There is reason to hope that with continued reductions in exposure to the harmful components of cigarettes, the decreases will follow through to older age groups.

Public health laws exclude tobacco from regulatory action because smoking tobacco is viewed as a personal decision, and one in which Congress has decided not to intervene. The Government limits its responsibility to informing smokers and potential smokers of the hazards of cigarettes, conducting behavioral studies on ways of affecting smoking habits, and supporting research on low-tar/nicotine cigarettes.

ALCOHOL

Alcohol is considered next because of the interaction between tobacco smoking and alcohol-related cancers. The National Institute on Alcohol Abuse and Alcoholism (NIAAA) (257) estimated that approximately one-third of adult Americans drink alcoholic beverages at least once a week and another third do not drink so regularly but drink primarily on special occasions. In addition, NIAAA estimated that there are 9.3 to 10 million "problem drinkers," including alcoholics, in the adult population. Alcohol consumption is influenced by numerous personal characteristics including sex, age, education, socioeconomic status, occupation, residence, ethnicity, and religious affiliation.

Alcohol's association with cancer was first suspected around the turn of the century. Today, as is the case with tobacco, there is indisputable evidence that alcohol consumption increases the risk of developing cancer at various body sites. The 1978 Department of Health, Education, and Welfare (DHEW) report, *Alcohol and Health* (257), states:

> In comparison to the general population, heavy consumers of alcohol always show a marked excess of mortality from cancers of the mouth and pharynx, larynx, esophagus, liver, and lung. In the United States, these cancers range from 6.1 to 27.9 percent of the total incidence of all cancer recorded in those locations where there are cancer registries.

Epidemiologic studies have demonstrated that cancers are more common in men employed in trades that encourage the consumption of large amounts of alcohol. A recent study showed that Danish brewery workers have a higher risk of developing cancer then the general population (193). Clinical evidence suggests that consumption of alcohol at levels sufficient to cause cirrhosis of the liver also increases the incidence of liver cancer (257).

Researchers have tried to determine whether the association between alcoholic drink and cancer is due to the alcohol itself or to other chemicals found in spirits, wines, and beers (348). Pure grain alcohol (ethanol) has not been shown to be carcinogenic in animal bioassays (93,277); however, both pure ethanol and methanol, a contaminant of many alcoholic beverages, are mutagenic in bacteria (160,277). Additionally, many alcoholic drinks are found to be mutagenic. The results from such experiments do not yet lead to firm conclusions, but it may be that components of alcoholic beverages as well as alcohol itself are related to increased cancer risk. Some evidence suggests that the risk of cancer is greatest when alcohol is consumed as spirits and that the apple-based drinks consumed in Northwest France are particularly harmful (93). However, the carcinogenic effect of alcoholic beverages is largely independent of the form in which it is drunk. In addition to a direct effect, alcohol may also exert a carcinogenic effect by facilitating contact between extrinsic carcinogenic chemicals and the contents of the stem cells that line the upper digestive tract and larynx.

Epidemiologic evidence supports the view that excessive alcohol consumption increases the risk of developing cancers of the mouth (excluding lip), larynx, and esophagus and that alcohol acts additively and even synergistically with tobacco in the pathogenesis of cancers of the upper digestive tract (257,367).

Most estimates of the percentage of cancer associated with alcohol fall in the 3- to 5-percent range. From data presented by Schottenfeld (233), alcohol appears to be associated with 4 to 5 percent of 1978 U.S. cancer deaths; Wynder and Gori (368) estimated 4 percent male and 1 percent female 1976 U.S. cancer incidence; and Higginson and Muir (166) estimated 5 percent male and 3 percent female 1968–1972 cancers in the Birmingham and West Midland region of England.

Rothman (313) (see table 14) and Doll and Peto (93) estimated that 3 percent of U.S. cancer mortality is related to alcohol. Rothman's calculations are based on attributing a proportion of 1974 cancer deaths at each alcohol-related body site to alcohol consumption. Doll

Table 14.—Proportion of Cancer Deaths Attributable to Alcohol Consumption by Site and Sex

	Males			Females		
Body site	Number of deaths[a] from cancer	Percent ascribed[b] to alcohol	Number of deaths ascribed to alcohol	Number of deaths[a] from cancer	Percent ascribed[b] to alcohol	Number of deaths ascribed to alcohol
Buccal cavity and pharynx ...	5,686	50	2,843	2,282	40	913
Esophagus ..	4,917	75	3,688	1,735	75	1,301
Liver	1,600	30	480	865	30	260
Larynx	2,826	50	1,413	436	40	174
Total......	15,029	–	8,424	5,318	–	2,648
Total cancer deaths	199,194	4.2		166,338	1.6	

[a] In 1974.
[b] Proportion of alcohol-caused cancer at each site from (313).

SOURCE: Adapted from Rothman (313).

and Peto assume that cancers at sites related to alcohol consumption account for 7 percent of all cancer deaths in men and 3 percent in women. They attribute to alcohol about two-thirds of these cancer deaths in men, about one-third in women, plus a small proportion of the liver cancer deaths (which constitute less than 1 percent of all cancer deaths) and derive overall estimates for the combined sexes of 3 percent (range: 2 to 4 percent). It should be emphasized that most of the cancer risk posed by alcohol

consumption is also related to cigarette smoking. Therefore, most of the cancer deaths caused by alcohol would be avoided in the absence of smoking even if alcohol consumption remained unchanged.

Table 15 shows annual incidence rates for alcohol-related cancer sites for several regions in the United States where cancer registries exist (348). Among the white population, the proportion of total cancer incidence associated with

Table 15.—Age-Adjusted Annual Incidence Rates for Selected Cancer Sites in Various Population Groups in the United States

Place	Population	Tongue	Mouth	Oropharynx	Hypopharynx	Esophagus	Liver	Larynx	Total for the 7 cancer sites	Proportion of all cancers (%)
California: Alameda	White	3.0	3.7	2.2	1.1	3.6	2.2	7.9	23.7	8.5
	Black	2.2	4.1	2.2	1.5	13.2	4.3	12.9	40.4	12.3
Bay Area	White	3.2	4.2	2.6	1.5	4.0	2.8	7.5	25.8	8.6
	Black	2.1	4.8	3.3	1.5	15.2	4.2	11.8	42.9	12.5
Connecticut		2.8	4.3	2.1	1.5	5.7	2.0	7.8	26.2	9.2
Iowa		1.4	2.6	1.1	1.2	3.0	1.6	5.8	16.7	6.7
Detroit	White	2.7	3.3	2.0	1.2	4.0	2.6	7.5	23.3	8.7
	Black	3.3	3.3	2.1	1.1	14.1	4.5	7.7	36.1	11.3
New Mexico	Spanish	0.4	0.7	0.4	0.2	2.2	3.0	2.7	9.6	6.1
	Other white	2.2	2.8	1.4	3.0	3.0	3.1	5.8	18.6	6.7
New York State		2.2	3.2	1.3	0.8	4.5	1.9	5.9	19.8	8.0
Puerto Rico		7.5	7.8	4.3	4.4	14.8	3.3	6.4	48.5	27.9
Utah		2.1	2.5	0.9	0.4	1.8	0.9	4.4	13.0	6.1

SOURCE: Tuyns (348).

alcohol varies from 6.1 to 9.1 percent but reaches 11.3 to 12.5 percent among blacks. The highest proportion, 27.9 percent, is found among people living in Puerto Rico. It should be noted that these data refer only to those cancers for which an obvious association with alcohol consumption has been demonstrated.

Estimating the proportion of cancer attributable to alcohol alone is hindered by the difficulty of obtaining accurate data on the amount of alcohol consumed. Results of studies must also be interpreted with caution in view of the fact that individuals who do not drink are often distinguished by behavioral characteristics very different from those seen in drinkers, many of which may affect cancer incidence.

Figure 18 depicts the relative risk of developing esophageal cancer in relation to different

Figure 18.—Relative Risks of Esophageal Cancer in Relation to the Daily Consumption of Alcohol and Tobacco

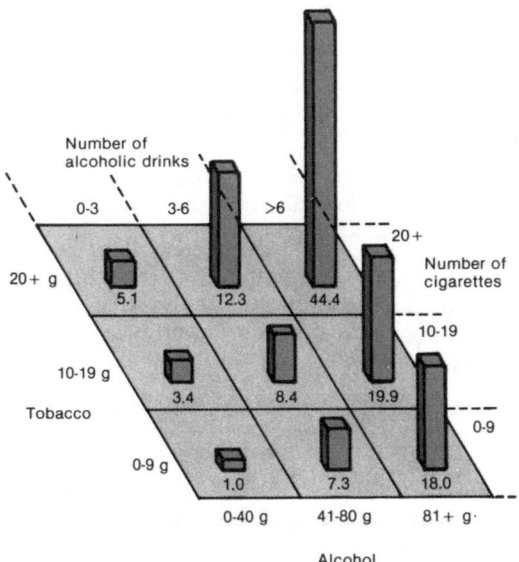

Note: The risk is 44.4 times greater for individuals consuming 20 g or more of tobacco and 80 g or more of alcohol per day (upper right block) than for individuals consuming little or none of either drug (lower left block). One ounce of ethyl alcohol is approximately 23.4 grams, thus 40 grams is 1.7 oz. or approximately equivalent to 3 drinks.

SOURCE: National Institute on Alcohol Abuse and Alcoholism (257).

smoking and drinking habits. The risk of the nonsmoker developing cancer from the consumption of even very large amounts of alcohol is small.

Feldman et al. (118) found that the risk of head and neck cancer was 6 to 15 times greater in heavy drinkers who smoked than in nondrinkers and nonsmokers. Nonsmoking drinkers had a "slightly" higher risk (around 1.5) than total abstainers while nondrinking or light drinking smokers had 2 to 4 times the risk.

Breslow and Enstrom (32) correlated average annual age-adjusted cancer mortality rates for the period 1950–1967 with per capita consumption of cigarettes, spirits, wine, and beer as estimated from 1976 tax receipts in 41 States. As expected, respiratory cancers were related to cigarette consumption. They also found a correlation between consumption of spirits and certain cancers of the upper alimentary tract. In addition, cancers of the stomach, large intestine, kidney, bladder (for men), and breast (for women), were correlated with spirits consumption. The strongest correlation was found between rectal cancer and beer consumption. This finding was also observed in a separate analysis involving 24 countries.

A retrospective study of male veterans by Rothman and Keller (315) demonstrated individual effects for smoking and drinking and synergistic effects for cancers of the mouth and pharynx. Both they and Schottenfeld (323) calculated that 76 percent of cancers at alcohol and tobacco-related sites, which represents 36 percent of total male cancer mortality, could be eliminated if drinking and smoking were avoided.

Examining trends of alcohol consumption permits some speculation about future cancer rates. Quantitative estimates cannot be made, but several factors highlighted in the *Third Special Report to the U.S. Congress on Alcohol and Health* (257) indicate that alcohol will increase in importance as a carcinogenic factor:

- Increased availability of alcoholic beverages has occurred as a result of the lowering of the drinking age in several States, a trend to longer hours of sales, and an increase in the number of retail outlets. (Recently, several States have raised drinking ages.)

- Around 1960, total per capita sales of absolute ethanol began to rise significantly registering a 30-percent gain between 1961 and 1971. Since 1971, there has been virtually no change in per capita sales. The effect of the overall increase may not yet have fully manifested itself in cancer rates.
- There is particular concern over increased alcohol consumption in youths. This is heightened by the observation that early drinking behavior predicts drinking habits in later life.
- The proportion of high school students who reported ever having been drunk increased dramatically from 19 percent before 1966 to 45 percent between 1966 and 1975. The proportion reporting being intoxicated at least once a month rose from 10 percent before 1966 to 19 percent between 1966 and 1975.

The importance of alcohol as a health hazard is not limited to its association with a relatively small percentage of cancer. Estimates of the annual number of deaths related to alcohol range from 37,000 to 205,000. Cirrhosis of the liver, the seventh leading cause of death in the United States, was responsible for 30,066 deaths in 1978. As an contributory cause of homicides, suicides, and accidents, alcohol's toll is even greater. The Institute of Medicine (178) recently completed a study of alcoholism and related problems and indicated several opportunities for research. These included further research on alcohol metabolism, development of appropriate animal models, and further efforts through epidemiologic studies to explore the link between alcohol and its adverse health consequences.

DIET

Introduction

Studying the relationship of diet and health is a continued source of frustration and excitement. Food affects all body functions and comes into direct contact with the digestive system and indirect contact with all other organs. Cancer rates for digestive sites vary considerably around the world and have prompted studies of diet's role in cancer causation.

As discussed here, diet encompasses those items ingested as food, including substances added to food, those produced during normal cooking, storage, and digestion, but excluding drinking water and alcohol (discussed in this chapter under *Air and Water Pollution* and *Alcohol*, respectively).

The amounts and balance of the major components of diet are generally believed to be responsible for the lion's share of diet-related cancers. Deficiencies or excesses of microelements, and the presence of additives or contaminants, are probably less important. The various means by which diet may influence the development of cancer are listed in table 16. Diet also plays a role in the treatment of cancer illustrating the pervasive role of diet with respect to all aspects of the disease.

Unfortunately, dietary studies are plagued with methodological problems and conflicting evidence exists for almost every specific question that has been investigated. The overall association of cancer with diet exists but there is no reliable indication of exactly what dietary changes would be of major importance in reducing cancer incidence and mortality.

The strongest positive associations identified through correlations of dietary patterns and cancer rates are those between total fat intake, particularly animal fat consumption and cancers of the breast and endometrium; and between total protein intake and cancer of the colon. The most dramatic change observed in a diet-related cancer site has been the reduction in incidence and mortality from stomach cancer. In the United States, the 1950 age-adjusted mortality rate from stomach cancer was 24.4/100,000 for males and 13.1/100,000 for females

**Table 16.—Some Currently Attractive Hypothetical or Actual Ways
in Which Diet May Affect the Incidence of Cancer**

Possible ways or means	Example[a]
Ingestion of powerful, direct-acting carcinogens or their precursors	Carcinogens in natural foodstuffs (plant products)
	Carcinogens produced in cooking
	Carcinogens produced in stored food by microorganisms (bacterial and fungal)
Affecting the formation of carcinogens in the body	Providing substrates for the formation of carcinogens in the body (e.g., nitrites, nitrates, secondary amines)
	Altering intake or excretion of cholesterol and bile acids (and hence the production of carcinogenic metabolites in the bowel)
	Altering the bacterial flora of the bowel (and hence the capacity to form carcinogenic metabolites)
Affecting transport, activation, or deactivation of carcinogens	Altering concentration in, or duration of contract with, feces
	Altering transport of carcinogens to stem cells
	Induction or inhibition of enzymes (which affect carcinogen metabolism or catabolism)
	Deactivation, or prevention of formation, of short-lived intracellular species (e.g., by use of selenium, vitamin E, or otherwise trapping free radicals; by use of b-carotene or otherwise quenching singlet oxygen; by use of other antioxidants)
Affecting "promotion" of cells (that are already initiated)[b]	Vitamin A deficiency (clinical or subclinical)
	Retinol [Binding Protein] (hormonal and other factors determine blood RBP, though vitamin A intake may not affect it much)
	Otherwise affecting stemcell differentiation (carotenoids? determinants of lipid "profile"?)
Overnutrition	Age at menarche
	Adipose-tissue-derived estrogens
	Other effects

[a]There may be considerable overlap between many of the entries in this table.
[b]Or, more generally, affecting the probability that a partially transformed stem cell will become fully transformed and will proliferate successfully into cancer.
SOURCE: Doll and Peto (93).

while in 1977 the rate was 8.8/100,000 for males and 4.0/100,000 for females. This decrease has occurred in many other countries, including those with high initial rates, such as Japan and Iceland, and those with lower initial rates, such as Canada and New Zealand. The factors believed to have contributed to these decreases include: reduction in use of salt and pickling, lower consumption of smoked foods, and increased use of refrigeration, increased consumption of milk, green vegetables, fruit, and antioxidants (237).

In general, as a result of increased intake of calories, proteins, and certain other nutrients, Americans have been growing taller and reaching sexual maturation earlier. A great improvement in the Nation's health has resulted from this change, but increased risk for certain cancer sites may accompany the improvement. For ex-

ample, earlier sexual maturation in women is associated with higher risk of breast cancer later in life, though as yet, no increases in breast cancer has been attributed directly to improved nutrition (see *Sexual Development, Reproductive Patterns, and Sexual Practices* for a more complete discussion of this topic).

Many estimates of the importance of diet to cancer have been put forth. Doll and Peto (93) estimated that altering dietary practices may reduce cancer by as much as 35 percent (stomach and large bowel cancer by 90 percent; endometrium, gallbladder, pancreas, and breast by 50 percent; lung, larynx, bladder, cervix, mouth, pharynx, and esophagus by 20 percent; others by 10 percent). The great uncertainty of this estimate is indicated by the range of 10 to 70 percent which they attach to their estimate. Wynder and Gori (368) estimate, by calculating the percent difference between U.S. mortality rates and the lowest rates reported worldwide and by considering specific case-control studies, that an even larger proportion of cancer, approximately 40 percent in males and 60 percent in females, could be attributable to diet.

In testimony before the Subcommittee on Nutrition of the Senate Committee on Agriculture, Nutrition, and Forestry, Dr. Arthur Upton (353), then-Director of the National Cancer Institute (NCI), succinctly discussed the extent of involvement of diet and cancer when he stated:

Despite the impression that cancers are linked with dietary patterns and the inability to pinpoint specific dietary carcinogens, scientists generally agree that factors in diet and nutrition—including drinking water contaminants—appear to be related to a large number of human cancers, perhaps approaching 50 percent.

Dietary Intake

Fat/Meat Intake

Examination of cancer rates in different countries show positive correlations between colon cancer and consumption of meat and animal protein and between cancer of the breast and endometrium with total fat consumption (17). These cancers are common in the United States, Canada, and Western Europe and rarer throughout the developing world.

The most widely held theory is that fat in the diet has a promotional effect on the development of cancer. One suggested mechanism is that fats affect hormone levels. Several cancers, including breast, ovarian, and endometrial are, in turn, influenced by hormones. This association of dietary fat with higher cancer rates is, however, not found uniformly. Breast and colorectal cancers are not uncommon among vegetarians, and the observed incidence in Seventh Day Adventists who are largely vegetarian, is matched by the same incidence in Mormons who eat meat (293). This finding and the fact that meat intake among Mormons is not markedly lower than among the general population is often cited as a rebuttal to the meat/fat cancer causation hypothesis. These interpretations

should be viewed cautiously for the studies may not have been adequate to reflect any promotional effect in these low risk groups who are less exposed to many other types of carcinogenic stimuli, such as, cigarettes and alcohol, than is the general population. Additional studies in this area are needed.

More and more, studies have focused on specific types of fat. Evidence suggests that diets with a high ratio of polyunsaturated fats (mainly of vegetable origin) to saturated fats (mainly of animal origin) may increase the risk of cancer. Paradoxically, this type of diet is recommended to lower the risk of heart disease. Results from epidemiological studies (98,290) and animal trials (53,305) have been inconsistent and confusing, and have shown different effects on different cancer sites. In rats, polyunsaturated fats need be only a small proportion of a total high fat intake to promote breast tumor incidence. If the animal model is applicable to humans, virtually all high-fat diets will exert a promotional effect (52).

Serum cholesterol has been investigated in many studies as a risk factor for various cancers. Serum levels are directly affected by intake of cholesterol and fat. A diet with a low saturated fat to polyunsaturated fat ratio decreases the amount of ingested cholesterol that will appear in the serum. The discovery that the stools of colorectal cancer patients contain an abnormally high proportion of acid steroids, derived from bile salts, and cholesterol, supports the hypothesis that certain types of fat play a role in the production of colorectal cancer.

A recent epidemiologic study found an association between high-density lipoproteins and cancer risk (199). On the other hand, in a prospective epidemiologic study of heart disease in Framingham, Mass., serum cholesterol levels were inversely associated with the incidence of colon cancer and other sites in men. Men with the lowest serum cholesterol levels experienced a colon cancer rate which was three times higher than men with the higher cholesterol levels (361). A similar negative association was reported in data from the Paris Prospective Study of Coronary Heart Disease (45).

The hypothesis that dietary cholesterol plays a direct role in the production of colon cancer is supported by some animal studies. For instance, the addition of cholesterol to the diet of rats on a cholesterol-free liquid diet, had a promotional effect and cholesterol enhanced the carcinogenic effect of a known carcinogen (1,2 dimethylhydrazine).

Fiber Intake

Burkitt (40) observed that several intestinal diseases that are common in developed countries are rare in rural Africa where unprocessed food is consumed, and the stools tend to be soft, bulky, and frequent. It is suggested that dietary fiber may reduce colorectal cancer by decreasing the time stools remain in the bowel, by increasing bulk (thereby decreasing the concentration of carcinogens in stool), or by perhaps altering the distribution of bacteria, some of which may produce or destroy carcinogenic metabolites.

The effects of fiber on cancer incidence have attracted much interest but remain problematical. As in the case of fats, dietary fiber is a term which covers a multitude of different substances, each of which may have different influences on carcinogenesis. The methods by which types of fiber are chemically characterized are still in a primitive state, and analyses of the composition of dietary fiber in many foods is lacking. Despite the drawbacks, some associations have emerged. A close inverse correlation has been found between the pentose fiber content of the diet and mortality from colon cancer in part of the United Kingdom (93). No correlation was shown with any other fiber types, or with dietary fiber as a whole.

Elements and Vitamins

Several metals and vitamins are linked with cancer development. They can either act as carcinogens themselves or they may biologically compete with other dietary constituents to enhance or suppress a cancerous response.

An iron-deficient syndrome was shown to be associated with a high risk of developing cancers of the pharyngeal and esophageal mucosa in northern Scandinavia. The incidence of gastric cancer is found to be 4 to 5 times higher in countries where iron deficiency is prevalent than in the United States (356).

Selenium, an effective antioxidant, is often found at higher levels in plants, milk, or human blood in sections of the United States with low cancer rates. Selenium deficiency in rats consistently increases the carcinogenic effect of known chemical carcinogens, particularly in animals fed on high polyunsaturated fat diets (190). Supplementation with selenium above dietary requirements decreases tumor yield in animals on both low- and high-polyunsaturated fat diets (188).

Stocks and Davies (24) found that a high zinc-copper ratio in soils was associated with elevated rates of human stomach cancer while Strain et al. (24) reported an association of elevated cancer rates with low zinc-copper ratios. Marginal zinc deficiency is associated with increased esophageal cancer in animals (122) and esophageal cancer patients had lower levels of zinc in their blood, hair, and tumor tissue than controls in a study of Chinese men (211). Zinc deficiency may interact synergistically with alcohol to enhance esophageal carcinogenesis (135).

The overall relationship between cancer and vitamins is not well understood. Vitamin C has been shown to reduce carcinogen formation in experimental animals (359), and this activity may be important in reducing cancer occurrence. Vitamin A (retinol) has been more exhaustively studied than any other vitamin (for review see 292) and it has been suggested that vitamin A, or, more particularly, its vegetable precursor, beta-carotene, may decrease the susceptibility of a variety of epithelial tissues to the development of cancer. Retinol (or its analogs retinoic acid and various retinoids) has been repeatedly demonstrated to diminish the risk of experimentally induced cancer in laboratory animals (93). These results are particularly intriguing because the protective effect is observed even when these substances are fed long after the animal is treated with an initiating carcinogen, and the vitamin and its analogs appear to be effective at a wide variety of sites.

People with a history of consuming above average amounts of provitamin A (beta-carotene) have a slightly lower incidence of several different types of cancer than people who give a history of consuming less. Beta-carotene is found in carrots, green leafy vegetables and in red palm oil which is used for cooking in many tropical countries. Further epidemiologic studies are now in progress in areas where red palm oil is habitually used. The role of beta-carotene in cancer prevention is still uncertain and this particular hypothesis has been mentioned to illustrate the potential importance of diet.

Local deficiency of folate (a B-complex vitamin) has been demonstrated in the abnormal cervical tissue of some women taking oral contraceptives. The observed abnormalities are often precursors of cervical cancer. Supplementation with folic acid in these women can reverse the abnormality and appears to prevent progression to carcinoma (41). Deficiencies of lipotropes (choline, methionine, and folic acid) increased the susceptibility of animals to a variety of environment carcinogens in several studies (311).

Dietary Balance

Studies in laboratory animals have shown that altering gross aspects of diet can have substantial impact on the risk of an animal developing cancer. Jose (195) reviewed several reports which demonstrate that restricting calorie intake without modifying the proportion of the individual constituents reduces the incidence of spontaneous tumors and of a variety of cancers produced by exposure to known carcinogens. Not only did calorie restriction result in decreased incidence of tumors, but it also delayed the time of appearance of tumors, and when tumors appeared, they grew and metastasized more slowly. The life spans of animals on restricted diets were often increased up to 50 percent compared to normally fed controls. However, decreased calorie intake, when accompanied by inadequate protein intake makes laboratory animals more susceptible to many environmental carcinogens (47).

A suspected association between obesity and the risk of cancer was strengthened in an epidemiologic study conducted by ACS which followed 750,000 people from 1959 to 1972 (207). Overall cancer mortality was found elevated for those individuals who were more than 40 percent heavier than average. Mortality from cancers of the colon and rectum were increased among men while mortality from cancers of the gallbladder and biliary passages, breast, cervix, endometrium, and ovary were increased among women. The meaning to be attached to the results is not entirely clear since weight is associated with a variety of social and behavioral characteristics that affect the risk of cancer in other ways, including smoking habits and socioeconomic status. Another concern is that diagnosing cancers may be more difficult in obese individuals, and cancers may generally be more advanced when they are detected.

In addition to the quantity and composition of food, the timing of intake has also been shown to be important. For example, Roe and Tucker (cited in 93) randomized mice with a high spontaneous incidence of mammary tumors, between continuous feeding, in which the mice were fed 6 g of food each day, which they consumed in frequent small amounts, and intermittent feeding, in which food was limited to 5 g per day which was eaten at once. No clear difference in longevity was observed, but nonfatal spontaneous mammary tumors arose in 64 percent of the continuously fed mice and in only 8 percent of those fed intermittently.

Immune function in both humans and animals can be severely compromised by deficiencies of certain dietary nutrients—in particular, protein, methionine, choline, folate, vitamin B_{12}, vitamin A, zinc, and pyridoxine (147). Deficiencies in certain of these nutrients, with a concomitant depression of immune system function have been demonstrated in animals and are suspected of increasing the susceptibility of developing certain cancers (356).

Naturally Occurring Carcinogens and Precursors

Along with the major components, thousands of chemical substances occur in small quantities in foods. Most naturally occurring carcinogens and mutagens are of plant origin, but an important class, nitrates and nitrites, occurs in both plants and animals.

Nitrates and Nitrites

Nitrate and nitrite salts naturally occur in vegetables, fish, and meat, are added to food for their preservative properties (see *Additives* p. 82), and are present in pesticide and drug residues in food (127). They react with other chemicals in the body to produce N-nitrosamines and N-nitrosamides. N-nitrosamines are among the most powerful chemical carcinogens in laboratory animals, producing tumors at a variety of sites including liver, kidney, lungs, esophagus, bladder, pancreas, trachea, nasal cavities, and peripheral nervous system (221). Experimentally, vitamin C has been shown to inhibit the formation of nitrosamines (359).

Epidemiological evidence linking nitrites and nitrates to cancer is fragmentary. Evidence for a relationship between gastric cancer and the nitrite content of the diet is not wholly consistent. It is notable that vegetables, which are usually the main source of dietary nitrates, appear to protect against the development of the disease, possibly because of their vitamin C content (93). On present knowledge, the possible contribution of dietary nitrates and secondary amines to the production of cancer is uncertain.

Other Substances

Cycasin in the cycad nut, safrole in sassafras, pyrrolizidine alkaloids in some plants, and extracts of coltsfoot and bracken fern are a few naturally occurring compounds which exhibit carcinogenic properties in animals. Only bracken fern has been demonstrated to cause cancer in man. Bracken fern is commonly eaten in Japan, and Japanese who eat it daily have three times the risk of developing cancer of the esophagus as Japanese who do not eat it at all (93). It has been postulated that the high bowel cancer rates in Scotland may be due to the ingestion of cattle fed on bracken fern or the leaching of the carcinogenic components into water or food (24). Range-fed cattle and sheep may pass pyrrolizidine alkaloids along to humans in their meat and milk (215).

Certain plant-derived preparations are associated with cancer. Extracts of some plants used to make herbal infusions, for use as home remedies, tonics or beverages, are carcinogenic in animals, and their tannin-containing fractions are particularly active. Some population groups who use these products have high rates of esophageal cancer, suggesting an association (297). Perhaps of greater concern, because of its widespread use, coffee has been associated with human bladder (24) and pancreatic cancer (220), but whether the associations are causal is not yet known. Studies in animal cell cultures have shown caffeine, a constituent of both coffee and tea, to potentiate the effect of carcinogenic substances (96).

Mutagenic substances have also been identified in cruciferous plants (cabbage, broccoli, etc.), from cereal grains, and some grazing range plants in the Southwestern United States (MacGregor, 1980). Other not-yet-identified carcinogens and mutagens may occur naturally in food, but on present evidence, naturally occurring carcinogens are not regarded as an important cause of cancer in the United States (93).

Carcinogens and Precursors Produced by Cooking

Another possible source of carcinogens is their production in cooking. Humans are the only animals that cook their food, and it has been known for many years that carcinogenic chemicals such as benzo(a)pyrene (B(a)P) and other polycyclic hydrocarbons are produced when meat or fish is broiled or smoked or when food is fried in fat which has been used repeatedly. Sugimura et al. (336) demonstrated that broiling also produces powerful mutagens that cannot be accounted for by the production of B(a)P alone. Few people eat more broiled foods than Americans and while the declining stomach cancer rate provides some assurance that cancer at that site is not related to broiled food, the possibility remains that colorectal cancer, which has not decreased materially, might be related. Recent evidence has shown that mutagens can in fact be produced by cooking at relatively low temperatures (100- 200C) (93).

Contaminants

Natural Contaminants

A less obvious source of carcinogenic activity and one that was overlooked altogether until the early 1960's, is the production of carcinogens by micro-organisms in stored food. Aflatoxin, a product of the fungus *Aspergillus flavus*, is the most powerful liver carcinogen known for some animal species. In addition, human liver cells contain the enzymes necessary to produce the metabolic products that appear to be responsible for its activity. There is evidence for believing that aflatoxin is a major factor in the production of liver cancer in certain tropical countries where it is a contaminant of carbohydrate foods, particularly grains and nuts. The incidence rates of primary liver cancer in different parts of Africa are approximately proportional to the amount of aflatoxin in the diet (212).

Liver cancer occurs more commonly in people who are chronically infected with hepatitis B virus and it seems probable that where aflatoxin is present in the diet, both aflatoxin and hepatitis B virus contribute to the risk of liver cancer, each multiplying the other's effects.

In the United States, primary cancer of the liver is a rare disease accounting for less than 1 percent of cancer deaths (2,796 deaths in 1978). The amount of aflatoxin in the American diet is small and is only one among several other possible causes of liver cancer. In the American context, the chief importance of the discovery of the dangers of aflatoxin is that it raises the possibility that other as yet unrecognized mycotoxins in food may be carcinogenic. Recently, there has been some evidence to suggest that a fungus may contribute to the high incidence of esophageal cancer in parts of China by increasing the nitrite content of contaminated food (209).

Environmental Contaminants

In late 1979, OTA (284) examined both regulatory approaches and monitoring strategies for coping with contaminated food. A wide variety of industrial products ranging from heavy metals and pesticide residues, to substances that leach out of packaging, such as polyinyl chloride, can pollute food. Organic compounds are felt to pose the greatest potential for environmental food contamination based on the number, volume, and toxicity of organics manufactured in the United States.

Polycyclic aromatic hydrocarbons (PAH) are found widely in all types of foods, sometimes at the same level which can be present in charcoal-broiled meats and smoked ham, i.e., up to 15 ug B(a)P/kg net weight. Some shellfish and finfish from polluted waters have been reported to contain up to 1,000 ug B(a)P/kg. The importance of ingested B(a)P in cancer induction is uncertain. Epidemiologically, no relationship has been established, and when cancer is produced experimentally in laboratory animals, it either affects an organ not represented in man or occurs by a mechanism that does not appear relevant (93).

Some chlorinated hydrocarbons that were used as pesticides (e.g., DDT, aldrin, dieldrin) produce liver tumors (hepatomas) in mice, and some have been shown to be carcinogenic in other species. These compounds accumulate in human fat, but no increase in liver tumors appears to have accompanied their introduction and use. However, the latent period is not known, and the possibility exists that effects may be seen some years from now. Pesticide residues in the form of secondary amines may constitute a hazard if the formation of nitrosamines in the stomach proves to be a cause of cancer in man.

Many other chemicals fall into this category of environmental contaminants. The extent to which these have contributed to the production of human cancers is difficult to evaluate, but believed to be small (328).

Additives

Chemicals are used to preserve food and give it color, flavor, and consistency. Food dyes were among the first chemicals investigated because of their structural similarities to accepted chemical carcinogens (24). Consumption of chemicals by consumers who are unaware of their presence is partially responsible for the food safety laws. The laws require that newly introduced direct food additives be carefully screened in the laboratory before they may be used.

Some definitely carcinogenic chemicals, which have now been withdrawn from foods, were used for a time before their carcinogenicity in animals was discovered. These include butter yellow, thiourea, and a food preservative used in Japan. The number of cancers, if any, which these additives produced is unknown. Doll and Peto (93) estimated an attribution of less than 1 percent of total cancer mortality to food additives.

Of the many food additives presently used in the United States, three require special consideration: the artificial sweeteners cyclamates and saccharin, butylated hydroxytoluene (BHT), and nitrites and nitrates.

Cyclamates were shown to produce bladder cancer in animals (24) and were removed from commerce in 1969. OTA (282) reviewed data that show saccharin caused cancer of the bladder in rats in two circumstances: 1) in straightforward feeding studies when given over two generations, and 2) when given following the administration of a powerful carcinogen. OTA also reported positive and negative results from a number of short-term tests. Therefore, some evidence supports the conclusion that saccharin causes cancer in defined conditions. The human evidence that has been collected over the last few years fails to distinguish clearly between saccharin and cyclamates, but it is more relevant to the former as the use of saccharin began earlier (in 1902) and has continued longer. An increase in incidence or mortality from bladder cancer could not be attributed to the introduction of saccharin (16).

One epidemiologic study (175) showed that ingestion of artificial sweeteners by males increased their relative risk of bladder cancer to 1.6. (The incidence of bladder cancer among men who did not consume saccharin was taken as relative risk equal to 1.0; saccharin users had a risk 60-percent higher). The results reported in the study were consistent with those from the

laboratory. In both cases cancer occurred in the bladder in males.

Subsequent epidemiologic studies have failed to confirm the relative risk of 1.6. The large case-control study of bladder cancer in the United States conducted by NCI revealed relative risks of 0.99 for males and 1.01 for females among users of artificial sweeteners in any form (174). However, Wilson (362) points out that one projection from animal studies suggests that only about 500 bladder cancer cases annually are to be expected from saccharin consumption in the United States (see also 282). The relative risk represented by 500 cases could not have been detected in the case-control study.

Doll and Peto (93) reviewed five case-control studies which examined saccharin consumption and bladder cancer. With the exception of Howe et al. (175), the relative risks in all the experiments lie very close to 1.0; some slightly higher; some lower. They conclude that the "human evidence could hardly be more null," at least for cancer of the bladder, which was the anatomic site affected by saccharin in rats (93).

BHT has been used extensively as an antioxidant for many years. It is not carcinogenic by itself, but has been reported to enhance the production of lung tumors by urethan in mice (93). Conversely, its antioxidant effect is found to inhibit the formation of active carcinogens in the laboratory (93), and similar effects might be expected to occur in vivo. It has been postulated that its use— and perhaps that of the more widely used butylated hydroxyanisole—have contributed to the decline in mortality from stomach cancer (24).

Nitrites have been used to preserve meat since the last century (also see above). According to Shubik (328), nitrites added to food constitutes only 10 percent of the total nitrite reaching the stomach in vegetables and saliva. However, if the formation of nitrosamines and nitrosamides in the intestinal tract proves to be of practical importance, dietary nitrite may play a role in cancer formation. The National Research Council's Panel on Nitrates (cited in 93) was unable to reach any conclusions about their quantitative effect, but advised that reasonable measures be taken to minimize human exposure to N-nitroso compounds, including the restriction of the amounts of nitrate and nitrite added to meat products.

There is great uncertainty regarding the contribution of the compounds discussed above to the formation of cancer. The possibility also exists that other additives might have detrimental effects.

Diet Summary

Dietary components discussed above, and many others, are currently the subjects of intensive research, from which some results should be known within the next few years. The outcomes may show diet to be a factor in determining cancer occurrence at many sites, particularly the stomach, large bowel, endometrium, gallbladder, and in tropical countries, the liver. Diet may also be shown to affect the incidence of cancers of the breast and pancreas, and, through the antipromoting effects of retinoids, to reduce incidence of epithelial cancers in many other tissues. If these or other hypotheses are proven, practicable means of dietary modifications may eventually be identified to reduce cancer rates.

Cairns (43) draws attention to the probable difficulty of changing cancer incidence even if a direct link is shown between a diet constituent and cancer incidence:

> Cancer of the lung is due to a pleasant and highly addictive habit, cancer of the large intestine and breast are most common in affluent countries and so are presumably associated with some desirable habit, such as a diet high in animal fats, that the rich nations can afford and the others cannot . . . . These are signs, therefore, that the campaign to prevent cancer may come into some conflict with people's immediate desires.

OCCUPATIONAL EXPOSURES

The last several years have seen a heated discussion concerning the contribution of occupational exposures to cancer in the United States. Since the formation of the Occupational Safety and Health Administration (OSHA) in 1970, 20 regulations have been promulgated and two more proposed relating to suspect carcinogenic factors in the workplace. Labor unions and public interest groups have criticized OSHA for moving slowly, while industry and their trade associations claim unnecessary irrational regulation and undue expense. In an effort to implement a comprehensive and rational policy for the regulation of carcinogens in the workplace, OSHA held 2 months of hearings in 1978 which attracted the participation of labor unions, environmental groups and spawned a major new trade association, the American Industrial Health Council (AIHC). Subsequently, OSHA promulgated "a general policy for the identification and regulation of physical and chemical substances that pose a potential occupational carcinogenic risk to humans" (278,279).

The first recognized industrial cancer was identified by Percival Pott, a British surgeon, who observed that scrotal cancer occurred more frequently in men who had been employed as chimney sweeps as boys. This led to the identification of soot as the first chemical and occupational carcinogen. In the ensuing years, many other groups of workers have been found to suffer from occupationally induced cancer. For the purpose of this assessment, occupational exposure is defined as exposure to a substance or physical agent through any route during the course of employment.

The workplace setting has proved to be the single most productive source of information in the discovery of carcinogenic substances. This is because of the defined populations involved and higher exposures which can be more easily monitored and identified. Table 17 lists carcinogens and processes found in the workplace which are associated with increased cancer risk. Occupations known to produce an elevated risk of cancer, though the specific agents responsible

Table 17.—Occupational Cancer Hazards

Agent	Cancer site or type	Type of workers exposed
Acrylonitrile	Lung, colon	Manufacturers of apparel, carpeting, blankets, draperies, synthetic furs, and wigs
4-aminobiphenyl	Bladder	Chemical workers
Arsenic and certain arsenic compounds	Lung, skin, scrotum, lymphatic system, hemangiosarcoma of the liver	Workers in the metallurgical industries, sheep-dip workers, pesticide production workers, copper smelter workers, vineyard workers, insecticide makers and sprayers, tanners, miners (gold miners)
Asbestos	Lung, larynx, GI tract, pleural and peritoneal mesothelioma	Asbestos factory workers, textile workers, rubber-tire manufacturing industry workers, miners, insulation workers, shipyard workers
Auramine and the manufacture of auramine	Bladder	Dyestuffs manufacturers, rubber workers, textile dyers, paint manufacturers
Benzene	Leukemia	Rubber-tire manufacturing industry workers, painters, shoe manufacturing workers, rubber cement workers, glue and varnish workers, distillers, shoemakers, plastics workers, chemical workers
Benzidine	Bladder, pancreas	Dyeworkers, chemical workers
Beryllium and certain beryllium compounds	Lung	Beryllium workers, electronics workers, missile parts producers
Bis(chloromethyl)ether (BCME)	Lung	Workers in plants producing anion-exchange resins (chemical workers)
Cadmium and certain cadmium compounds	Lung, prostate	Cadmium production workers, metallurgical workers, electroplating industry workers, chemical workers, jewelry workers, nuclear workers, pigment workers, battery workers
Carbon tetrachloride	Liver	Plastic workers, dry cleaners
Chloromethyl methyl ether (CMME)	Lung	Chemical workers, workers in plants producing ion exchange resin
Chromium and certain chromium compounds	Lung, nasal sinuses	Chromate-producing industry workers, acetylene and aniline workers, bleachers, glass, pottery, pigment, and linoleum workers
Coal tar pitch volatiles	Lung, scrotum	Steel industry workers, aluminum potroom workers, foundry workers
Coke oven emissions	Lung, kidney, prostate	Steel industry workers, coke plant workers
Dimethyl sulphate	Lung	Chemical workers, drug makers, dyemakers
Epichlorohydrin	Lung, leukemia	Chemical workers
Ethylene oxide	Leukemia, stomach	Hospital workers, research lab workers, beekeepers, fumigators
Hematite and underground hematite mining	Lung	Miners
Isopropyl oils and the manufacture of isopropyl oils	Paranasal sinuses	Isopropyl oil workers
Mustard gas	Respiratory tract	Production workers
2-naphthylamine	Bladder, pancreas	Dyeworkers, rubber-tire manufacturing industry workers, chemical workers, manufacturers of coal gas, nickel refiners, copper smelters, electrolysis workers
Nickel (certain compounds) and nickel refining	Nasal cavity, lung, larynx	Nickel refiners
Polychlorinated biphenyls (PCBs)	Melanoma	PCBs workers
Radiation, ionizing	Skin, pancreas, brain, stomach, breast, salivary glands, thyroid, GI tract, bronchus, lymphoid tissue, leukemia, multiple myeloma	Uranium miners, radiologists, radiographers, luminous dial painters
Radiation, ultraviolet	Skin	Farmers, sailors, arc welders
Soots, tars, mineral oils	Skin, lung, bladder, GI tract	Construction workers, roofers, chimney sweeps, machinists
Thorium dioxide	Liver, kidney, larynx, leukemia	Chemical workers, steelworkers, ceramic makers, incandescent lamp makers, nuclear reactor workers, gas mantle makers, metal refiners, vacuum tube makers
Vinyl chloride	Liver, brain, lung, hematolymphopoietic system, breast	Plastics factory workers, vinyl chloride polymerization plant workers
Agent(s) not identified	Pancreas	Chemists
	Stomach	Coal miners
	Brain, stomach	Petrochemical industry
	Hematolymphopoietic system	Rubber industry workers
	Bladder	Printing pressmen
	Eye, kidney, lung	Chemical workers
	Leukemia, brain	Farmers
	Colon, brain	Pattern and model makers
	Esophagus, stomach, lung	Oil refinery workers

SOURCES: Institute of Medicine (179), International Agency for Research on Cancer (185), and the Occupational Safety and Health Administration (279a).

have not yet been identified, are also included. Many of these exposures represent substantial hazards, and it is likely that other human carcinogens exist which have not yet been detected in the workplace. This may be because the added cancer risk is small in comparison to other causes of cancer, because only a few workers have been exposed, or simply because a hazard has not been suspected and therefore not looked for. Besides the substances listed, many other industrial chemicals have been found to cause cancer in laboratory animals. It must also be borne in mind that human cancer seldom develops until one or more decades after exposure to a carcinogen, and thus it is too early to ascertain whether chemicals introduced into industry during the last few decades will affect cancer rates.

Epidemiologically demonstrating an increased risk of developing cancer from an occupational exposure generally involves results from examining large numbers of exposed people, the existence of relatively large risks, or sometimes a rare cancer, which facilitates drawing associations. Even then, years may pass before a hazard is identified. As the workplace changes, workers will be exposed to additional substances, some of which may turn out to be carcinogenic.

Estimating the proportion of today's cancers that can be attributed to occupational hazards is difficult. Determining how many future cancers may arise from past and present occupational exposures is even more speculative. As with all studies of carcinogenesis, the latent period makes it extremely problematic to associate a particular occupational exposure with an increased cancer risk. Individuals frequently change jobs which can result in exposure to numerous substances, several of which may interact with each other either to promote or to inhibit tumor formation. With rapidly changing technologies, new exposures emerge while others cease. Often, the available information is based on studies which have inadequate exposure information. Exposure data are generally poor because they are usually not collected until a hazard is recognized, or at least suspected. OSHA requires monitoring only for some of the substances which it regulates. Oftentimes employees, and even in some cases employers, are unaware of specific chemical exposures.

Certain occupational diseases are difficult to diagnose and this can lead to underreporting, as exemplified by recent letters to the *New England Journal of Medicine* concerning the inability of board-certified pathologists to identify cases of asbestosis (1,318). Studies can be designed to obtain exposure data and continuously monitor workers' health, but they are expensive. Even though no system has yet been adopted to gather these types of information, such an approach may be feasible in some industries.

Many estimates have been made of the percentage of human cancers associated with occupational exposures, most ranging from 1 to 10 percent. In most instances the bases for these estimates are not presented and the estimates themselves appear little more than informed guesses. Since epidemiologic studies do not always follow individuals for their full lifetimes, calculated risks may be underestimates. The magnitude of a detected risk is dependent upon the time elapsed between exposure and the time individuals are studied.

Higginson and Muir (165) estimated the impact of environmental factors in human cancer. They stated:

> Although occupational cancers recognized so far provide some of the most satisfactory data for identifying external agents, the absolute number of cancers due to occupational exposures would appear to be relatively small, probably 1 to 3 percent of all cancers.

Wynder and Gori (368) estimated the percent of 1976 cancer incidence in the United States attributable to occupation. From their summary figure, it appears that they estimated that the fraction of cancers attributable to occupational factors was 4 percent for men and 2 percent for women. Their explanation for these estimates is as follows:

> The data presently available are, at best, educated estimates of the relationship between specific cancers and specific occupational groups. Cole et al.[2] (1972) suggested that 20%

[2]P. Hoover, R. Cole, and G. H. Friedell, "Occupation and Cancer of the Lower Urinary Tract," *Cancer* 29: 1250-60, 1972.

of bladder cancers occurring in males in the Boston area are related to occupational exposure. In certain counties of New Jersey, the increased risk for this cancer appeared to be high among workers in certain chemical industries. General estimates of the percentage of all human cancers related to occupational exposure range between 1 and 10 percent.

Cole (62) estimated slightly higher figures for workplace-caused cancer:

> My estimates are less than 15 percent for men and less than 5 percent for women. These rather low figures emphasize that we are not dealing with a single major public health problem. Rather, we are dealing with a series of modest problems which are, however, of great importance in the specific industries where they occur.

Cole does not describe the data used to derive the estimate.

Higginson and Muir (166), in a later study estimated that 6 percent of male cancers, skin cancer included, in the Birmingham and West Midland region of England in 1968 through 1972, could be attributed to occupational exposures. Their paper describes some of the information considered.

Fox and Adelstein (126) reviewed 1970-72 British vital statistics and found that 12 percent of the differences in cancer mortality among different occupational classifications could be explained by variations associated with work and the remaining 88 percent by lifestyle factors. They describe their estimate as an "oversimplified calculation, ignoring interactions between direct and indirect influences . . . clearly very crude."

Recently, a different approach was used to generate an estimate of workplace cancers by 10 distinguished research workers of NCI, the National Institute of Envronmental Health Sciences, and the National Institute for Occupational Safety and Health (82). The report calculated the proportion of cancers "for the near term and future," from quantitative estimates of risk and the numbers of workers exposed to six known carcinogens—asbestos, arsenic, benzene, chromium, nickel oxides, and petroleum fractions. This paper (82) concludes: ‚

Reasonable projections of the future consequences of past exposure to established carcinogens suggest that . . . occupationally related cancers may comprise as much as 20% or more of total cancer mortality. Asbestos alone will probably contribute up to 13-18% and the data (relating to five other carcinogens) suggest at least 10-20% more.

The total of occupationally related cancers from those six exposures is then 23 to 38 percent of the overall cancer total, to which must presumably be added the effects of other occupational carcinogens not included in the calculation. This report has been widely misquoted as an assessment of the contribution of occupational exposures to present cancer rates and is frequently discussed and criticized because of the magnitude of the estimates and their divergence from previous estimates.

While this report has not been submitted for publication, it has been widely circulated and reviewed (c.f., 9,93,332,345). The two reviews that have been published are discussed below.

Toxic Substances Strategy Committee (TSSC) Review

TSSC (345) identified several methodological aspects which might have caused the HEW (82) paper to overestimate or to underestimate the contribution of occupational factors to the overall cancer rate.

Overestimating

1. The number of cases of lung cancer associated with asbestos may have been overestimated by attributing all cases of lung cancer among asbestos workers to asbestos exposure.
2. Exposures to the examined carcinogens were probably higher in the past than they have been recently.
3. Estimates of the number of workers exposed may have been too high since: a) workers who were employed in more than one of the six industries, a likely possibility in the chromium and nickel industries, might have been counted twice, and b) estimates of the

number of exposed persons still alive and thus at risk may be exaggerated. This is particularly so with regard to the asbestos industry.

Underestimating

1. The six industries examined are not the only ones believed to have carcinogens in the workplace.
2. Epidemiologic data on which the estimates are based do not reflect total lifetime risk.
3. Identifying unexposed groups to use for comparison is difficult and the comparison group used may be at a higher risk then the least exposed members of the population.

The TSSC report concludes (345):

> Because it is difficult to quantify the impact of all these factors, one cannot tell whether the factors which lead to overestimation and those which lead to underestimation balance each other out.

Doll and Peto Review

Doll and Peto (93) examined the calculations in the OSHA paper and in their view, the estimates:

> . . . could not be regarded as having any validity, primarily because the implicit assumption was made that the industrial conditions that had been recognized as giving rise to gross hazards of occupational cancer were typical of the condition to which 11.9 million workers in the United States were currently exposed.

Doll and Peto (93) used a different approach to estimate the proportion of cancers associated with occupational exposures. Rather than focusing on individual occupational hazards, they based their assessment on the contribution of occupational factors to individual cancer sites and arrived at an estimate of approximately 4 percent with an acceptable range from 2 to 10 percent.

Lung cancers caused by asbestos contribute the largest proportion to the estimates made both by Doll and Peto (93) and by HEW (82). Hogan and Hoel (171) have completed a careful analysis of asbestos and cancer and conclude that it may be associated with as much as 3 (range: 1.4 to 4.4) percent of all cancers now or likely in the near future. This inference is considerably less than the 13 to 18 percent estimated by HEW (82).

Occupational Exposure Summary

Despite all of the arguments that have surrounded the estimates of workplace associated cancers, almost every estimate fits comfortably in the range of 10 ± 5 percent. Uncertainties about unknown carcinogens confound the estimates. Regardless of the exact number of cancers associated with the workplace, the identification of causes is most important. Preventive measures can reduce exposures only to identified risks. Recently, an unusual number of melanomas in a nuclear research installation (89) and of brain tumors among oil industry workers (55) have triggered further studies. These examples emphasize the value of workplace monitoring.

AIR AND WATER POLLUTION

Determining the health effects of pollution is difficult, particularly from low-level chronic exposures. The absolute risk from each pollutant is likely to be low and the resulting disease may not appear for many decades, as is the case with cancer. Direct measurement of the incremental risk from these pollutants using epidemiologic methods, against the background of more potent carcinogens, for instance tobacco, presents extreme methodological problems. There is often little variation between individuals in the type and extent of exposure to pervasive pollutants, and where measurable differences do exist, confounding variables often hinder adequately demonstrating an effect or the lack of one. It is therefore often necessary to rely on indirect sources of evidence that a pollutant is carcinogenic: short-term laboratory experiments that demonstrate mutagenicity or other toxic effects, animal bioassays, and epidemiologic data derived from groups exposed to high levels of pollutant chemicals. The latter are often obtained in special situations, usually occupational, where people are exposed to much larger amounts than the general public.

Air Pollution

Air pollution is primarily a problem of major cities but it can move in and out of different areas and affect everyone. The Census Bureau (35) estimates that over 70 percent of the U.S. population lives in urban centers and that this number is increasing with each passing year. The amount and type of air pollution in a given region changes not only with the time of day, but from day to day and year to year, making meaningful measurement difficult. Air pollution can be generally classified as a secondary environmental stressor, aggravating existing disease conditions or increasing the risk of disease in those predisposed to ill health (326).

A variety of carcinogenic substances has been identified in air—e.g., asbestos, arsenic, PAH—and EPA has promulgated several regulations under section 112 of the Clean Air Act to limit exposure to these substances. Table 17 (see *Occupational Exposures*) lists several recognized occupational carcinogens which may escape into the atmosphere in the course of industrial activity and constitute a potential cancer hazard.

Morbidity and mortality due to chronic obstructive lung disease—asthma, bronchitis, and emphysema—are probably the most important long-term health effects of air pollution. Urban areas generally have a higher death rate from chronic obstructive lung disease and lung cancer than more rural environments (54,205). This has been used as the basis for suggesting that atmospheric pollution is an etiologic factor in the development of cancer. However, like many apparently simple observations, this one is plagued by conflicting and confounding factors. Individuals residing in urban centers generally have smoking, drinking, and eating habits different from their rural counterparts, and their

risk of infection and exposures to industrial environments also varies. In addition, urban areas tend to have more accurate death certification and disease diagnosis which might bias collected statistics. Epidemiologic studies that examine the health effects of air pollution must deal with these factors.

Many airborne carcinogens are believed to interact synergistically with tobacco and occupational exposures. Since cigarette smoking is the predominant cause of lung cancer, it is a primary suspect for explaining the observed urban/rural gradient. There have been numerous attempts to disentangle the health effects of smoking from environmental pollution. Unfortunately, many studies have compared broad categories of smoking habits, such as "smokers" versus "nonsmokers" or "never smoked" versus "ever smoked" which reduces the probability of discerning any effects. More specific categories—e.g., taking into account number of years smoked, age at which smoking began, number of cigarettes smoked per day—are necessary to evaluate any urban/rural variation. In addition, other important differences may exist in smoking habits between urban and rural dwellers, for instance, in the tar and nicotine content, inhalation habits, and other factors contributing to differences in effective dose of carcinogen received (see *Tobacco*). Most studies concentrating on nonsmokers have failed to demonstrate, or found only a slight difference, in lung cancer rates between nonsmokers in urban and rural environs, suggesting that airborne carcinogens by themselves can be responsible for only a small portion of the disease. Several have suggested that the effects of smoking a given amount may be greater in urban than rural areas (for review, see 91).

One of the most extensive investigations into the effects of air pollution is a cohort study conducted by ACS. Data concerning men without known carcinogenic occupational exposure produced "little or no support to the hypothesis that urban air pollution has an important effect on lung cancer death rates" (154). When lung cancer rates for men with occupational exposure were compared to those for men without occupational exposures, the authors found a relative difference of 26 percent in large metropolitan areas, 18 percent in smaller metropolitan areas, and 7 percent in nonmetropolitan areas. These differences, as Hammond and Garfinkel suggest, may be due to different types of occupational exposures in the different areas. However, an alternative explanation is that the higher ratio of lung cancer may be due to an attribute of the place of residence, air pollution being one possible factor. In a reevaluation of these data, it was estimated that approximately 10 percent of lung cancer in the ACS population could be attributed to an "urban effect" after accounting for smoking and occupation (61). Studies which concentrate on nonsmokers or the nonoccupationally exposed do not permit investigating any interactive effects.

Another method for estimating the influence of pollution on the cancer rate is to extrapolate from instances of high exposure. Occupational studies that include measurements of the concentration of carcinogens in the respired air are especially useful for this purpose. Measurements of the concentration of B(a)P are frequently used because it appears to be a good indicator of the concentration of PAH. However, it should be noted that B(a)P is not a perfect indicator of PAH in air, nor does it accurately reflect the carcinogenic potential of total air pollution. For instance, some non-PAH fractions of air pollution are as active as PAH in causing changes in cell cultures, which is a measure related to carcinogenicity (294).

Pike and his colleagues (294) concluded that 1 ng B(a)P per m^3 in city air causes 0.4/100,000 extra cases of lung cancer per year. In 1977, an international symposium at the Karolinska Institute in Stockholm, reached a similar conclusion (54):

> . . . combustion products of fossil fuels in ambient air, probably acting together with cigarette smoke, have been responsible for cases of lung cancer in large urban areas, the numbers produced being of the order of 5 to 10 cases per 100,000 males per year . . . The actual rate will vary from place to place . . . depending upon local conditions.

These estimates must be used with caution since they are directly dependent on the concentration of the different air pollutants, many of which have been changing over time. In 1959, BaP concentrations ranged from 1 ng/m^3 to approximately 60 ng/m^3; most nonurban areas had levels below 1 ng/m^3. Recent monitoring by EPA found that the average concentration of B(a)P in 26 urban areas decreased from approximately 4 ng/m^3 in the late 1960's to 0.5 ng/m^3 in 1977 (70). Doll and Peto (93) estimated that the current contribution of atmospheric B(a)P and associated combustion products to the production of lung cancer is unlikely to account for more than 1 percent of future cases of lung cancer.

Similar calculations have been made for other carcinogenic substances including airborne arsenic and asbestos (93). These suggest that contributions to the overall cancer rate from these agents should be small. Higher levels of pollutants and therefore greater risk may exist around particular sources of pollution as exhibited by the significantly increased mortality from lung cancer found in residents of counties with copper, lead, or zinc smelters or refineries (28). The amount of asbestos commonly present in urban air is 1,000 to 10,000 times less than the most stringent occupational regulations, although the general public is exposed continuously to this low level. At present, there is no evidence to indicate that the risk to the general public from these sources is measurable.

Also included under the heading of atmospheric pollution is the effect on the general population of mining and milling of uranium and other radioactive ores and of radioactive fallout due to testing of nuclear weapons. The HEW Interagency Task Force on the Health Effects of Ionizing Radiation (182) estimated that for 1978 the U.S. population collective dose was 1 million to 1.6 million person-rem. Based on the risk estimates derived from the linear model of the NAS Committee on the Biological Effects of Ionizing Radiation (BEIR) III (158 to 403 excess cancer deaths per million persons from continuous lifetime exposure to 1 rad/yr) one can estimate that atmospheric radiation accounts for an upper limit of 645 fatal cancers per year. The lower limit of risk can be considered to approach zero.

The other class of atmospheric agents given considerable attention because of a potential effect on cancer rates are the chlorofluorocarbons. Chlorofluorocarbons, used extensively as refrigerants and aerosol propellants, persist in the atmosphere and, it is argued, eventually reach the stratosphere where they react with ozone, reduce its concentration, and hence permit more ultraviolet light to reach the surface of the Earth. This occurrence would result in an increase in the incidence of skin cancer, including melanoma. The issues involved, which are complex and based on a number of unproved assumptions about physical and chemical processes, have been reviewed by the National Academy of Sciences (NAS) (70,264). They found that if global release of chlorofluorocarbons were to continue at 1977 rates, the ozone concentration would eventually decline by 16.5 percent, with a reduction of about 8 percent by the year 2030 (70). A 16-percent ozone depletion is predicted to eventually cause several thousand more cases of melanoma each year in the United States and several hundred thousand more cases of other less serious skin cancers (70). This is approximately the same order of magnitude predicted by Urbach (354). The present contribution of chlorofluorocarbons to overall cancer incidence is likely to be much less.

Until recently, air pollution was a problem believed to be limited to outside air or dirty workplaces. Several studies have found that indoor air pollution may be a more serious health hazard than outdoor air pollution (140). It has been shown that a single smoker can pollute indoor air with around 1-1.5 ng/m³ B(a)P (260). NAS was asked by EPA to examine the variables which are contributing to indoor air pollution, their sources, and possible health hazards. To date, this issue has not been looked at in a systematic way though many people spend a large percentage of their time in the indoor environment. The General Accounting Office (140) suggested that the Clean Air Act be amended to provide EPA the responsibility and necessary authority to address indoor air pollution in the nonworkplace.

In sum, determining the proportion of the total cancer rate attributable to air pollution is not possible with the available data. In most studies, air pollution and smoking are seen as interactive in cancer production. Whatever the correct percentage of cancer associated with air pollution, most researchers in this area believe that it is small. Doll and Peto (93) estimated that 2 percent of cancer mortality, representing approximately 8,000 cancer deaths, can be attributed to industrial pollution of air, water, and food, principally accounted for by the uncertain effects of combustion products of fossil fuels in urban air. This relatively small percentage does not mean that efforts to control air pollutants should be minimized. Air pollution is responsible for many serious detrimental health effects other than cancer and uncontrolled pollution might someday be found to impact more dramatically on cancer rates. Greater attention should be directed at discerning whether atmospheric pollutants act as initiating and/or promoting agents. If air pollution is acting as a secondary stressor, then its role as a promoter may prove to be most important.

Drinking Water Pollution

The extent to which water pollution is a causative agent for cancer is even less certain and more debated than is the role of air pollution. The passage of the Safe Drinking Water Act, Public Law 93–523, December 1974, was prompted by the recognition that organic and inorganic chemicals, including substances identified as known or suspect carcinogens and mutagens were present in drinking waters. The sources for these contaminants are numerous: industrial pollution, agricultural runoff, leachate from waste disposal sites, and of particular recent interest, byproducts of the disinfection of drinking water.

In the mid 1970's, EPA set up various programs, such as the National Organics Reconnaissance Survey, to evaluate the nature and extent of organics in drinking water. Primary emphasis was on detecting a class of organics, the trihalomethanes, formed during water treatment with chlorine and believed to be the most ubiquitous group of organics found in drinking water. Levels have been found to range from below 1 ug/liter to above 300 ug/liter. The Federal Government has recently sought to reduce exposure to trihalomethanes by promulgating a regulation establishing a "maximum contaminant level" of 100 ug/liter total trihalomethanes for all community water systems serving 10,000 persons or more that add a disinfectant in the treatment of their water (107).

Much attention has been centered on the relatively high concentrations of synthetic organics found in untreated drinking water from ground water sources in certain areas of the United States. The extent to which these waterborne pollutants contribute to human carcinogenesis has been evaluated by the examination of both laboratory and epidemiologic data. Many of these studies were reviewed by the NAS Safe Drinking Water Committee (266,270) as mandated by the Congress. (These reports stand as references for many issues concerning the health effects of drinking water contaminants.)

The numerous epidemiologic studies that have examined the association between drinking water and cancer have been of varying reliability and have taken many forms. These studies suggest an association between constituents in drinking water and cancer mortality (169). However, the degree and extent of the association is disputed. NAS discussed and evaluated 10 of the studies which focused on the relationship of trihalomethanes and cancer mortality. All but one of the studies were found to demonstrate a statistical association between exposure and excess cancer rate, but excess cancer at no single anatomical site was associated with exposure. The epidemiologic analyses do not have the extrapolation difficulties of animal experiments, but they are plagued by confounding variables such as exposures to other sources of carcinogenic stimuli, including smoking, which were generally not accounted for. Many of the studies utilized the cancer deaths rates of a

region and related them to the water quality of that region. The difficulty with this approach is twofold: 1) an individual's place of death may differ considerably from where that person resided during most of his water-drinking life, and 2) the data on water quality are extremely limited, often reflecting the water quality of only one water source in a region.

Prior to 1970, about 100 different organic compounds has been identified in water (169). In the past, organic pollutants were measured by crude, nonspecific methods such as biochemical oxygen demand and total organic content. Today, analytical techniques permit detection of chemicals in minute quantities, and many are found in concentrations of parts per trillion. NAS (270) found that over 700 volatile organic compounds contaminate U.S. drinking water. Volatile substances make up only 10 percent of the total organic content of water and approximately 90 percent of this component has been identified and quantified. On the other hand, only 5 to 10 percent of the nonvolatile constituents of drinking water have deen characterized (266). As technology improves and detection methods become more sensitive, an ever-increasing number of compounds may be detected in drinking water.

In a report for the Council on Environmental Quality, Crump and Guess (74) reviewed five of the recent case-control studies on cancer risk associated with drinking water quality in this country. While inadequacies were identified in each of the studies (74):

> . . . increased risks . . . are large enough to be of concern yet small enough to be very difficult to separate from confounding risks associated with other environmental factors.

Rectal cancer risk ratios for chlorinated v. unchlorinated water were found to range from 1.13 to 1.93. In three of the studies the risk ratios were statistically significant. Statistically significant risk ratios were also found in three of the studies for colon cancer and in two studies for bladder cancer. Although the studies did not indicate a consistently increasing cancer risk with increasing exposure to organic contaminants, one study did show such a relationship for rectal cancer and another was suggestive for colon cancer.

Crump and Guess made crude estimates of the possible range of carcinogenic risks from consuming ground water (from wells) containing various levels of synthetic organic chemicals. They computed an upper risk limit of 7.5 × 10^{-4} or about one case per 1,300 persons from consuming water from a hypothetical well containing the highest detected concentrations of commonly found contaminants. Levels to which most Americans are exposed are typically much lower. The estimate is based on summing the individual upper limits on human risk derived by a procedure which tends to produce exaggerated estimates of human risk. On the other hand, only risks from chemicals known to be present in the wells and for which positive carcinogenicity data exist, were considered in the estimate (74). Crump and Guess also computed an upper limit on the lifetime total cancer risk associated with an average concentration of chloroform to be 1.8 × 10^{-4} or about one case per 5,000 persons. The actual risk is probably much lower.

The NAS Safe Drinking Water Committee lists 19 carcinogens and 3 suspected carcinogens identified in or thought to be in drinking water (266). NAS estimated the 95-percent upper confidence limit of cancer risks to humans from lifetime exposure to water containing 1 ug/l of each of these compounds. These estimates are displayed in table 18 and are compared with risk estimates computed by EPA's Carcinogen Assessment Group. It is interesting to note that in many cases a tenfold to hundredfold difference exists between the two estimates. These differences are due to the use of different extrapolation models and the use of point rather than interval estimates.

The problem of evaluating the effects of multiple exposures is acutely relevant to waterborne pollutants because of the multitude of compounds found in drinking water. Bioassays have rarely attempted evaluation of synergistic or antagonistic effects. Therefore, these estimates may not accurately reflect the human carcinogenic risk from these compounds.

Table 18.—Concentration of Drinking Water Contaminants and Calculated Excess Cancer Risk

	NAS[a]	CAG[b]
	10^{-6} ug/l[c]	10^{-6} ug/l[c]
Acrylonitrile	0.77	0.034
Arsenic	—	0.004
Benzene	—	3.0
Benzo (a) pyrene............	—	—
Beryllium	—	0.02
Bis (2-chloroethyl) ether	0.83	—
Carbon tetrachloride	9.09	0.086
Chlordane..................	0.056	0.012
Chloroform	0.59	0.48
DDT	0.083	—
1,2-Dichloroethane	1.4	1.46
1,1-Dichloroethylene	—	.28
Dieldrin	0.004	—
Ethylenedibromide	0.11	0.0022
ETU	0.46	—
Heptachlor	0.024	2.4
Hexachlorobutadiene	—	1.4
Hexachlorobenzene	0.034	—
N-nitrosodimethylamine	—	0.0052
Kepone	0.023	—
Lindane	0.108	—
PCB	0.32	—
PCNB	7.14	—
TCDD.....................	—	5.0 × 10^{-6}
Tetrachloroethylene	0.71	0.82
Trichloroethylene	9.09	5.8
Vinyl chloride	2.13	106.0

[a]Standardized to 10^{-6} risks from National Academy of Sciences, *Drinking Water and Health* (266) for consumption of 1 l/water/day.
[b]Recalculated to exclude aquatic food intake from Cancer Assessment Group, *Ambient Water Quality Criteria* (104). Standardized to 1 l/water/day intake.
[c]Average adult water consumption is 2 l/day.

SOURCE: Office of Technology Assessment.

As more chemicals are tested, additional substances found in drinking water will be shown to be carcinogenic. Two substances identified in drinking water, toxaphene and 1,2 dichloroethane, not considered carcinogenic by NAS in 1977, have since been shown by NCI to be carcinogenic in animals. Two additional compounds, bromodichloromethane and chlorodibromomethane, found in most drinking water systems surveyed by EPA, have not been appropriately tested for carcinogenic properties but have been shown to be mutagenic in the Ames test (169). In 1978, NCI (203) published a list of 23 recognized or suspected carcinogens, 30 mutagens and 11 tumor promoters which have been found in American drinking water.

Turning from the organics to inorganics, several studies have attempted to correlate levels of carcinogenic trace metals in water supplies, with cancer rates. Associations of high levels of arsenic in drinking water with cancer of the skin and other sites were found in Taiwan and Argentina (203,370). Berg and Burbank (25) compared concentrations of eight carcinogenic metals in water supplies with State cancer mortality rates. They found strong correlations with cadmium concentrations and cancer mortality; no significant correlations with iron, cobalt, and chromium; a low but not biologically interpretable level of significance with nickel and arsenic; and some correlations with lead and beryllium which correspond to known biological activities.

Asbestos, an established human carcinogen, is also of some concern since it has been found to contaminate water supply systems. No relationship between asbestos in drinking water and cancer has been found but available data are very limited.

Experimental and epidemiologic data provide some evidence that a carcinogenic hazard exists from drinking water contaminants, but does not permit adequate quantification. Most attention on quantifying risk estimates from waterborne carcinogens has focused on chloroform, since it alone has consistently generated dose-response data sufficient for extrapolating human risk. An ad hoc study group of the EPA's Hazardous Material's Advisory Committee (158) estimated the risk as follows:

> The level of risk, estimated from consideration of the worst case [Miami, 311 ppb] and for the expected cancer site for chloroform (the liver), might be extrapolated to account for up to 40% of the observed liver cancer incidence.

The results of a large NCI case-control study which is examining possible relationships between water quality and bladder cancer are expected in 1981. Information was obtained in that study on a wide range of demographic and exposure factors and a data bank on water quality was created for more than 1,000 utilities serving many of the people in the study. That information will hopefully permit linking an individual's risk factors with disease state. In addition, a case-control interview study to investigate relationships between drinking water and colorectal cancer is being conducted (74).

CONSUMER PRODUCTS

Consumer products are a class of agents that are so numerous that it is only possible to echo the uncertainty with which pollutants were discussed in the previous section. Detergents and other surfactants, hair dyes and other cosmetics, solid or foam plastics, paints, dyes, polishes, solvents, fabrics, and even the processed paper and the printer's ink in this report are but a few. It is likely that some of these products are already causing, unnoticed, a number of today's cancers, and it is quite possible that after prolonged exposure substantial risks might be detected in the future.

The difficulty in assessing cancers associated with exposure to consumer products is that the dose is usually low, and the exposed population tends to be very large. An adequate assessment of the carcinogenic effect of a consumer product might require a study of a million people, whereas a study of only 1,000 workers might be adequate in an occupational setting. Further, while occupational exposure to a carcinogen is frequently limited to a group of relatively healthy workers, consumer exposure includes subpopulation groups usually considered to be "at high risk," such as infants, small children, the elderly, and the infirm.

For most consumer products, available laboratory and human evidence is insufficient to determine whether they pose a cancer risk. The magnitude of the potential health hazard becomes apparent when one begins to examine population exposure to different consumer products. In 1973, U.S. production of aerosol products was estimated at 2.9 billion units. A recent Consumer Product Safety Commission (CPSC) study indicated that manufacturers removed trichloroethylene (TCE), a widely used solvent in aerosol formulations, from consumer aerosol product formulas after TCE was shown to be carcinogenic in tests at NCI (117). The extent to which aerosol products containing TCE has impacted on today's cancer rates or how many future cancers will result from past exposures is difficult to evaluate.

Attempts at quantifying potential adverse effects associated with consumer exposure to carcinogens are relatively new. In 1977, CPSC estimated that exposure of children to TRIS-treated clothing could result in an excess risk of cancer of up to 180 cases per million exposures. Other examples of estimated consumer risk include up to 2,000 lifetime excess respiratory cancer deaths per million persons exposed to asbestos-containing patching compounds; paint stripper containing 52 percent benzene may present an excess risk of death from leukemia of up to 50 per million people exposed; and people living in a residence insulated with urea-formaldehyde foam may be at an excess cancer risk of up to 290 per million people exposed (117).

At this time it is impossible to assess the contribution of consumer products to the overall cancer rate. Many industrial products have been introduced so recently that even if they do prove hazardous their effects would not yet be apparent. Doll and Peto (93) attribute "less than 1 percent" of all cancer deaths to such products, but stress that there is too much ignorance for complacency to be justified.

MEDICAL DRUGS AND RADIATION

Medical practices have resulted in some devastating health crises, from the fatal puerperal fevers of the 19th century maternity wards to the millions who were exposed in utero to diethylstilbestrol (DES) and are now experiencing a variety of adverse health effects, including at least one type of cancer. Only drugs which have been associated with cancer in humans will be discussed in detail, but limited or inconclusive evidence exists for many others, and still others have not been investigated (see table 19).

The production of cancer, although always an undesirable side effect, is not necessarily a bar to the use of a drug if the risk of cancer development is materially less than the medical gains brought about by the treatment—e.g., by the use of alkylating agents, immunosuppressive drugs and radiotherapy in the treatment of cancer. The risks in some cases are known, as with some cancer chemotherapy agents, but more often are not suspected. Detection of disproportionate adverse effects through case reports and epidemiologic studies have caused the abandonment of certain agents and treatments for particular uses, for instance, inorganic trivalent arsenic, chlornaphazine, DES during pregnancy, and the radioactive agents thorium and thorotrast.

The causal link between in utero exposure to DES, a synthetic estrogen, and subsequent development of a rare type of vaginal cancer in females (and possibly testicular cancer in males) about 20 years later is a well-publicized example of unsuspected risk. Between 4 million and 6 million Americans (mothers, daughters, sons) were exposed to DES since about 1945 (258) in efforts to prevent spontaneous abortions. As later became evident, DES was an ineffective therapy (90).

In this case, in spite of the long latency between in utero exposure and cancer development two or three decades later, the connection was made between exposure and disease. The facilitating factor in this case was the near non-existence of the cancer type in the general population at the ages in which the disease was seen. However, had the effect been a small excess of a common cancer, it is doubtful that the association would have been uncovered. Since the original association was uncovered, other possible adverse effects have been suspected in DES mothers, daughters and sons.

In cases of agents for which some risk is known or suspected, the use of the agent is continued under controlled conditions, in the belief

Table 19.—Drugs Associated with Cancer in Humans

Drugs established as human carcinogens

Drug	Malignancy

Radioactive drugs:
  Phosphorus (P^{32})
  Radium
  Mesothorium
  Thorotrast
	Organs where concentrated:
	  Acute leukemia, osteosarcoma,
	  nasal sinus carcinoma, angiosarcoma
	  of the liver

Chlornaphazine	Bladder cancer
Arsenic	Skin cancer
Methoxypsoralen	Skin cancer

Alkylating agents:
  Melphalan, chlorambucil,
  dihydroxybusulfan, busulphan, and others
	Acute nonlymphocytic leukemia
	  other sites?

Cyclophosphamide	Bladder cancer

Immunosuppressive agents—Azothioprine	Lymphoma, skin cancer, soft-tissue sarcoma
	  melanoma? liver and gallbladder?
	  lung adenocarcinoma?

Androgenic-anabolic steroids	Hepatocellular carcinoma

Steroid contraceptives	Endometrial carcinoma, liver tumors (benign)
	  breast cancer? cervical cancer? ovarian cancer?
	  choriocarcinoma? melanoma?

Estrogens:
  DES (prenatal)
  Conjugated estrogens
	
	Vaginal adenocarcinoma
	Endometrial carcinoma
	  breast cancer? ovarian cancer?

Phenacetin-containing drugs	Renal pelvis carcinoma bladder cancer?

Suspect drugs for which human evidence of carcinogenicity is either inconclusive or conflicting

Drug	Malignancy
Chloramphenicol	Leukemia
Iron Dextran	Soft tissue sarcoma (site of injection)
Dilantin	Lymphoma
Phenobarbital	Brain tumors, liver cancer
Amphetamines	Lymphoma
Reserpine	Breast cancer
Progesterone (Depo-Provera)	Cervical cancer
Phenylbutazone	Leukemia
Crude tar ointment	Skin cancer
Clofibrate	Gastrointestinal and respiratory malignancies

Suspect drugs for which human studies have as yet not yielded evidence of carcinogenicity

Isoniazid

Metronidazole

Antimetabolites (Methotrexate, 5-Fluorouracil)

Suspect drugs as yet unevaluated in humans

Dapsone

Griseofulvin

Phenothiazines

Oxytetracycline

Chloroquin

SOURCE: Hoover and Fraumeni (173).

that the benefit will prove to outweigh the harm. Many of the known hazardous drugs are used in the treatment of relatively uncommon serious conditions and the sum of the cancers caused by them can amount to no more than a few score throughout the entire country each year. However, some drugs, including oral contraceptives, and estrogens are or have been used extensively. These and the medical use of ionizing radiation, also known to be carcinogenic, are discussed below.

Oral Contraceptives

Oral contraceptives are taken by over 80 million healthy women the world over (366), spurring international concern about possible health effects. Not surprisingly, the possibility of increased cancer risk after long-term use and a long latent period has been the focus of major epidemiologic efforts.

The evidence to date has clearly implicated one type of sequential oral contraceptive (an estrogen and a progestin taken separately during the first and second halves of the monthly cycle), the use of which has been abandoned, with some cases of endometrial cancer in young women. Conversely, there is some evidence that users of combination type oral contraceptives (an estrogen and a progestin taken together in the same pill) may be at slightly lower risk for endometrial cancer (360).

In animal tests, both breast and liver cancers have been induced by components of oral contraceptives. A small number of benign liver tumors in humans have been associated with certain types of oral contraceptives, and though not cancers in the usual sense, they can cause fatal internal hemorrhage. No controlled study has yet evaluated the possible risk of malignant liver tumors (173).

Studies of breast cancer in oral contraceptive users have thus far yielded no clear-cut evidence for either increased or decreased risk, except perhaps some increase for women already at high risk (see p. 99, *Sexual Development, Reproductive Patterns, and Sexual Practices* for a full discussion of risk factors). Cervical cancer

also has been studied extensively with no consistent findings.

There is some evidence to suggest that oral contraceptives may reduce the risk of ovarian cancer. The reduction may be related to lowered levels of ovulatory activity, since high levels have been associated with an increased risk of ovarian cancer.

Because oral contraceptives have been part of the American lifestyle for a relatively short period, large numbers of users have not reached old age, the period of greatest cancer risk. Until such time, perhaps within the decade, the full effects cannot be known. Even then, because there are many types of oral contraceptives, some of which already have been shown to have different effects, and because formulations and dosage levels have changed significantly over time, risks identified for that first cohort may not apply to today's users. Overall, evaluating the evidence available at this time, oral contraceptives do not appear to be a major cause of cancer, but do require continued epidemiologic attention.

Menopausal Estrogens

The use of "replacement estrogens" to relieve menopausal symptoms became widespread in the 1960's. A sharp rise in the incidence of endometrial cancer followed through the mid-1970's in what has been termed "one of the largest epidemics of iatrogenic disease . . . in this country" (194). A cause-and-effect relationship was established through epidemiologic studies, precipitating a decline in the use of these agents. Shortly after the levels of use dropped, incidence began to fall toward previous levels, and the "epidemic" appears to be largely over. Fortunately, these endometrial cancers have a relatively good prognosis, and while morbidity increased sharply, mortality attributable to estrogen therapy has not paralleled the incidence trend. Estrogen therapy is still prescribed for some women, generally for shorter periods of time than previously. Used in this way, the risk of endometrial cancer appears much lower, though some cases may still occur, but the benefits of therapy are thought to outweigh the residual risk.

Evidence has been accumulating that breast cancer risk may be increased by menopausal estrogen therapy (173), particularly among women who develop benign breast disease while taking estrogens (93). Unlike the case of endometrial cancer and estrogen therapy, where increased and decreased risk follow closely the temporal pattern of usage, change in breast cancer risk appears to require many years to manifest itself.

Other associations between menopausal estrogens and cancer have been suggested. The Boston Collaborative Drug Surveillance Program (30) reported increased gallbladder disease, which is a strong risk factor for cancer of the gallbladder, among women who had estrogen therapy. Some studies have suggested an increased risk of ovarian cancer; others a decreased risk of some reproductive-site cancers (173). Because of these uncertainties and the long latent periods associated with many cancers, continued long-term followup is required to determine if associations exist, and if so, the magnitude of the risks.

Other Drugs of Known Carcinogenicity

Certain alkylating agents, a class of drugs used primarily in the treatment of cancer, have been convincingly associated with acute non-lymphocytic leukemia, known to have a relatively short latent period, and one agent in particular, cyclophosphamide, with bladder cancer. As survival improves for some treated cancers, increases may be seen in some other solid tumors, which generally have longer latent periods than leukemia.

Immunosuppressive agents, used widely in transplant patients, greatly increase the risk of lymphoma, and result in moderate increases in tumors at several other sites. The sites which show an increase are similar to those encountered with genetically determined immune deficiency syndromes and other conditions associated with immunodeficiency.

The initial report of a program designed to screen large numbers of commonly used drugs for carcinogenicity has recently appeared (133). The followup period has been only 4 years, and 53 possible associations have been identified, some with increased risk and some with decreased risk of cancer. Until a longer followup period has elapsed, no conclusions of causality can be reached. The importance of this type of surveillance mechanism lies in its long-term utility, in identifying carcinogens and generating hypotheses.

The Interagency Task Force on the Health Effects of Ionizing Radiation (182) estimated that the collective dose of radiation received by the U.S. population for medical purposes, mainly diagnostic, amounts to about 18 million person-rem per year. Using the linear model from BEIR III (268), which produces a conservatively high estimate, the risk of all types of cancer ranges from 158 to 403 fatal cancers per million person-rem. Applying these values to the total population yields an estimate of between 2,844 and 7,254 fatal cancers per year. Using the least conservative model, the lower risk estimate approached zero. However, some of the medically associated radiation would have been received by people with an expectation of life that was too short for any significant chance of developing radiation-induced cancer (because of illness or age) and the total effect may be somewhat less.

Although well over half of the total population receives some medical radiation, the most susceptible members of the population—unborn fetuses—are of particular concern. Stewart, et al. (333) in England and MacMahon (216) in the United States first identified a risk to children who had been exposed in utero, which has been corroborated by numerous studies since. There is also evidence that the risk of childhood cancer is increased by X-rays of the mother even before pregnancy (327), suggesting that both germ cell (in this case, ovum) mutations as well as somatic (in the cells of the developing child) may be important.

Pelvimetry, a radiographic examination used to determine the pelvic dimensions of the mother and the fetal headsize, is the major source of ionizing radiation to fetuses. It has been estimated that in recent years, 6 percent (about 200,000/yr) of all births have received routine pelvimetry, and rates are much higher in some places (46,198). The Food and Drug Administration (FDA) panel on X-ray pelvimetry, in a statement adopted by the American College of Radiology concluded that, "Pelvimetry is not usually necessary or helpful in making the decision to perform a cesarean section." A similar statement approved by the American College of Obstetricians and Gynecologists states that: "X-ray pelvimetry provides little additional information to physicians involved in the management of labor and delivery." Both groups recommend that pelvimetry be limited to individual cases meeting specific criteria for usefulness, and should not be used as a routine examination (39). Although the actual numbers of childhood cancers caused by medical radiation may be modest, the number could easily be reduced by reductions in irradiation at least during and probably prior to pregnancy.

Unnecessary and unproductive radiation is not limited to pelvimetry. The Bureau of Radio-logical Health (FDA) has addressed this issue by beginning to prepare a series of documents addressing patient selection, conduct of examinations, and interpretation of results in radiographic procedures (38).

Doll and Peto (93) have estimated that about 1 percent of 1977 cancer deaths probably are attributable to medical practice. They go on to say that the number of ways in which drugs might in principle increase or decrease cancer incidence rates is almost limitless.

Higginson and Muir (163) attributed about 1 percent of all cancers in the Birmingham and West Midland region of England (1968–72) to iatrogenic causes. They note that the widespread use of estrogen therapy in the United States might indicate a higher proportion for U.S. women. Wynder and Gori (368) estimated that about 4 percent of 1976 U.S. cancer incidence was associated with exogenous hormones.

SEXUAL DEVELOPMENT, REPRODUCTIVE PATTERNS, AND SEXUAL PRACTICES

Sexual development and reproductive patterns affect the development of a number of cancers, affecting females to a greater degree than males. The course of sexual development itself may be heavily influenced by such factors as diet and body composition (fat-to-lean ratio), and reproductive patterns are often influenced by economic and social conditions. Reproductive and dietary factors might well interact multiplicatively in the production of these cancers and there will be overlap between what is preventable through diet and through reproductive factors. Doll and Peto (93) have estimated that about 7 percent (6 percent from breast, ovarian, and endometrial cancers and 1 percent from cervical cancer) of all cancers might be prevented by measures affecting the mechanisms of reproduction and sexual factors.

Some evidence is consistent with cervical cancer in women being associated with infectious agents and less certain evidence associating other genitourinary cancers with infection. If this is true, some cancer-causing agents may be transmitted as venereal diseases.

Cancers of the Breast, Ovary, and Endometrium

The probability that environmental factors contribute heavily to cancer of the breast, endometrium, and ovary is supported by international comparisons and studies of migrants. The highest rates are found in white women in the United States and Western Europe and the lowest among Asian women (see table 20) (184). Lifestyle differences, particularly in diet and reproductive patterns, are probably important contributors to the rate differences. Migrant studies in the United States have shown that the

Table 20.—Selected International Age-Standardized Incidence per 100,000 for Cancers of the Breast, Corpus Uteri, Cervix Uteri, Ovary, Prostate, Testis and Penis

	Females			
	Breast	Corpus uteri	Cervix uteri	Ovary
Oxford, United Kingdom	54.5	9.4	11.4	11.7
Alameda County, Calif., blacks........	56.6	13.6	28.0	10.3
Alameda County, Calif., whites........	76.1	33.3	12.3	13.5
Osaka, Japan	12.1	0.9	16.2	2.8
Ibadan, Nigeria	15.3	1.6	21.6	7.0

	Males		
	Prostate	Testis	Penis
Oxford, United Kingdom	19.2	2.6	0.7
Alameda County, Calif., blacks	75.0	0.5	1.2
Alameda County, Calif., whites	40.4	4.4	0.6
Osaka, Japan	2.7	0.7	0.5
Ibadan, Nigeria	10.0	0.1	0.2

SOURCE: Data from International Agency for Research on Cancer (184).

initially lower rates for Mexican-Americans (234) move toward the higher rates for whites in the United States after a generation or two, owing to shifts in lifestyle toward those of the American population.

ACS (6) estimates that 110,000 women in the United States will develop breast cancer in 1981, and that 37,000 women will die from the disease. Breast, the leading site of cancer death in women today, will account for approximately 19 percent of all female cancer deaths in 1981. A host of studies has established a set of factors that characterize women at high risk for breast cancer (219). Age, geographic area of residence, age at first childbirth, age at menarche (beginning of menstrual function), age at menopause (cessation of menstrual function), history of benign breast disease, and familial history of breast cancer are the major predictors.

International comparisons of breast cancer risk by age has provided the basis for hypotheses which have been examined in further epidemiologic studies. In areas where incidence is high (e.g., North America and Western Europe) the rate increases throughout life, often with a break, where incidence decreases or at least ceases to rise, at about 50 to 55 years of age, after which it increases steeply once again. In areas of low incidence (e.g., most areas of Asia and Africa), rates increase through middle age, decreasing after about age 50. Intermediate patterns occur in areas of intermediate incidence (e.g., Southern Europe and South America) (219).

One basic hypothesis following from the study of age-specific rates is that breast cancer is best described as two diseases: one occurring premenopausally and the other postmenopausally, each with different causes. De Waard (79) presents some additional arguments from epidemiologic research favoring this hypothesis. Paffenbarger, Kampert, and Chang (289) have recently added weight to the arguments against the hypothesis, based on a large case-control study of breast cancer, concluding that overall the evidence supports a "common cause subject to modifying influences" for all breast cancer. The weight of evidence does not yet allow concluding whether breast cancer should be described as one disease or two.

Age at first childbirth is a strong predictor. Giving birth to the first child after age 30, or having no children at all place one at a greater risk than giving birth to the first child before age 20 (238). A pregnancy must go to full term for any protective effect. It is widely believed that the first stimulus to lactation, whether or not breast feeding is carried out, may be the factor of consequence. Miller and Bulbrook (238), reporting on a meeting of the Multi-Disciplinary

Project on Breast Cancer of the International Union against Cancer, speculate:

A population that achieved a 5-year reduction in age at first delivery might achieve a 30-percent reduction in incidence of breast cancer.

An analysis of population-based cancer mortality rates (27) supports the correlation between nulliparity and higher rates. The data suggest that, if the current pattern continues, the decreasing fertility trends of the 1960's and 1970's may foretell increased breast cancer rates for women in this decade.

Age at menarche has also been shown to have some degree of predictive value in nearly all breast cancer studies, with a lower age indicating a higher risk. Tulinius et al., (346) in their study of Icelandic women, found a "slight influence" remaining after adjustment for parity and age at first pregnancy. Henderson et al. (162) found that women with menarche before age 13 had 1½ times the breast cancer risk of a woman with later menarche.

Age at menarche, itself, may be influenced by environmental factors, notably nutrition. Population-based data reveal a steady decline in the age at menarche for American women, thought to be attributable to improved nutritional status (238). The effect of this on future breast cancer rates is uncertain. Early studies in rats correlated body size, more than age, with onset of menarche (121). Similarly, observations in humans, including a recent look at menarche and disturbances in the menstrual cycle of ballet dancers (134), provide evidence that lean body mass is related to later menarche. Later age at menopause brings increased risk. Women with natural menopause after age 55 have about twice the risk of developing breast cancer as do women with natural menopause before age 45 (219).

Breast cancer risk has a strong familial component that has not been entirely explained by lifestyle similarities among relatives. First-degree (sisters, mothers and daughters) and second-degree (nieces and aunts) relatives of women with breast cancer have two to three times the risk of the general population. Relatives of women with bilateral breast cancer are at higher risk, and are more likely to be diagnosed at an earlier age and to develop bilateral disease than are relatives of women with unilateral disease (15).

Gray, Henderson, and Pike (144) looked at the higher rate of breast cancer in U.S. white women compared with U.S. black women. They found that the relationship between black and white rates is not constant. Below age 40, black women have higher rates than whites, while after age 45, black rates were 20 to 30 percent lower than those for whites. This can be only partially explained by differences in age at menarche, but a full explanation has not been demonstrated.

Cancers of the endometrium and ovary share at least two important risk factors with breast cancer. They are all associated with high-fat diets and women who have not borne children are at an increased risk for all three types compared to women who have borne children. Occurrence of either breast or ovarian cancer increases the risk of a cancer developing at the other site. Breast cancer also increases the risk of future endometrial cancer (324). Ovarian hormonal activity may be the influencing factor in all of these sites.

Cancer of the Cervix

There is a striking association between cancer of the uterine cervix and the number of sexual partners a woman has had. The death rate for this cancer among nuns is much lower than it is for the general population (129), suggesting the involvement of a venereally transmitted agent. A possible candidate is a virus (Herpes simplex type II) which has been found in association with both cervical cancer and other cervical cell abnormalities (244). Some study results support this hypothesis, but the data are considered only suggestive at this point, and no conclusion of causality can be drawn.

The number of deaths from cervical cancer (ACS projects 7,200 in 1981) has decreased and continues to decline, partially due to the more widespread use of cervical screening (6). Based on the assumption that the majority of cervical cancers are caused by infective processes, Doll and Peto (93) estimate that prevention or treatment of infection might reduce total cancer mortality by 1 percent.

Cancers of Male Reproductive Organs

International comparison and a study of Ugandan men has shown a correlation of higher rates of penile cancer in areas where circumcision is not generally practiced and where penile hygiene is poor (163).

Age-standardized incidence rates for prostate cancer vary between about 3/100,000 in Japan and 40/100,000 in U.S. whites, to a high of about 75/100,000 for some U.S. blacks (184), suggesting an environmental etiology. Feminella and Lattimer (119) found an increase in cervical carcinomas among wives of cases. A common, perhaps viral, etiology is suggested; however it is not substantiated by some population-based rates, for instance, a lower rate of prostatic cancer and a higher rate of cervical cancer occurs among Mexican-Americans as compared to U.S. blacks (163).

Testicular cancer is highly associated with abnormalities of sexual development, particularly cryptorchidism (failure of the testes to descend into the scrotum) (208). Cancer occurs in 11 to 15 percent of undescended testes (5). The association may be direct or a third factor, perhaps endocrinological, may predispose individuals to both conditions.

NATURAL RADIATION

One would like to think that at least Mother Nature would not place a carcinogenic burden on the people of this planet. This unfortunately is not the case. Several types of natural radiation cause concern regarding carcinogenicity, the most important of which, ultraviolet radiation and ionizing radiation, were among the first factors recognized as human carcinogens.

Ultraviolet Radiation

Ultraviolet radiation (or ultraviolet light) is associated with some lip cancers, with a large proportion of squamous-cell carcinomas and is the principal cause of basal-cell carcinoma of the face and neck in light-skinned people. The evidence for the association includes prevalence on sun-exposed areas, increased incidence in lightly pigmented people, and increased incidence with greater insolation and greater time outdoors. Basal-cell carcinomas account for over 75 percent of all skin cancers, but appropriate treatment cures about 95 percent (159). The squamous- and basal-cell carcinomas are referred to as nonmelanoma skin cancer. Approximately 400,000 cases occur annually— as many cancers as occur at all other sites combined (66). Fortunately, most are not fatal.

NCI conducted a nonmelanoma skin cancer survey in eight locations in the United States during the period 1977-78, as mandated by the Clean Air Act Amendments of 1977. Men were found to be at greater risk of cancer than were women. The average age-adjusted incidence rate for white males was 310/100,000 and for white females 172/100,000 (250). An increase of 15 to 20 percent was reported in incidence as compared to the rate estimated from the Third National Cancer Survey (TNCS). This increase may be due, in large part, to changes in clothing styles and greater exposure to sunlight than was customary years ago.

Ultraviolet radiation has also been associated with the far more serious skin cancer, malignant melanoma. However, the data are less convincing since the distribution of cancers on the body does not directly correspond to the degree of exposure. In 1978, there were approximately 6,000 deaths from malignant melanoma in the United States. ACS (6) estimates that there will be 14,300 new cases and 6,700 deaths from melanoma in 1981. Melanoma is the leading cause of death from all diseases of the skin and is unquestionably increasing in frequency.

Incidence and mortality rates from skin cancer in different countries correlate fairly closely with the intensity of ultraviolet radiation. The disease is most prevalent in people receiving large amounts of sunlight, and it is a recognized occupational hazard for individuals working outdoors. The maps prepared by Mason, et al. (223), which depict average age-adjusted cancer mortality rates on a county-by-county basis, convincingly demonstrate higher risk of skin cancer in the Southeast United States. TNCS found the annual incidence rate for nonmelanoma skin cancer to be 539/100,000 in the Dallas-Fort Worth, Tex., area as compared to 174/100,000 in Iowa.

An individual's risk of developing skin cancer is strongly influenced by genetic makeup. A higher risk exists for those with phenotypic characteristics such as fair complexion, light eye and hair color, and poor ability to tan. By contrast, skin cancer is very rare in deeply pigmented populations. In addition, several different types of chemicals can augment the carcinogenic properties of ultraviolet radiation, including some used as medications and in cosmetics.

As discussed in the *Air Pollution* section, the use of chlorofluorocarbons has been restricted in the United States because of the belief that they may react in the stratosphere to reduce the thickness of the ozone layer and cause an increase in ultraviolet radiation reaching the surface of the Earth. NAS (70) estimated that global release of chlorofluorocarbons at 1977 rates could result in several hundred thousand additional cases of nonmelanoma skin cancer and several thousand melanomas in the next century. (For additional information on the possible carcinogenic impact from release of chlorofluorocarbons, see *Air Pollution.*)

Higginson and Muir (166) estimated that 10 percent of male and female cancers in the Birmingham and West Midland region of England could be attributed to sunlight. Doll and Peto (93) attribute 90 percent of lip cancers (in conjunction with smoking), 50 percent or more of melanomas, as well as 80 percent of other skin cancers to ultraviolet radiation. This accounts for between 1 and 2 percent of all cancer deaths if these proportions are applied to 1978 U.S. cancer deaths.

Ionizing Radiation

About half of the average U.S. exposure to ionizing radiation comes from natural sources. Of the remainder, most comes from diagnostic medical exposures, and smaller amounts come from medical therapy, occupational exposures, and from radioactive pollutants. (Those exposures are discussed in *Medical Drugs and Radiation, Occupation,* and *Air Pollution,* respectively.) Cosmic rays and the minute amounts of radioactive isotopes that occur in our bodies and in all natural materials are the major sources of natural background radiation.

The quantitative dose-response relationship between cancer and low-level ionizing radiation has been the cause of much debate. Until 30 years ago, it was commonly assumed that ionizing radiation did not cause cancer unless the exposures were high enough to cause clinically detectable damage to the irradiated tissue. This assumption is now known to be false, although the dose-response relationship at low levels is still not known with certainty.

Organs and tissues differ in their susceptibility to carcinogenic effects induced by radiation. Leukemia was the first form of cancer associated with exposure to ionizing radiation, but we now know that cancer may be induced by radiation in many tissues of the human body and that the risk of inducing solid tumors exceeds that of leukemia (268). The major cancer sites affected are the breast in women and the thyroid, lung, and digestive organs in both sexes. Solid tumors have a longer latency period (10 to more than 30 years) than the few years before the excess risk for leukemia manifests itself. The total cancer risk from radiation is greater for women than men, principally because of the contribution of breast cancer.

More information is available on the dose-response relationship between radiation and cancer than any other, but there is still much controversy over the appropriate extrapolation model to use for estimating the cancer risk from ionizing radiation. In July 1980, NAS officially released BEIR III (268). The estimates for the risks from ionizing radiation used by BEIR III were derived principally from human experiences with much higher doses than most people receive. The most important of these are data from populations exposed to atomic blasts in Hiroshima and Nagasaki, patients exposed to therapeutic radiation, and various occupational groups such as uranium miners and radium watch dial painters. Disagreement persists in the field of radiation carcinogenesis over the appropriateness of these high-exposure populations for estimating low-level risks.

The development and release of the BEIR III report illustrates the diverging and changing opinions concerning the appropriate methodology for extrapolating from the measured effects of high doses of ionizing radiation to the most probable effects of low doses. A draft of the BEIR III report was released for public comment in May 1979 but was retracted when it was learned that a majority of the committee supported a model different from the one presented.

Some members of the committee felt that for low doses, a linear model overestimated the risk and a pure quadratic model, which estimates a lower risk, could be used as a lower bound. However, others felt that the linear model was more accurate. Because of this disagreement, a consensus panel was assembled and it adopted the linear-quadratic model: the pure quadratic model produces the lowest estimate, the linear the highest, and the linear-quadratic estimates an intermediate risk. Depending on which model is used, estimates of mortality from all forms of cancer will differ by about one order of magnitude.

The committee also could not agree on whether the cancer risk from radiation would have an additive or multiplicative effect on the general cancer rate. Throughout the report, excess risk is given as both an *absolute* (additive) and as a *relative* risk. The relative approach assumes that the excess risk increases gradually and continuously, proportional to the spontaneous risk, which increases with age for nearly all cancers. The absolute approach assumes a constant number of additional cancers throughout life.

The BEIR III report (268) makes various attempts at estimating cancer risk from different types of exposure but does not quantify the risk from low-dose radiation:

> . . . the degree of risk is so low that it cannot be observed directly and there is great uncertainty as to the dose-response function most appropriate for extrapolating in the low-dose region.

It further states:

> It is by no means clear whether dose rates of gamma or x radiation of about 100 mrads/yr are in any way detrimental to exposed people . . .

For the purpose of this assessment, the risks derived for continuous lifetime exposure to 1 rad/yr of low-dose (gamma or X-ray) radiation is the most relevant, though it is an order of magnitude higher than average natural background radiation. Table 21 displays both absolute and relative risk estimates generated by BEIR III.

The BEIR III report estimated that the average whole body dose of natural background radiation in the United States is approximately 100 mrem/yr. The dose of radiation received varies with altitude and geographical location. Using a figure of 220 million Americans, one can estimate that the population as a whole would be exposed to 22 million person-rem of background radiation.[3] Although BEIR III did not attempt to estimate the risk of cancer induced by low-dose radiation, it would not be incorrect to compute an upper limit of risk from the linear model since this is the only model which assumes that dose and effect are proportional. Using the range of risk estimates, 158–403 excess cancer deaths per million persons per rad, yields estimates of 3,476 and 8,866 cancer deaths per year attributable to background radiation. These figures represent between 0.9 and 2.2 percent of all cancer deaths, and are comparable with 3-percent estimates by Doll

---

[3]In 1972, EPA estimated that the average dose of natural background radiation for a person living in the United States is 130 mrem. Based on this estimate, the Interagency Task Force on the Health Effects of Ionizing Radiation estimated that the U.S. population is exposed to 20 million person-rem, but this is in error because dividing 20 million person-rem by 130 mrem produces a quotient of 154 million people. The population is nearer 220 million.

and Peto (93) and Jablon and Bailar (191). The lower estimate can be considered to approach zero, in keeping with risks derived from other models, including the quadratic model.

Table 21.—Estimates of Excess Cancer Mortality From Continuous Exposure to 1 Rad/Year of Low-Level (background-type) Radiation by Three Dose-Response Models and Two Risk Projection Models

Estimates of excess annual cancer mortality from continuous exposure to 1 rad/year of low-level (background-type) radiation (excess deaths/million exposed and percentage of normal expectation of cancer deaths)

Dose-response model		Risk projection model	
		Absolute	Relative
Linear quadratic	Normal expectation of cancer deaths	167,300	167,300
	Excess deaths: number	4,751	12,920
	Percent of normal	2.8	7.7
Linear	Excess deaths: number	11,250	30,520
	Percent of normal	6.7	18.2
Quadratic	Excess deaths	a	a

aNot calculated because estimates very close to zero.

Estimates of excess lifetime cancer mortality from continuous exposure to 1 rad/year of low-level (background-type) radiation (excess deaths/million exposed)

Dose-response model	Risk projection model	
	Absolute	Relative
Linear quadratic	67	182
Linear	158	403
Quadratic	—	—

SOURCE: Tables adapted from (270).

INFECTION

Infection, particularly viral infection, has long been thought to be a cause of cancer. This idea is partially based on the observation that neoplasms appear in many animal species following viral infections, and specific animal tumor viruses have been convincingly indentified. However, epidemiologic evidence indicates that cancer is not a contagious disease. People who come into close contact with cancer patients, such as nurses, doctors, and spouses of patients, are at no higher risk of developing the disease than others. Reports are occasionally published of the occurrence of an unusually large number of cases of rare cancers, but such clusters can be expected to occur periodically by chance. It is more plausible that certain viruses exist which are important in the development of

some types of cancer, but that they are widespread in the community. It is probably not the virus itself, but a variety of other factors which determine whether the virus will lead to the development of the disease. These may include genetic and hormonal factors, chemical carcinogens, and defective immune mechanisms, which appear to exert an effect in only a small proportion of those exposed.

The strongest evidence implicating a viral infection in human cancer causation concerns Epstein-Barr virus (EBV) and hepatitis B virus, believed responsible for several cancer types which are relatively rare in the United States. Epstein-Barr is a herpesvirus which is strongly associated with Burkitt's lymphoma and nasopharyngeal carcinoma (93,304). EBV occurs ubiquitously and is known to be the specific cause of infectious mononucleosis. It is postulated that the viral DNA integrates into the genetic material of a human stem cell and that cell becomes the parent of a malignant clone. Epidemiologic data and the detection of Epstein-Barr viral DNA in lymphoma cells supports the association between the virus and these two cancers. The association with nasopharyngeal carcinoma, found in the Far East, is not so strong as with Burkitt's lymphoma, which occurs mainly in children in central Africa and New Guinea. Nasopharyngeal carcinoma is believed to involve a stronger genetic component, since Chinese migrating to the United States have a much higher incidence of the disease than U.S. whites and blacks, but the rate is lower than among Chinese remaining in the Far East (128). The unusual geographical distribution suggests that the virus may act as a cocarcinogen and that additional factors, such as immunosuppression as a result of malaria, may be involved.

Hepatitis B virus is associated with chronic liver infection which often advances to hepatocarcinoma. A greater prevalence of active hepatitis B infection has been demonstrated in patients with primary hepatocellular carcinoma as compared with matched controls and the general population (304). The virus is believed to be the initiating agent, but promoting agents such as aflatoxin may be important cofactors (304). Two other herpesviruses are suspected of being associated with cancer: herpes simplex virus type 2 with cervical cancer, and less closely, cytomegalovirus with prostatic and cervical cancers.

The vast majority of human cancers are not characterized by the presence of viral DNA in the genetic material of cells. This may, of course, be because the methods currently used to detect the presence of a virus are not sufficiently sensitive, or it may be that viruses are not often associated with cancer.

Doll and Peto (93) suggest that viral infection may eventually be shown to be an essential factor in the production of some cancers:

- cancer of the uterine cervix—women with multiple partners are at high risk (see *Sexual Development, Reproductive Patterns, and Sexual Practices*);
- cancer of the penis—wives of penis cancer patients are at high risk for cancer of the uterine cervix;
- acute lymphatic leukemia in children—disease may recur in donor cells after a marrow transplant; and
- reticulosarcoma—occasional appearance shortly after receiving doses of immunosuppressive drugs.

If all of the above cancers depended on viral infection, the proportion of cancers attributable to infection would be about 4 percent (93). The proportion may be considerably larger if, like diet, infectious agents act by indirect means to contribute to the production of cancers. Viruses may promote the development of cancer by causing tissue death, thereby stimulating the division of stem cells and sensitizing them to the action of chemical carcinogens. It is possible for instance, that this is the mechanism whereby hepatitis B virus is associated with the development of liver cancer.

Infection with bacteria or parasites may also contribute to the production of cancer. The *Diet* section discusses the possible role of intestinal bacteria in producing or destroying carcinogenic metabolites in the large bowel and of salivary duct bacteria in converting nitrates into nitrites and hence facilitating the formation of N-nitroso compounds in vivo. Bacterial infection associated with the development of chronic bronchitis has been thought to increase the risk of lung cancer in cigarette smokers (93), possibly by impairing the efficiency of the mechanism for clearing the bronchi and hence permitting more prolonged contact between inspired carcinogens and the bronchial stem cells. A similar role for infection may also explain the association between ulcerative colitis and colorectal cancer, and that between schistosomiasis, a parasitic infection of the bladder common in parts of Africa, and the development of bladder cancer.

The examples cited are unlikely to be the only ways in which infection affects the risk of developing cancer; but even if they were, the range of estimates for its contribution to the overall cancer rate would be large. Rapp (304) speculated that if herpesviruses are eventually shown to be involved in all cancers of the male and female genitourinary systems, then those with active venereal disease would have a 1 per 70-100 risk of developing the disease:

> This estimate is based on the number of new genitourinary cancer cases per year in the United States (100,000 for females and 70,000 for males) in a population containing about 14 million active cases . . . of venereal disease due to herpesviruses.

If one applies this reasoning to 1978 U.S. cancer deaths, approximately 15 percent of all cancer mortality would be associated with infection. This estimate is extremely tentative—there is much more certainty around the association with cervical cancer than other genital sites. Doll and Peto (93) suggested a figure about 10 percent as a very uncertain best estimate, within a very wide range of acceptable estimates, of the proportion of cancer deaths attributable to infection, distributed as follows:

> . . . 5% perhaps attributable to the action of viruses and a token figure of 5% to allow for the possible role of other infective agents in determining the conditions under which cancer is produced in vivo. The likely role of infectious agents in the etiology of cancer of the uterine cervix provides a lower limit of at least 1%, but we can at present make no useful guess at the upper limit.

OTHER OR UNKNOWN ASSOCIATIONS

Two basic classes of "other" associations will be considered:

1. Associations with cancers which as yet remain unidentified, but which, when elucidated, will most likely fall into categories that have been discussed in this chapter.
2. Associations of agents or exposures with cancers of the future. These may have been introduced recently, but have not yet produced cancers, or may be introduced in the future.

Causes of Cancers Occurring Today

The agents associated with and/or responsible for many of today's cancers have not been identified. For example, although cancers of the breast, colon, rectum, and stomach are associated in some way with dietary factors, a causal relationship has not been found for cancers at those sites. Additionally the incidence of some cancers, myelomatosis and non-Hodgkins lymphoma, for example, appear to be increasing but no evidence associates those cancers with even a broad category of factors.

The search for environmental factors associated with cancer will undoubtedly continue. Observed differences in rates between populations, within countries, and through international comparisons will result in advancing new hypotheses and promoting further studies.

Some suggested associations that were not discussed above are likely to be further investigated, but currently few data exist about them. Biological factors, like immunologic control, may normally limit the onset of disease, and a breakdown of this mechanism which may be brought on by an environmental agent, could increase the propensity for cancer development. Similarly, psychological factors such as stress may create an internal milieu suitable for tumor growth. There is some animal evidence to support this hypothesis but it is limited. Studies of patients in mental hospitals are not supportive of an increased risk (93). Psychological stress does have a recognized role in causing people to smoke, drink, overeat, and take part in other harmful activities which may directly or indirectly increase their risk of cancer.

New Cancer Associations

Hazards exist today which may not have caused any cancers, but which may do so in the future. A timely example is hazardous wastes that have been improperly disposed of in areas commonly termed "dumps." EPA has estimated that there are more than 50,000 improperly operated dump sites containing hazardous waste that are not being properly operated. Of these, they estimate that 30,000 pose a significant health risk. The carcinogenic potential of the myriad chemicals in these dumps is unknown at present. (An OTA assessment about nonnuclear industrial wastes, which will look at health risks, among other things, is to be completed in late 1982.)

Hundreds of new chemicals are introduced into commerce each year. Some of these may present cancer risks. Exposures may be through many routes—pollution, occupation, consumer products, foods, or others.

Table 22.—Estimates of the Percentage of Total Cancer Associated with Various Factors

Factor Estimate	Time period to which estimate applies	Author
Tobacco		
30% U.S. mortality, males and females combined	1977	Doll and Peto (93)
25–35% U.S. male mortality population	1960–72	Hammond and Seidman (155)
5–10% U.S. female mortality	1960–72	Hammond and Seidman (155)
24–38% various populations	—	Enstrom (100)
43% U.S. male incidence	1980	U.S. Surgeon General (287)
18% U.S. female incidence	1980	U.S. Surgeon General (287)
51% U.S. male mortality	1980	U.S. Surgeon General (287)
26% U.S. female mortality	1980	U.S. Surgeon General (287)
30% male cancers, England[a]	1968–72	Higginson and Muir (166)
7% female cancers, England[a]	1968–72	Higginson and Muir (166)
28% U.S. male incidence[b]	1976	Wynder and Gori (368)
8% U.S. female incidence[b]	1976	Wynder and Gori (368)
Alcohol		
4–5% of mortality, males and females combined	1978	OTA based on Schottenfeld (323)
14% U.S. male mortality	1974	Rothman (313)
12% U.S. female mortality	1974	Rothman (313)
3% U.S. mortality, males and females combined (approximately 4.6% for males and 1% for females)	1977	Doll and Peto (193)
4% U.S. male incidence[b]	1976	Wynder and Gori (368)
1% U.S. female incidence[b]	1976	Wynder and Gori (368)
5% male cancers, England[a] (tobacco/alcohol)	1968–72	Higginson and Muir (166)
3% female cancers, England[a] (tobacco/alcohol)	1968–72	Higginson and Muir (166)
Diet		
40% U.S. male incidence[b]	1976	Wynder and Gori (368)
60% U.S. female incidence[b]	1976	Wynder and Gori (368)
35% U.S. mortality, males and females combined	1977	Doll and Peto (93)
Occupation		
4% U.S. male incidence[b]	1976	Wynder and Gori (368)
2% U.S. female incidence[b]	1976	Wynder and Gori (368)
6% male cancers, England[a]	1968–72	Higginson and Muir (166)
2% female cancers, England[a]	1968–72	Higginson and Muir (166)
<15% U.S. male cancers	Not specified	Cole (62)
< 5% U.S. female cancers	Not specified	Cole (62)
23–38% U.S. incidence, males and females combined	Near term and future	HEW (82)
6.8% U.S. male mortality	1977	Doll and Peto (93)
1.2% U.S. female mortality	1977	Doll and Peto (93)

Table 22.—Estimates of the Percentage of Total Cancer Associated with Various Factors (Continued)

Factor Estimate	Time period to which estimate applies	Author
Asbestos		
13-18% U.S. cancers	Near term and future	HEW (82)
3% (1.4-4.4%) U.S. cancers	Now or likely in near future	Hogan and Hoel (171)
Air pollution		
2% U.S. mortality	Future	Doll and Peto (93)
Consumer products		
< 1% U.S. mortality, males and females combined	1977	Doll and Peto (93)
Infection		
5%?-10%?? U.S. cancers	Present and future	Doll and Peto (93)
15% U.S. mortality	1978	Rapp (304)
Lifestyle		
30% male cancers, England[a]	1968-72	Higginson and Muir (166)
63% female cancers, England[a]	1968-72	Higginson and Muir (166)
Radiation, natural and medical:		
Ultraviolet		
10% male cancers, England[a]	1968-72	Higginson and Muir (166)
10% female cancers, England[a]	1968-72	Higginson and Muir (166)
Unspecified radiation		
1% male cancers, England[a]	1968-72	Higginson and Muir (166)
1% female cancers, England[a]	1968-72	Higginson and Muir (166)
Ultraviolet and X-ray		
8% U.S. male incidence[b]	1976	Wynder and Gori (368)
8% U.S. female incidence[b]	1976	Wynder and Gori (368)
Natural ionizing		
0-(0.9-2.2%) U.S. mortality	1978	OTA based on BEIR III (268)
3% U.S. mortality	1978	Doll and Peto (93)
3% U.S. mortality	1978	Jablon and Bailar (191)
Medical drugs and radiation		
1% U.S. mortality, males and females combined	1977	Doll and Peto (93)
1% male and female cancers combined, England[a]	1968-72	Higginson and Muir (166)
4% U.S. incidence, males and females combined (refers only to exogenous hormones)	1976	Wynder and Gori (368)
Sexual development, reproductive patterns and sexual practices		
7% U.S. mortality, males and females combined	1977	Doll and Peto (93)
Other or unknown		
?%	Present and future	Doll and Peto (93)
15% male cancers, England[a]	1968-72	Higginson and Muir (166)
11% female cancers, England[a]	1968-72	Higginson and Muir (166)

[a]Birmingham and West Midland Region.
[b]Estimated from graphic presentation.

SOURCE: Office of Technology Assessment.

4.
Methods for Detecting and Identifying Carcinogens

Contents

LIST OF TABLES

LIST OF FIGURES

4.
Methods for Detecting and Identifying Carcinogens

Beginning with this chapter, the focus of this report shifts from all causes of cancer to only chemicals. This shift does not represent a decision that chemicals, in the workplace or in the general environment, are more important in cancer causation than dietary elements, personal habits, radiation, or certain aspects of human biology. However, it does reflect the major legislative and regulatory emphasis recently placed on chemicals, and the greater ease with which chemical carcinogens can be detected by present-day methods.

Different methods are available, employing different techniques, using different test organisms, and producing different types of information about carcinogenicity. This chapter discusses a variety of those methods, their strengths and weaknesses, some results from each, and the tools they require.

METHODS

There are four major methods for detecting and identifying carcinogens:

1. molecular structure analysis,
2. short-term tests,
3. long-term chronic bioassays in laboratory animals (termed "bioassays" or "animal tests" hereafter), and
4. epidemiology.

The first two methods produce information about potential carcinogenicity; the third provides direct evidence of carcinogenicity in animals; the fourth produces direct evidence about cancer in man. These categories are briefly described in table 23.

Probably no statement made in the last column of table 23 is free from dispute. Results may be, and frequently are, challenged for several reasons: because the test was incorrectly designed or executed (all methods); because the method does not directly measure carcinogenicity (methods 1 and 2); because the test is too sensitive and produces false positives (methods 2 and 3); because the test is too insensitive and produces false negatives (method 4); and because the test does not measure human experience (all methods but 4), etc.

Knowledge about tests and about the validity of test results increases as the tests are more often used, more discussed, and more refined. The state of scientific knowledge plays an important role in decisions to test or not to test a chemical, decisions about which tests are appropriate, and decisions about interpretation of the test results. As will be discussed, "policy statements," sometimes issued as guidelines or standards, detail the methods that an organization will use in making decisions. A certain tension is apparent in all the policies. Tests cost money and take time; bigger and better tests cost more and take more time; compromises are necessary in the design of each test so that a reasonable number of chemicals can be tested.

An equally important issue is the amount of information necessary to decide that a chemical is or is not a carcinogen that requires some control action. The fact that some regulations are based on nonhuman test systems shows that proof that a chemical is a human carcinogen is not demanded. This illustrates that prevention of cancer is seen as so important that it is appropriate to make decisions to restrict exposures before human damage is observed.

Table 23.—General Classification of Tests Available To Determine Properties Related to Carcinogenicity

Method	System	Time required	Basis for test	Result	Conclusion, if result is positive
Molecular structure analysis	"Paper chemistry" Basic laboratory tests	Days Weeks	Chemicals with like structures interact similarly with DNA	Structure resembles (positive) or does not resemble (negative) structure of known carcinogen	Chemical may be hazardous. That determination requires further testing.
Short-term tests	Bacteria, yeast, cultured cells, intact animals	Generally few weeks (range 1 day to 8 months)	Chemical interaction with DNA can be measured in biological systems	Chemical causes (positive) or does not cause (negative) a response known to be caused by carcinogens	Chemical is a potential carcinogen.
Bioassay	Intact animals (rats, mice)	2 to 5 years	Chemicals that cause tumors in animals may cause tumors in humans	Chemical causes (positive) or does not cause (negative) increased incidence of tumors	Chemical is recognized as a carcinogen in that species and as a potential human carcinogen.
Epidemiology	Humans	Months to lifetimes	Chemicals that cause cancer can be detected in studies of human populations	Chemical is associated (positive) or is not associated (negative) with an increased incidence of cancer	Chemical is recognized as a human carcinogen.

SOURCE: Office of Technology Assessment.

ANALYSIS OF MOLECULAR STRUCTURE AND OTHER PHYSICAL CONSTANTS

Some information about the likelihood of a chemical being a carcinogen may be obtained by comparing its structure and chemical and physical characteristics with those of known carcinogens and noncarcinogens. This first stage in an orderly determination of whether or not a chemical is a carcinogen requires the gathering of all available information about it. The information can be obtained from sources as diverse as results from testing a chemical in animals to anecdotal stories about human disease, but the most readily available information is often about the molecular structure and physical and chemical properties of the suspect chemical.

Certain molecular structures have been associated with carcinogenicity, and structural similarity is used in making decisions about which agents are more or less suspect. For instance, 8 of the first 14 carcinogens regulated by the Occupational Safety and Health Administration (OSHA) are aromatic amines. The Environmental Protection Agency (EPA) relies heavily on structural analysis in determining whether or not "new" chemicals, described in premanufacturing notices, may present an unreasonable risk to health or the environment. Chemical and physical properties which are useful in evaluating a chemical's carcinogenic potential include solubility, stability, sensitivity to pH, and chemical reactivity. Often this type of information is generated by the manufacturer of the chemical.

A number of proposals have been made that chemicals be divided up into classes depending on their structural similarities and that testing be done on a number of members in each class. Unfortunately, carcinogens are known in several chemical classes, and " . . . the dozen or more known classes of these agents [carcinogens] share no common structural features" (239). Furthermore, even within classes, closely related chemicals may differ with respect to carcinogenicity—e.g., 2-acetylaminofluorene (2-AAF) is a well-documented carcinogen; its chemical relative, 4-acetylaminofluorene (4-AAF), is not a carcinogen (see figure 19).

Figure 19.—Molecular Structures of Two Closely Related Chemicals: One a Carcinogen and One a Noncarcinogen

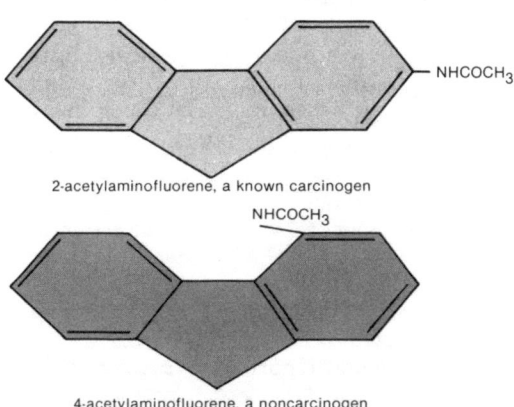

2-acetylaminofluorene, a known carcinogen

4-acetylaminofluorene, a noncarcinogen

SOURCE: Office of Technology Assessment.

EPA recently based a regulatory decision on molecular structural analysis. Under section 5(e) of the Toxic Substances Control Act (TSCA), EPA prohibited the entry of six new chemical substances into the marketplace unless the manufacturer provided additional information about toxicity. A National Cancer Institute (NCI) bioassay had shown a related chemical to be carcinogenic, and based on that result, EPA decided that more information was needed before manufacture could begin (88). The manufacturer decided not to proceed with the testing and did not market the chemicals.

SHORT-TERM TESTS

Short-term tests are so named because of the relatively short time needed to conduct the experiments. Some studies involving micro-organisms require less than 1 day to complete (87), most require a few days to a few weeks, and the longest, using mice, requires 8 to 9 months (172). These times may be compared to the more than 3 years required to complete a bioassay and the months to years required to complete epidemiologic studies.

A number of reasons account for the growing interest in using short-term tests to predict a chemical's carcinogenic potential:

- shorter time period required for the tests;
- low cost ($100 to a few thousand dollars for each test compared to $400,000 to $1 million for a bioassay);

- evidence that the majority of chemical carcinogens are mutagens and that many mutagens are carcinogens;
- growing opinion that short-term tests can predict which chemicals may be carcinogens.

The third point is important because many short-term tests determine whether or not a chemical causes mutations (mutagenicity) rather than if it causes cancer (carcinogenicity). The postulated relationship between mutagenicity and carcinogenicity stems from biological properties common to all living organisms. The genetic information in both germ cells (egg and sperm) and somatic cells (nongerm or "body cells") is composed of deoxyribonucleic acid (DNA), and agents that cause mutations in germ cells are also expected to cause mutations in somatic cells. A germ cell mutation may prevent the formation of viable offspring, cause a genetic malformation, or produce subtle defects in the progeny, such as minimal depression in intelligence or increased susceptibility to disease.

The consequences of somatic cell mutations are quite different from those in germ cells. Somatic cells do not contribute genetic information to succeeding generations, but as each somatic cell grows and divides, copies of its DNA are passed on to its two "daughter" cells. Some somatic cell mutations result in uncontrolled cellular growth: The normal tightly controlled growth pattern of the somatic cell is broken down, the cell grows and divides more quickly than it should, progeny cells exhibit the same uncontrolled growth, and cancer results.

The hypothesis that assigns genetic changes in somatic cells a role in cancer initiation is referred to as "the somatic mutation theory of cancer." Cairns (42) discusses the origin and development of this theory, which provides intellectual support for associating mutagenicity and related changes measured in short-term tests with potential carcinogenicity.

The short-term tests that depend on mutagenicity can detect only materials that interact with DNA. Some cancers may be caused by other, "epigenetic," pathways that may not involve alterations in genetic information (317). Short-term tests cannot detect such activities. Additionally, short-term tests do not detect promoters that do not interact with DNA. The generally good correlation between mutagenic and carcinogenic activity as well as the bulk of results from basic cancer biological research support the notion that carcinogens generally interact with DNA.

The Ames Test

The most widely used and best-studied short-term test, the "Ames test," is named for its developer, Bruce Ames, a molecular biologist. The test measures the capacity of a chemical to cause mutations in the bacterium *Salmonella typhimurium*, a favorite tool for laboratory investigations since the 1940's. Salmonella's genetics and biochemistry are well understood: it is quickly and easily grown; it presents few

manipulative problems in the laboratory, and test results are easily interpretable and reproducible between laboratories.

Basically, the Ames test involves mixing the chemical under test with a bacterial culture and then manipulating the culture so that only mutated bacteria will grow. The number of mutated bacteria is a measure of the potency of the tested material as a mutagen.

It is well known that some chemicals must be altered before they interact with DNA and that in humans and other mammals these changes are often accomplished by enzymes in the liver. The addition of liver extracts to the Ames test system and to other short-term tests provides a mechanism for these metabolic activation changes to be accomplished. Generally, extracts are prepared from rats, hamsters, or other laboratory animals. The source of the extracts and the amount used in the tests affect results, and careful experiments report these specifics so that others can replicate the tests. Some chemicals are "activated" by bacteria normally present in the intestine rather than by the liver. The addition of extracts of such bacteria to Ames test mixtures has been shown to activate some chemicals to mutagenic forms (338).

As of early 1979, more than 2,600 Ames test results had been published (172). The interested reader is referred to Hollstein et al. (172) and Devoret (87) for more detailed descriptions of the tests, to Ames (11) for a description of the problems of carcinogen identification addressed by short-term tests, to a series of papers in the April 1979 issue of the *Journal of the National Cancer Institute* and to Bartsch et al. (22) about experiments to validate the reliability of short-term tests.

Short-term tests are still in their infancy; development of the Ames test began about 15 years ago (11). The major factor influencing the acceptance or rejection of any short-term test as a method for identifying carcinogens is a demonstration that the test can discriminate between carcinogens and noncarcinogens.

The crux of validation experiments is determining: 1) how frequently carcinogens are correctly identified by short-term tests (sensitivity) and 2) how frequently noncarcinogens are correctly identified (specificity). Ideally the frequency for both sensitivity and specificity would be 100 percent. If the Ames test worked perfectly, every tested carcinogen would be a mutagen; every tested noncarcinogen would be a nonmutagen in the test.

The difference between the ideal and the measured performance can be expressed in terms of sensitivity. If the test identified 90 of 100 carcinogens as mutagens, it would have a sensitivity of 90 percent. The same observation can be described in terms of its false-negative rate. In the example, 10 carcinogens were falsely negative in the mutagenicity test, so it had a 10-percent false-negative rate.

Similarly for noncarcinogens, the test's success can be expressed as a specificity rate. If it identified 90 of 100 noncarcinogens as nonmutagens, its specificity was 90 percent. Alternatively, the result can be expressed in terms of the false-positive rate, which is 10 percent in the example.

Ames and his associates tested agents that had been classified as carcinogens or noncarcinogens in bioassays. They found that 156 of 174 animal carcinogens (90 percent) were mutagenic, and, equally important, 96 of 108 (88 percent) chemicals classified as noncarcinogens were not mutagenic (227). Ames has suggested that some of the "noncarcinogenic" chemicals that were detected as mutagens might have been incorrectly classified as noncarcinogens on the basis of bioassay results (11,227). His suggestion points up a problem inherent in "validating" any test against the results of other tests: There is no guarantee that the results of the tests that are used as standards are completely accurate.

Other researchers have investigated the correlation between Ames test mutagenicity and animal carcinogenicity in efforts to validate the mutagenicity test for predicting carcinogenicity. The good correlation between mutagenicity and carcinogenicity found by McCann et al. (227) was "confirmed in a smaller . . . study by the Imperial Chemical Industries" (34). (In addition, see for instance 13,22,226,309,335). There is general agreement that the tests are predictive,

but some disagreement about whether they are 70-, 80-, or 90-percent sensitive. A number of factors contribute to the observed differences in sensitivity. For instance, better correlations may reflect testing chemical classes on which the Ames test performs well. Ames has shown that his test does not work well with certain classes of chemicals, e.g., halogenated hydrocarbons and metals, and including those in validation tests decreases the sensitivity of the tests.

Bartsch et al. (22) report on 89 chemicals studied in the Ames test for mutagenicity. The 89 were chosen because sufficient data existed to classify each of them as a carcinogen or noncarcinogen in animal tests. Results from the Bartsch et al. (22) study along with those from an earlier study by McCann et al. (227) are shown in table 24.

It can be seen that 76 percent of the tested carcinogens were mutagenic in the Bartsch experiments as compared to the 90 percent that were reported mutagenic in McCann et al. (227). The sensitivity in the former study was lower, but comparable to the other report. The comparison of specificity is somewhat deceiving. The 57-percent specificity recorded by Bartsch et al. (22) is much lower than the 88 percent from the earlier study, but results from only seven noncarcinogens were reported by Bartsch et al. (22). McCann et al. (237) tested 108 noncarcinogens. The 57 percent is subject to much larger error than the higher estimate of specificity.

In both reports, the predictive value was found to be over 90 percent. The predictive value is calculated by comparing the number of carcinogens identified as mutagens to the total number of both carcinogens and noncarcinogens that were mutagenic. This means that more than 90 percent of the substances detected as mutagens were carcinogens.

An important qualifier must be applied to the predictive value of a test. It depends strongly not only on sensitivity and specificity but also on the proportion of carcinogens in the collection of substances tested for mutagenicity. The proportion of carcinogens in both validation experiments shown in table 24 was well above 50 percent.

Table 24.—Results Obtained in Two Validation Studies of the Ames Test When Known Carcinogens and Noncarcinogens Were Tested

	Calculation[a]	Results from:	
		Bartsch et al. (22)	McCann et al. (227)
Sensitivity	$\dfrac{C^+ M^+}{C^+ M^+ + C^+ M^-}$	76% (62/82)	90% (156/174)
Specificity	$\dfrac{C^- M^-}{C^- M^+ + C^- M^-}$	57% (4/7)	88% (96/108)
Predictive value	$\dfrac{C^+ M^+}{C^+ M^+ + C^- M^+}$	95% (62/65)	92% (156/168)
Proportion of carcinogens	$\dfrac{C^+ M^+ + C^+ M^-}{\text{all chemicals tested}}$	92% (82/89)	62% (174/282)

[a] C^+ chemicals known to be carcinogens; C^- chemicals known to be noncarcinogens
M^+ chemicals identified as mutagens; M^- chemicals identified as nonmutagens
$C^+ M^+$ carcinogens "correctly" identified as mutagens
$C^- M^-$ noncarcinogens "correctly" identified as nonmutagens
$C^- M^+$ noncarcinogens "incorrectly" identified as mutagens
$C^+ M^-$ carcinogens "incorrectly" identified as nonmutagens.

SOURCE: Office of Technology Assessment; adapted from Bartsch et al. (22).

Table 25 shows the expected results from examining two hypothetical collections of chemicals. The first collection of 1,000 chemicals contains 10 carcinogens (1 percent); the second contains 100 carcinogens in 1,000 total chemicals (10 percent). The short-term test in both cases is assumed to be 90-percent sensitive and 90-percent specific. The predictive value in the two collections differs more than sixfold because of the higher contribution of false positives to the total positives in the 1-percent carcinogen collection. This example illustrates the important role played in predictive value computations by the percentage of carcinogens included in validation experiments.

McMahon, Cline, and Thompson (233) developed a modification of the Ames test and used it to assay 855 chemicals. To validate their own test system, the authors included 125 chemicals that had been tested previously in the Ames test. They reported "excellent agreement" between results in their tests and those reported by McCann et al. (227). Among the other chemicals tested by McMahon, Cline, and Thompson (233) the 299 chosen from manufacturing or laboratory synthesis provided the largest per-

centage of mutagens; 60 of 299 (20 percent) were mutagenic. In contrast, chemicals developed as potential agricultural or pharmaceutical products were less often mutagenic; 29 of 361 such compounds (6 percent) were positive. The authors state (233):

> Very few of the chemical mutagens detected in this study had chemical structures uniquely different from known carcinogens. Further study in other test systems will be required to assess the significance of results with the few unique compounds encountered. The results of the study do suggest, however, that as testing continues on more and more compounds it will be found that most of the new mutagenic compounds detected will be related to known carcinogens and mutagens and that new unique chemical structures possessing these properties will be found rarely.

The McMahon, Cline, and Thompson paper (233) illustrates that large numbers of chemicals can be tested quickly. Furthermore, their results, which are in "excellent aggreement" with those earlier reported by McCann et al. (227) for chemicals tested in both studies, illustrate that the test is reproducible in different laboratories. Whether the prediction that most

Table 25.—Expected Results of Examining Two Collections of Chemicals for Mutagenicity Using a Short-Term Test That is 90-Percent Sensitive and 90-Percent Specific: One Collection of Chemicals Contains 1 Percent Carcinogens; the Other Contains 10 Percent

	Calculation[a]	Collections of chemicals with	
		1% carcinogens	10% carcinogens
Proportion of carcinogens in sample of 1,000 chemicals	$\dfrac{C^+ M^+ + C^+ M^-}{\text{all chemicals tested}}$	1% (i.e., 10 carcinogens)	10% (i.e., 100 carcinogens)
Carcinogens identified as mutagens	$\dfrac{C^+ M^+}{C^+ M^+ + C^+ M^-}$	90% (i.e., 9 of the 10 carcinogens)	90% (i.e., 90 of the 100 carcinogens)
Carcinogens identified as non-mutagens—false negatives in the test	$\dfrac{C^+ M^-}{C^+ M^+ + C^+ M^-}$	10% (i.e., 1 of the 10 carcinogens)	10% (i.e., 10 of the 100 carcinogens)
Noncarcinogens identified as nonmutagens	$\dfrac{C^- M^-}{C^- M^- + C^- M^+}$	90% (i.e., 891 of 990 noncarcinogens)	90% (i.e., 810 of 900 noncarcinogens)
Noncarcinogens identified as mutagens—false positives in the test	$\dfrac{C^- M^+}{C^- M^- + C^- M^+}$	10% (i.e., 99 of 990 noncarcinogens)	10% (i.e., 90 of 900 noncarcinogens)
Summary:			
Carcinogens identified as mutagens		9	90
Noncarcinogens identified as mutagens		$\dfrac{99}{108}$	$\dfrac{90}{180}$
Predictive value— carcinogens identified as mutagens/total carcinogens plus noncarcinogens identified as mutagens	$\dfrac{C^+ M^+}{C^+ M^+ + C^- M^+}$	8.3% (i.e., 9/108)	50% (i.e., 90/180)

[a] C$^+$ chemicals known to be carcinogens; C$^-$ chemicals known to be noncarcinogens
M$^+$ chemicals identified as mutagens; M$^-$ chemicals identified as nonmutagens
C$^+$ M$^+$ carcinogens "correctly" identified as mutagens
C$^-$ M$^+$ noncarcinogens "incorrectly" identified as mutagens.
C$^+$ M$^-$ carcinogens "incorrectly" identified as nonmutagens.

SOURCE: Office of Technology Assessment; adapted from Bartsch et al. (22).

mutagens will have structures related to those of known carcinogens awaits further testing.

The International Program for the Evaluation of Short-Term Tests for Carcinogenicity (partially supported by the National Toxicology Program (NTP), the National Institute of Environmental Health Sciences (NIEHS), and EPA) is analyzing the accuracy of about 30 short-term test systems including the Ames test. The program distributed 42 coded carcinogens and noncarcinogens to 66 investigators, and the results of those studies will be published in 1981. The accuracy of the Ames test in the 12 laboratories which examined it is comparable to the higher accuracy figures (about 80 percent) in the literature (188).

The largest program in genetic toxicology (mutagenicity) is EPA's Genetox Program (357). It is not now engaged in validating short-term tests for predicting carcinogenicity, but it is examining correlations among various short-term tests. Beginning in early 1982, the program expects to publish recommendations for batteries of tests most appropriate for measuring particular mutagenic effects.

How much reliance is to be placed on the results of short-term tests continues to be discussed. Leon Golberg, former President of the Chemical Industry Institute of Toxicology (CIIT), for instance, compared the results from Ames tests to bioassay results for hair dye components. He found little agreement and cautions against using the Ames test as a substitute for bioassays (142,143). However, a recent paper found good correlation between the mutagenicity and carcinogenicity of phenylenediamine hair dye components (330).

In summary, the Ames test is reported to detect known carcinogens as mutagens with a frequency as high as 90 percent. Although a breakthrough in understanding of the correlation between mutagenicity and carcinogenicity is required before more definitive conclusions can be drawn from the Ames test, a positive Ames test result shows that the agent is a mutagen and suggests that it may be a carcinogen.

Other Short-Term Tests

The number of short-term tests has proliferated rapidly. Purchase et al. (301) included only six short-term tests in a 1976 review of the published literature; less than 1 year later, OTA had saccharin tested in 12 short-term tests (282). Two years after that, in the summer of 1979, a review by Hollstein et al. (172) reported that over 100 short-term tests had been described in the scientific literature. The proliferation of tests reflects the great interest in cheaper, faster tests for identifying chemical carcinogens.

Hollstein et al. (172) divided short-term tests into eight classes, according to what they can detect:

1. mutagenesis in bacteria (including Salmonella) and bacterial viruses;
2. mutagenesis in yeast;
3. mutagenesis in cultured (laboratory-grown) mammalian cells;
4. mutagenesis affecting mouse hair color;
5. mutagenesis in fruit flies (Drosophila melanogaster);
6. effects on chromosomal mechanics in intact mammals and in mammalian cells in culture;

7. disruption of DNA synthesis and DNA repair mechanisms in bacteria and other organisms; and
8. in vitro transformation of cultured cells.

One of the powerful tools available to biology is the use of cell culture systems, which allows cells obtained from animal or human tissues to be grown and manipulated in the laboratory. Cell cultures can be manipulated to serve as assays for mutagens (#3 above) and for chemicals that interfere with chromosomal mechanics (#6 above), but the most directly applicable use of cultured cells for carcinogen identification involves in vitro transformation (#8 above).

Cells grown in culture exhibit characteristic morphologies and growth patterns. Exposing cultured cells to known tumor-causing viruses or to chemical carcinogens causes changes in morphology and growth characteristics. The changes are collectively called "transformation." Transformed cells resemble cells from tumors and have the important property of causing tumors when they are injected into animals, thus demonstrating a direct relationship between transformation and oncogenicity (tumor formation). Transformation of cell cultures is biologically more closely related to oncogenicity than is mutation, and transformation assays may take on major importance in testing programs. The NTP 1979 Annual Plan (271) stated:

A lifetime bioassay in rodents is the current procedure utilized to determine carcinogenic potential of a chemical. The NTP does not propose alternative methods but acknowledges a need in the longer term, to develop or validate less expensive and more rapid methods that may in some instances supplant the need for lifetime bioassays. Mammalian cell transformations are potential short-term assays that indicate carcinogenic potential of a chemical . . .

And less than a year later, a more optimistic comment appeared in the Department of Health, Education, and Welfare (DHEW) Health Research Planning document of December 1979 (130):

The dimensions of NTP, and the significant demands it places on the funds and personnel of the participating agencies, should diminish by 1985, as the fiscal projections suggest . . . . It is our hope that, by then, better test systems will begin to replace the tedious and costly animal assays now required.

Not everyone is so optimistic as to think a replacement for animal assays will be available in 4 or 5 years. Transformation tests are probably the best bet for the replacement, but they require more development and validation.

Transformation assays are technically more difficult than the Ames test, but not so difficult as to preclude their use on a routine basis. Validation studies are being carried out on a number of in vitro transformation systems to determine how accurately they identify carcinogens and noncarcinogens (271,272).

NTP is conducting additional validation studies of a test that uses whole animals. This test, which has been in limited use for about 30 years, requires about 6 months to complete. Exposure of a particular strain of mice to known carcinogens causes an increase in the frequency of lung tumors (adenomas) and causes earlier appearance of the tumors. The test takes much less time than the standard assay, and NTP (272) has found this test accurately predicts results in bioassays. NTP tested 60 chemicals in this system in 1980 and plans to test another 30 in 1981.

The British publication *The Economist* (97) singled out a transformation assay, using Chinese hamster ovary cells, as having promise for carcinogen identification. Discussion of short-term tests in that publication, which seldom publishes articles about biology, reflects the increasing importance of the tests. A more authoritative source, the NCI National Cancer Advisory Board's Subcommittee on Environmental Carcinogenesis (245) said: " . . . this subcommittee is enthusiastic about the possible future use of in vitro [short-term] tests as part of a screening system for potential carcinogens and believe that their further development and validation deserve high priority."

Use of Short-Term Test Results and Policy Statements About the Tests

How best to utilize short-term tests in carcinogen identification is hotly debated. The majority view is that the tests are most useful as a screen to determine a chemical's potential carcinogenicity. As a new chemical is developed or as an old one comes under suspicion, an inexpensive short-term test or battery of tests can provide information about whether it is or is not likely to be a carcinogenic hazard. If the results of the test are negative, the chemical is considered less likely to be a hazard than a chemical that is positive. In the case of a chemical being commercially developed, a positive result might suggest that the chemical not be produced or that the cost of testing it in a bioassay should be considered in deciding whether or not to produce it. A positive short-term test result on a commercially produced chemical most likely causes more of a problem. The manufacturer is faced with having to begin other tests and to warn his employees and customers of potential hazard.

Opinions differ about the weight to be placed on short-term test results. Peter Hutt, former General Counsel at the Food and Drug Administration (FDA), and now in private law practice says that he advises his clients not to continue the development of a product which is positive in a short-term test. He maintains that, "life is too short" to invest time and effort in a chemical that is more likely than not to be considered a suspect carcinogen. Near the other end of the spectrum of opinion, Leon Golberg, in reviewing poor correlations between results of Ames testing and bioassays of components of hair dyes, concludes " . . . it is very hard to accept the fact that the Ames test is a predictor of carcinogenic potential" (143).

The OSHA document "Identification, Classification and Regulation of Potential Occupational Carcinogens" (279), accepts the results of short-term tests as supportive evidence for deciding whether a chemical will be classified as a carcinogen or noncarcinogen. TSCA test standards (106) and Federal Insecticide, Fungicide, and Rodenticide Act (FIFRA) guidelines (102) accept short-term tests as measures for mutagenicity but do not consider them in making decisions about carcinogenicity. However, they mention that test developments are promising.

An important step in making decisions about the use of short-term tests are the ongoing validation studies which compare predictions made from short-term tests to knowledge about carcinogenicity from bioassays or epidemiology. These studies, although limited by the quality and quantity of data about carcinogenicity, are producing valuable information. In addition, studies of molecular mechanisms of mutagenicity and carcinogenicity are important in deciding about the applicability of short-term tests.

BIOASSAYS

Chemicals cannot be tested for carcinogenicity in humans because of ethical considerations. A substantial body of experimentally derived knowledge and the preponderance of expert opinion support the conclusion that testing of chemicals in laboratory animals provides reliable information about carcinogenicity. Animal tests employ whole mammal systems, and although they differ one from another, all mammals, including humans, share many biological features (266):

Effects in animals, properly qualified, are applicable to man. This premise underlies all of experimental biology and medicine, but because it is continually questioned with regard to human cancer, it is desirable to point out that cancer in men and animals is strikingly similar. Virtually every form of human cancer has an experimental counterpart, and every form of multicellular organism is subject to cancer, including insects, fish, and plants. Although there are differences in susceptibility between different animal species, and between individuals of the same strain, carcinogenic chemicals will affect most test species, and there are large bodies of experimental data that indicate that exposures that are

The problem of the carcinogens that are not detected (false negatives; lack of sensitivity) and the noncarcinogens that are falsely detected (false positives; lack of specificity) by any one test might be solved with additional short-term tests. The great attractiveness of a battery of short-term tests is that it might correctly identify all carcinogens and noncarcinogens. Unfortunately, no such battery has yet been defined. The composition of the battery will depend on validation studies and acceptance of each component test.

The growing use of short-term tests shows that short-term tests have moved to an important position in toxicology. The speed with which they have been incorporated into Government and private sector programs reflects the importance of the need to which they are addressed.

carcinogenic to animals are likely to be carcinogenic to man, and vice versa.

In comparison to short-term tests and epidemiology, bioassays have had a longer development period and enjoy greater acceptance than the short-term tests; they are more easily manipulated to produce evidence linking a particular substance to cancer than epidemiology, and they can predict human risks rather than relying on cases of human cancer to demonstrate risk. On the other hand, they take longer and cost much more than short-term tests.

The bioassay's apparent simplicity belies the difficulty of executing such experiments. Briefly, the suspect chemical is administered to a population of laboratory animals. As animals die or are killed during the course of the study, they are examined for the presence of tumors. At the end of the treatment and observation period (generally about 2 years), the surviving animals are killed and examined. A control group of animals is treated exactly the same except that they are not exposed to the suspect substance. The type and number of tumors and other relevant pathologies present in the exposed animals are compared with those in the control group, and statistically analyzed.

A statistical expression commonly used to describe a positive result is ". . . it has a p value less than 0.05" (5 percent). The p value is the probability that the observed effect might be explained by chance; in this case, the expression means that the probability of the observed carcinogenic effect being due to chance is less than 5 percent. A p value of 0.05 or less is commonly required to decide that a test result was statistically positive.

Finally a conclusion is drawn about whether or not the evidence indicates that the substance caused cancer in the exposed animals. An excellent discussion of experimental design and analysis is available from the International Agency for Research on Cancer (IARC) (187).

The first successful experimental induction of cancer in animals (in 1915) showed that painting rabbits' ears with coal tar produced tumors which morphologically resembled human tumors associated with exposure to the same agent (cited in 342). Most chemicals which are presently known to cause cancer in humans are also carcinogens in animals.

Verification of the predictive power of bioassays would require that the agent be shown to be a human carcinogen. Currently, IARC maintains that convincing evidence for human carcinogenicity is available for only 18 exposures, including 14 chemicals. At the same time, it lists 142 substances for which data are "sufficient" to conclude that they are carcinogenic in animals. It is difficult to demonstrate human carcinogenicity. Once a substance is shown to be an animal carcinogen, regulatory restrictions on and voluntary reductions in the use of the chemical may reduce human exposures, making those demonstrations more difficult. Reductions in exposure in such cases are far more important to human health than the foregone opportunities to verify the predictive powers of bioassays.

Standard Protocols for Bioassays

An important event in bioassay design was the development of NCI's Guidelines for Carcinogenic Bioassay in Small Rodents (331). The guidelines describe minimum requirements for the design and conduct of a scientifically valid bioassay and discuss important considerations in undertaking such studies. They are written to provide flexibility in experimental design while setting certain minimal requirements:

1. Each chemical should be tested in at least two species and both sexes. Rats and mice are usually the species of choice.
2. Each bioassay should contain at least 50 animals in each experimental group. When both sexes of two species are used and two treatment levels are administered and a third group is used as controls, a total of 600 animals is needed (see table 26).
3. Exposure to the chemical should start when the animals are 6 weeks old or younger and continue for the greater part of their lifespan. Mice and rats are usually exposed for 24 months.
4. One treatment group should receive the maximum tolerated dose (MTD), which is defined as the highest dose that can be given that would not alter the animals' normal lifespan from effects other than cancer. The other treatment group is treated with a fraction of MTD.
5. The route by which a chemical is administered should be the same or as close as possible to the one by which human exposure occurs.
6. Animals are closely monitored throughout the study for signs of toxic effects and other causes affecting their health.
7. Examination of animals is conducted by or under the direction of a pathologist qualified in laboratory animal pathology.

The guidelines also specify that special procedures (e.g., organ function tests, body burden determinations, absorption and excretion tests) may be needed for evaluating certain chemicals.

**Table 26.—Distribution and Number of Animals in
a Typical Bioassay Study of Carcinogens**

Experimental groups	Species A		Species B	
	Males	Females	Males	Females
Dosage MTD[a] group	50	50	50	50
Dosage MTD/x group	50	50	50	50
Control group	50	50	50	50

[a]Maximum tolerated dose.

SOURCE: National Cancer Institute.

A National Research Council report (262) suggested a two-generation bioassay when there is special concern with prenatal and perinatal effects of a substance. In the suggested two-generation experiment, the first generation is exposed from 6 weeks of age through their adult life, including periods of reproductive activity and pregnancy, and the offspring are exposed for their lifespans. The most important two-generation experiments, from the standpoint of public policy, were the three showing saccharin to be a bladder carcinogen in second generation rats (282). The advantage of the two-generation experiment is that it exposes fetuses and very young animals, which may represent the most sensitive stages of life. This procedure costs more and requires more time to complete than the one generation experiment. Probably because of those disadvantages, it has not often been used.

Table 27 compares some specifics of NCI guidelines with those proposed by EPA for testing under FIFRA (102) and TSCA (106). NCI guidelines state that at least two-dose levels be tested; EPA requires three test doses. The highest dose, high-dose level (HDL), for TSCA is defined as being "slightly toxic" and is to be determined in a 90-day-feeding study to precede the oncogenicity experiment. The other two doses are to be fractions of HDL. EPA prefers the term HDL, which is less specifically defined than MTD, because of the controversies which have erupted over defining MTD. Three-dose levels are proposed by EPA because a review of many NCI bioassays revealed that tumor incidence was sometimes higher at a dose of MTD/2 than at MTD because the higher dose killed some animals before tumors might have developed. The third-dose level will also provide additional information about the dose-

response curve (102). The text which accompanies the proposed EPA guidelines for carcinogen testing under FIFRA (102) contains additional information about alternative approaches considered and subsequently discarded for the guidelines.

Three to five years are required to complete a bioassay. A subchronic test, to set dose levels, requiring 2 to 6 months, is followed by an average 24 months of exposure to the agent, and sometimes an additional 3 to 6 months observation period. Pathological examination of tissues from the animals and evaluation of the pathological and other data may take an additional year.

The cost of a bioassay has been variously estimated: NCI estimates about $400,000, TSCA guidelines (106) estimated $400,000, and EPA (112) later estimated a range from $390,000 to $980,000.

Some changes have been made in protocols since the NCI guidelines were published, but in contrast to the situation in spring 1977, when OTA reviewed carcinogen testing (282), apparently much less confusion and contention now exist about what constitutes an adequate bioassay. NCI guidelines are for minimal standards; certainly larger populations of animals can be tested. For very important bioassays, larger numbers of animals or more dosage groups might be specified.

Objections to the Usefulness of Bioassays

Some general aspects of test design are seldom disputed. Examples of such provisions are the requirement of a minimum number of animals in the test groups and that (generally) both sexes

Table 27.—Guidelines for Bioassay in Small Rodents

	NCI (331)[a]	FIFRA (102)	TSCA (106)
Endpoint	Carcinogenicity	Oncogenicity	Oncogenicity
Study plan:			
Animal species	2, rats and mice	2, rats and mice	2, rats and mice
Number of animals at each dose	50 males, 50 females	50 males, 50 females	50 males, 50 females

Dosages	2, MTD
	  MTD/2 or MTD/4
	plus no-dose control
		3, MTD
		  MTD/2 or MTD/4
		  MTD/4 or MTD/8
		plus no-dose control
			3, HDL
			  HDL/2 or HDL/4
			  HDL/4 or HDL/10
			plus no-dose control

Dosing regimen			
Start	At 6 weeks of age	In utero or at 6 weeks	At 6 weeks of age
End	At 24 months of age	Mice, 18-24 mos; rats, 24-30	At 24–30 months of age
Observation period	3–6 months after end of dosing	N.s.	N.s.
Organs and tissues to be examined	All animals: external and histopathologic examination (ca. 30 organs and tissues)	All animals: external examination; some animals: pathologic exam of 30 organs and tissues, other animals, fewer organs and tissues	All animals: external and histopathologic examination (ca. 30 organs and tissues)[b]
Personnel qualifications:			
Study director	N.s.	N.s.	Responsibilities detailed
Pathologist	Board-qualified	N.s.	Board-certified or equivalent
Animal husbandry	N.s.	N.s.	Board-certified vet. or equivalent
Cost estimate	N.s.	N.s.	$400,000 ± 160,000

Abbreviations: MTD, Maximum tolerated dose, causes minor acute toxicity
              HDL, high dose level, causes some acute toxicity
              N.s., not specified

[a] The NCI Guidelines specify the indicated minimum requirements. They allow for flexibility in experimental design so long as the minimum requirements are met.
[b] EPA estimates that the 40,000 microscope slides produced in this examination will require more than 3/4 of a year of a pathologist's time for analysis.

SOURCE: Office of Technology Assessment.

be tested. On the other hand, consensus does not exist about some aspects of experimental design, for instance: How high a dose is to be administered? The policy of the agency that draws up the guidelines is reflected in what it says about the arguable aspects of experimental design. Tomatis (341) has discussed five debated issues about bioassay.

1. **Doses of chemicals to which test animals are exposed are too high and are not predictive for effects at levels of human exposure.**

High doses of suspect carcinogens are necessary to increase tumor incidence to a level that can be detected in the limited number of animals used for tests (180). A chemical causing tumors at a rate of 0.5 percent in the U.S. population would result in over 1 million cancer cases. But an incidence of 0.5 percent would very probably go undetected in the usual test population of 50

male plus 50 female rats or mice. Administration of the chemical at a 10-times higher dose might increase the response to a detectable level given comparable sensitivity between the test animals and humans. High doses are necessary to increase the sensitivity of the tests, but arguments arise over whether or not a dose is so high that it is not predictive of what happens at lower doses.

The biological argument against depending on results at high doses centers on the contention that such doses may alter metabolism or cause local irritations or other toxic response and cause cancer through a pathway that would not exist at lower doses (60,139,278). A solution sometimes offered to the problems raised by high doses is to run bioassays with many more animals tested at lower doses. The most spectacular attempt at this was the National Center for Toxicological Research (NCTR) ED_{01} study which used 24,000 mice and was designed to detect one cancer in 100 animals. Unfortunately, neither it nor (probably) any experiment can eliminate the necessity for testing chemicals at doses significantly higher than those experienced by humans. Even 24,000 is a small number compared to the number of people exposed to many chemicals.

2. Routes of exposure in animal tests do not correspond to routes of human exposure.

Chemicals are administered to laboratory animals in either food, water, by inhalation, force-feeding (gavage), skin-painting, or injection. Few objections are raised to administration in food, water, or by inhalation when the chosen route mimics the route of human exposure. More objections are raised to gavage, skin-painting, injection, or ingestion when that is not the normal human exposure route. However, such methods are sometimes necessary and, furthermore, carcinogens appear to be distributed throughout the body regardless of the route of exposure. EPA (106) stipulates that "to the extent possible, route(s) of administration should be comparable to expected or known routes of human exposure." Adherence to such suggestions will reduce the frequency of this objection.

3. Some animals used for testing are so biologically different from humans that results from them have no value.

Choice of animals for bioassays represents a compromise. Most current guidelines require or suggest that chemicals be tested in two rodent species, generally rats and mice. The advantages of these species are their small size, reducing the space necessary for housing, short lifespans (2 to 3 years), reducing the time needed for a lifetime study, and a large amount of information about the genetics, breeding, housing, and health of these animals. Rats and mice are cheap to buy, feed, and house, as compared with larger animals.

Primates are sometimes used for certain toxicological testing. They are certainly more like humans than rodents but their supply is limited. They are expensive, live up to 25 years, and require large areas for housing. Despite these difficulties, NCI now maintains about 600 monkeys for carcinogenicity testing at a cost of about $500,000 per year (2). Dogs are thought to be between rodents and monkeys in their apparent likeness to humans, but they are more like primates in costs.

Differences in metabolism, bioaccumulation, and excretion between rodents and humans should be considered in interpreting the significance of animal results for humans. There is no question that further research in the comparative biochemistry and physiology of man and rodents is necessary, but the comparisons will ultimately be limited by restrictions on what can be determined by experimentation in humans. Moreover, metabolic studies have shown that most differences between humans and experimental animals are quantitative rather than qualitative and support the idea that animal results can be used to predict human responses.

4. Some test animals or organs of test animals are exquisitely sensitive to carcinogens, and such sensitivity invalidates use of results from such animals.

Griesemer and Cueto (146) have analyzed the results of testing 190 chemicals in the NCI Bioassay Program (see discussion in *Expert Review of Bioassay Results* and app. A). They identified 35 chemicals that were "strongly carcinogenic" in either the rat or the mouse and noncarcinogenic in the other species. Of the 35, 18 were positive in the mouse and negative in the rat, and 17 were positive in the rat and negative in the mouse, which indicates that neither animal was much more often the sensitive species. However, 12 chemicals caused mouse liver tumors, no other lesion in the mouse and no lesions in rats. Taken by themselves these results suggest that the mouse liver is a sensitive organ.

Liver tumors are often found in mice but are infrequently found in U.S. citizens, although they occur frequently in human populations in other parts of the world. Should a chemical that causes mouse liver tumors be considered a hazard? An approach to resolving the mouse liver question was to review how predictive such results are for tumors in other animals. Tomatis, Partensky, and Montesano (343) showed positive correlation between a chemical's being oncogenic in the mouse liver and its being oncogenic either in the liver or at some other site in rats or hamsters. (Griesmer and Cueto (146) presented data only from rats and mice, and some mouse liver carcinogens in their compilation might be positive in animals other than rats.)

Despite the finding of Tomatis, Partensky, and Montesano (343) that mouse liver carcinogens were often positive at other sites or in other animals, IARC (185,187) considers mouse liver and lung tumors as "limited evidence" for carcinogenicity. However, OSHA (272) accepts mouse liver tumors as "indicators of carcinogenicity" if "scientific experience and judgment" are used in interpreting the data.

Crouch and Wilson (72) have analyzed some of the NCI Bioassay Program data. They calculated the potency and the standard error associated with potency of a chemical in causing a tumor at a particular site in either the rat or the mouse. In their analysis of 35 tested chemicals, they found that in 31 cases the potency in both rats and mice agreed within a factor of 10. Their analysis and similar analysis by Ames et al. (14), which consider the inherent error in experiments and the sensitivity of experiments, significantly reduces the number of chemicals that are positive in one species and negative in another. However, those analytical methods have not been generally applied to bioassay results.

5. Finding benign tumors in test animals has no value in defining carcinogenicity.

Tumors can be divided into two classes, benign and malignant. Benign tumors do not metastasize, the tumor cells remain in contact with each other and do not invade other tissues or organs. Malignant tumors can invade other tissues and metastasize, spreading to distant parts of the body and causing other tumors. Both types of tumors are found in experimental animals.

Hearings on pesticide regulations have been marked by repeated arguments about the importance of benign tumors. Should benign tumors found in experimental animals be taken as evidence that a chemical causes cancer?

The position that a benign tumor may later become malignant, that the line of demarcation between benign and malignant is unclear, and that benign tumors can also be life-threatening has prevailed in regulatory agencies. Therefore, no distinction is made in regulatory decisions between benign and malignant tumors. This is clearly reflected in FIFRA guidelines (102) and TSCA test standards (106) in which the endpoint is oncogenicity (tumor causation) rather than carcinogenicity (which emphasizes malignancy) (see table 27).

Griesemer and Cueto (146) reported no difficulty in deciding between benign and malignant tumors in the NCI Bioassay Program and that their conclusions about carcinogenicity were unaffected by including or excluding benign tumors. IARC statements reflect difficulties in the interpretation of benign tumors. As mentioned above, it considers the occurrence of some benign tumors as "limited evidence" for concluding that a chemical is a carcinogen (185). It also states that "preneoplastic lesions" may progress to "frank malignancy." Furthermore, IARC (186,187) considers that the occurrence of both preneoplastic and neoplastic lesions in the same organ strengthens conclusions about carcinogenicity.

Expert Review of Bioassay Results

In addition to the general objections to bioassay procedures that have been discussed, specific objections may be raised to particular tests. For instance, animals may have been inadvertently exposed to more than one chemical, to pathogenic micro-organisms, to extreme temperature, or to temporary deprivation of food or water, any one of which might influence results. Another frequent item of contention is whether or not a particular pathologic lesion indicates carcinogenicity. Critical reviews can reduce concern that flaws in experimental design or conduct mar the experiment or bring its results into question.

IARC periodically calls together panels of experts to review the worldwide literature about the carcinogenicity of particular chemicals or exposures. The IARC Monograph Program, begun in 1970, had published reviews of bioassays of 422 chemicals and processes by 1979. For 60 of the 422 chemicals and processes, IARC was able to evaluate both human and animal evidence for carcinogenicity. Those 60 are described in the epidemiology section below.

For the remaining 362 chemicals and processes (185),

> . . . there was no information available from studies in humans [but] the IARC was asked repeatedly to consider making an assessment of the carcinogenic risk for humans which was based only on animal data.

In response to those requests, the IARC working group recommended (185):

> . . . that in the absence of adequate data in humans it is reasonable, for practical purposes, to regard chemicals for which there is *sufficient evidence* of carcinogenicity (i.e. a causal association) in animals *as if they presented a carcinogenic risk for humans* (emphasis in original).

An IARC working group defined five categories of evidence—sufficient, limited, inadequate, negative, and no data—against which experimental data are to be compared (see app. A). The working group decided that for 142 chemicals there was sufficient evidence, for about 100 there was limited evidence, and for the remainder there was inadequate evidence for carcinogenicity. The IARC exercise is especially important because it shows that experts from both the private and public sectors, sitting on IARC panels, can consider experiments and results and reach decisions about their meaning.

Griesemer and Cueto (146) analyzed the results of NCI's testing 190 chemicals. IARC (185) and Griesemer and Cueto (146) classifications of chemicals included 33 chemicals in common. Analysis of the classification of those 33 (see app. A) shows that there was good agreement about the more carcinogenic of the chemicals. Such agreement lends credence to the idea that tests carried out in different laboratories and analyzed by different experts can lead to similar conclusions about carcinogenicity.

Policy Considerations About Bioassays

General acceptance of bioassays as predictors of human risk is sometimes obscured by controversies about particular test results. The Federal Government, in response to controversies arising from testing artificial sweeteners or pesticides, has asked a number of expert panels to consider bioassay designs, results, and usefulness. In all cases, the panels endorsed bioassays while reserving judgment about particular tests and attaching caveats to some results. Table 28 is a listing of some Government-affiliated panels and reports plus two trade associations, the American Industrial Health Council (AIHC) and the Food Safety Council, and a union organization which have commented on bioassays.

The Office of Science and Technology Policy (OSTP), in the Executive Office of the President (281) produced a good, brief exposition of methods, a well-crafted list of recommendations about carcinogen testing, and suggestions for a Federal carcinogen policy. About bioassays, the report says,

> . . . it would seem prudent to view a positive test result in a carefully designed and well-conducted mammalian study as evidence of potential human carcinogenicity.

As indicated by the quote, some organizations urge consideration of experimental design and execution before drawing conclusions about carcinogenicity. AIHC (8), in commenting on OSHA's (278) proposed cancer policy, endorsed bioassays as predictors of human risk:

> There is agreement further that a substance which is a confirmed oncogen in two mammalian species should be subject to regulation as a probable human carcinogen.

All Federal regulatory agencies accept animal test results as predictors of carcinogenic risk for humans. The Interagency Regulatory Liaison Group (IRLG) was formed in 1977 to aline the policies of the Consumer Product Safety Commission (CPSC), FDA, the Food Safety and Quality Service of the Department of Agriculture, EPA, and OSHA. IRLG stated (180):

Table 28.—Some Organizations That Have Considered and Endorsed Animal Tests as Predictors of Human Risk From Chemical Carcinogens

Organization	Publication
The Secretary's (HEW) Committee on Pesticides and their Relationship to Environmental Health	Report (325)
National Research Council	— Evaluating the Safety of Food Chemicals (259) — Safety of Saccharin and Sodium Saccharin in the Human Diet (261) — Pest Control: An Assessment of Present and Alternative Technologies (262) — Principles for Evaluating Chemicals in the Environment (263) — Food Safety Policy (269)
Office of Technology Assessment	— Cancer Testing Technology and Saccharin (282) — Environmental Contaminants in Food (284)
National Cancer Advisory Board, Subcommittee on Environmental Carcinogenesis	— General Criteria for Assessing the Evidence for Carcinogenicity of Chemical Substances (245) — The Relation of Bioassay Data on Chemicals to the Assessment of the Risk of Carcinogens for Humans Under Conditions of Low Exposure (246)
American Industrial Health Council	— AIHC Recommended Alternative to OSHA's Generic Carcinogen Proposal (8)
Food Safety Council	— Proposed System for Food Safety Assessment (125)
Occupational Safety and Health Administration	— Identification, Classification and Regulation of Potential Occupational Carcinogens (279)
Interagency Regulatory Liaison Group	— Scientific Bases for Identification of Potential Carcinogens and Estimates of Risks (180)
Office of Science and Technology Policy	— Identification, Characterization and Control of Potential Human Carcinogens: A Framework for Federal Decision-making (281)
American Federation of Labor, Congress of Industrial Organizations, and United Steelworkers of America	— Post-Hearing Brief on OSHA's Proposed Standard on the Identification, Classification and Regulation of Toxic Substances Posing a Potential Occupational Carcinogenic Risk (7)

SOURCE: Office of Technology Assessment.

Evidence of the carcinogenic activity of an agent can be obtained from bioassays in experimental animals.

and,

Positive results, obtained in one species only are considered evidence of carcinogenicity. Positive results in more limited tests (e.g., when the observation period is considerably less than the animal's lifetime), but by experimentally adequate procedures, are acceptable as evidence of carcinogenicity. Negative results, on the other hand, are not considered as evidence of lack of a carcinogenic effect, for operational purposes, unless minimum requirements have been met.

As these quotes show, both AIHC and IRLG accept bioassays as predictors of potential human risk. However, they differ in the weight of evidence each requires. AIHC wants positive test results in two species before making decisions about carcinogenicity, while IRLG will consider making a decision on the basis of positive results in one species. Labor organizations (e.g., American Federation of Labor, Congress of Industrial Organizations, and United Steelworkers of America (7)) and environmental groups also consider positive results in a single animal as sufficient to make a judgment about carcinogenicity.

How Many Chemicals Are Carcinogens in Animal Tests?

The number of chemicals that are carcinogenic in humans or animals is uncertain. A few estimates have been made, but the bases for the estimates are poor.

OSHA (279) states: "Most substances do not appear to be carcinogenic," and uses information from two lists of test results to support the statement. OSHA cites the study of Innes et al. (176), which tested 120 industrial chemicals and pesticides. Eleven (less than ten percent) were reported to be carcinogenic, 20 were considered to require further study, and 89 "did not give significant indication of tumorigenicity." A National Academy of Sciences review of pesticides (262) also drew attention to the low number of positive results reported in the Innes study. The small number was judged to be especially significant because of the large number of biologically active pesticides included in the test. Certain reservations must be attached to these conclusions. The maximum dose tested and the number of animals used in the experiments were smaller than now required, and consequently, the experiments were less conclusive than more recent ones.

A more direct criticism of relying on the Innes et al. (176) document as a measure of how many chemicals are carcinogens is that it was a preliminary report. Based on the complete report (26), Barnard (21) states that 29 percent of the tested compounds were carcinogenic.

The second source cited by OSHA (279) is the seven-volume Public Health Service (PHS) list of chemicals tested for carcinogenicity (298). OSHA (279) reported that about 17 percent of the 7,000 tested chemicals were tumorigenic. However, OSHA concluded that these data "overstated the true proportion of carcinogenic substances in the human environment" because suspicious chemicals are selected for testing.

Despite such reservations, the Task Force on Environmental Cancer, Heart and Lung Disease (339) said:

> Of the upwards of 100,000 known chemicals of potential toxicity, only approximately 6,000 have been tested for carcinogenicity. It is estimated that 10 to 16 percent of the chemicals so tested provide some evidence of animal carcinogenicity.

To treat the reported 10 to 16 percent of tested chemicals as carcinogens as a reliable number is probably an error because many of the 7,000

tests are clearly inadequate when measured against current testing guidelines. Scientists employed by the General Electric Co. (141a) have also examined the lists from the seven volumes (298). Using a relaxed criterion for carcinogenicity " . . . any listing that reported an incidence of tumors in the test animals higher than in the control animals was scored as 'positive,' " upwards of 80 percent of the listed chemicals were found to be positive. It is important to recognize that this relaxed criterion would not be accepted in any regulatory decision, and it exaggerates the number of positives. Furthermore, biases toward testing chemicals that are likely to be carcinogenic and toward reporting positive results push the percentage of positives upward.

OSHA (279) had a contractor analyze a list of 2,400 suspect carcinogens compiled by the National Institute of Occupational Safety and Health (NIOSH). The contractor estimated that for 570 (24 percent of the total) there were sufficient data to permit initiation of rulemaking to classify them as category I or II carcinogens under the proposed OSHA policy.

Neither the Innes study nor the PHS list provides information as reliable as that which is more recently available from NCI, IARC, and NTP. Fifty-two percent of NCI-tested and reported chemicals were carcinogens (146). Either "sufficient" or "limited" data existed to classify about 65 percent of IARC-listed chemicals as carcinogens (186,344). NTP (273) reported that 252 (including the 190 reported by Griesemer and Cueto (146)) tests have been completed in the NCI Bioassay Program. Under conditions of the tests, 42 percent were positive, 9.5 percent were equivocal, 36 percent were negative, and 13 percent were inconclusive.

The biases toward testing likely-to-be-positive chemicals cannot be ignored, and the fact that negative test results are less likely to be published and included in any compilation (279) further complicates analysis of lists of tested chemicals. These factors tend to increase the percentage of positive chemicals, and consequently may inflate the estimates of the percentages of chemicals that are carcinogens.

A definitive answer to questions about how many chemicals are carcinogens would depend on testing every chemical, and that is beyond the capacity of the bioassay system. Tomatis (341) reported that 828 chemicals were under test worldwide in governmental programs in 1975, and that 317 were repeat tests of chemicals for which, in his opinion, adequate data already existed. He did not estimate the number of chemicals under test in private or commercial laboratories.

Finding more and more chemicals to be carcinogenic in bioassays raises important policy questions and may force a decision to rank carcinogens for possible regulation or voluntary reductions. It is not apparent how to deal with a large number of carcinogens without ordering them according to their riskiness.

SELECTION OF CHEMICALS FOR TESTING IN BIOASSAYS AND SHORT-TERM TESTS

Tests develop information to aid in making decisions about chemicals, and the most important step in information development is placing the chemical on test. Limited testing capacity makes it necessary to pick and choose among chemicals. Not all can be tested. The second NTP Annual Report (272) underlines this point in discussing bioassays:

> It is unreasonable even to attempt to study all 48,000 chemicals in this way. Current known world capacity permits the initiation of perhaps 300 such chemical tests each year, and the results published this year are from the tests begun 4 or more years ago. This capacity—even if financial resources were not limiting—could be no more than doubled in the next 5-10 years. At this rate, it would take an additional 80 years to study all currently existing chemicals. Further, approximately 500 new chemicals are introduced into commerce each year, and this would result in an additional backlog of some 40,000 untested chemicals.

The same report pinpoints Federal Government testing capacity:

> In carcinogenesis testing the NTP proposes to start 75 new chemicals on the lifetime carcinogenicity bioassays in fiscal year 80. This is the same as the level achieved in fiscal year 79 and is a two-fold increase over the rate of testing prior to the establishment of the program. [In fact, 50 were started in fiscal year 1980; 30 are expected in fiscal year 1981.]

By spring 1980, the Federal Government had centered its selection activities on two programs, the Interagency Testing Committee (ITC), and the NTP Chemical Nomination and Selection Committee. ITC recommends chemicals for testing to the EPA Administrator under jurisdiction of section 4 of TSCA (the ITC list) and NTP selects chemicals for testing by the Federal Government. In addition, NCTR and CIIT have also published criteria for testing substances.

The Interagency Testing Committee

Section 4(a) of TSCA stipulates that EPA issue a rule to require testing if an individual chemical or category of chemicals "may present an unreasonable risk of injury to health or the environment . . . or will be produced in substantial quantities and . . . enter the environment in substantial quantities or there is or may be significant or substantial human exposure." The vagueness of such terminology, "unreasonable risk," "substantial quantities," "significant or substantial human exposure," requires EPA to generate interpretations within scientific, legal, and policy contexts.

Section 4(c) of TSCA established ITC to recommend chemical substances or mixtures which should be given priority consideration for testing. ITC is composed of eight members, one each from EPA, OSHA, the Council on Environmental Quality (CEQ), NIOSH, NIEHS, NCI, the National Science Foundation (NSF), and the Department of Commerce.

ITC is to give priority to those chemical substances which are known or suspected to cause or to contribute to the causation of cancer (carcinogens), mutations (mutagens), or birth defects (teratogens). The total number of chemical substances or mixtures recommended for testing at any one time is not to exceed 50. TSCA specifies that ITC must update, as necessary, the testing priority list at least every 6 months. The EPA Administrator is directed to respond to a chemical's being placed on the list within 12 months. The Administrator must either initiate rulemaking to require testing or publish reasons for not initiating a testing rule.

ITC's initial selection of chemicals for consideration was made by combining about 20 Government-compiled lists of potentially hazardous substances. Chemicals that did not come under TSCA's purview were eliminated from further consideration, and the remaining substances were ranked against two measures: exposure and biological activity. The bases for determining exposure were explicitly specified by Congress in section 4(e)(i)(A) of TSCA:

- general population exposure (number of people exposed, frequency of exposure, exposure intensity, penetrability);
- quantity released into the environment (quantity released, persistence);
- production volume; and
- occupational exposure.

In general, chemicals which were ranked high on the exposure scale were further ranked against biological activity measurements. TSCA specified the first three factors, and the others were included because of their significance in characterizing biological effects (183):

- carcinogenicity,
- mutagenicity,
- teratogenicity,
- acute toxicity,
- other toxic effects,
- ecological effects, and
- bioaccumulation.

ITC examined the biological activity score and the individual biological and exposure factors, and weighed the biological scores against the exposure scores to select chemicals for detailed reviews. After the reviews, chemicals were recommended to the EPA Administrator for consideration. A detailed description of the scoring system can be found in the initial ITC report to the Administrator of the EPA (183).

As of November 1980, ITC had filed seven reports to the EPA Administrator. Each report has updated and revised the list of chemicals eligible for promulgation of test rules under section 4(a) of TSCA.

Chemical Categories

An important consideration in selecting chemicals for testing is how to deal with chemical categories or classes. Section 26(c) of TSCA specifies that any action authorized or required under the act "may be taken by the Administrator . . . with respect to a category of chemical substances or mixtures [and] shall be deemed to be a reference to each chemical substance or mixture in such category." In making its recommendations ITC selected some categories of chemicals for testing. EPA must determine whether to evaluate the scientific, economic, and regulatory consequences of every present or potential member of a category of chemicals or to evaluate selected representatives from the category. If the decision is made to test representatives, EPA has to assess whether it could "reasonably" extrapolate test results to chemicals within the group that have not been studied. Some industry representatives have questioned the validity of using categories for chemical testing, particularly the categories recommended by ITC. They express concern that it would be unrealistic to establish a general policy for choosing which chemicals should be tested for every possible category. Charles Holdsworth, of the American Petroleum Institute, recommended that EPA select members of a category once the "metabolic actor" for the group is determined. Another possible approach would be to select chemicals of interest because of exposure or production volume.

Disposition of the ITC List

As of May 1981, 3½ years after completion of the first ITC list, EPA had issued no final rule requiring testing of any ITC-identified chemicals. However, EPA (110) in the summer of 1980 proposed its first health effects test rule on chemicals nominated by ITC. The proposed rule would require testing of chloromethane and representative members of the category of chlorinated benzenes for oncogenicity and other health effects. Support documents describing the reasons for deciding to require testing and an economic impact analysis of the tests were also released (110,112). As of April 1, 1980, draft copies of test rules for four additional chemicals and groups of chemicals from the 21 identified on the first three ITC lists were available from EPA.

The General Accounting Office (141) reported that EPA estimates it will take 5 years to issue a final test rule for an ITC-nominated chemical. That time is required for the agency to evaluate the published information about the chemical. EPA further estimates that an additional 4 years will be required for execution of bioassay and analysis of their results. At a minimum, then, 9 years will pass between the decision to test an ITC-selected chemical and completion of testing. Certainly the long time between the decision to require testing and the production of results is of concern to EPA, and the agency is working to reduce it (141).

There is a suggestion that many ITC-selected chemicals are currently under test in other arms of the executive branch. NTP (273) reported that of 20 single chemicals and 15 classes recommended by ITC (as of April 1980), 16 of the 20 chemicals and representative chemicals from 14 of 15 classes were then under test or scheduled for test by NTP. NTP (273) did not make a comparison between the types of tests recommended by ITC and the types of tests being carried out or planned by NTP. The NTP report draws attention to a problem common to an active field such as toxicology. ITC judgments about whether or not to require a test are based on what it knows about in-progress and completed tests. It is important that NTP and other testing

organizations share their latest information and plans with ITC. Accordingly, a liaison representative of NTP attends and participates in ITC meetings and related activities.

Responsibility for Testing Under TSCA

Once a chemical or category is selected for testing, EPA must determine who should bear the responsibility and burden of testing. TSCA requires EPA to indicate whether manufacturers, processors, or both manufacturers and processors bear the responsibility. EPA is presently evaluating exposures that occur at various points in a chemical's life cycle. If EPA finds that the chemical's manufacture may present a risk, only the manufacturers must test. If processing may pose a hazard, only the processors are required to test. However, if distribution in commerce, use, or disposal of the chemical may present a risk, both the manufacturers and the processors are required to test. This determination has substantial economic and legal ramifications since it will establish the universe of firms which must bear the cost of testing. Some of the chemicals for which test rules have been drafted are manufactured by more than one company. EPA is urging that firms cooperate to sponsor single tests of the chemicals rather than have each company sponsor its own test.

National Toxicology Program

NTP was established within DHEW (now Department of Health and Human Services (DHHS)) on November 15, 1978, to further the development and validation of integrated toxicological test methodologies. The NTP Executive Committee is composed of the heads of FDA, OSHA, CPSC, EPA, National Institutes of Health (NIH), NIOSH, NCI, and NIEHS.

NTP's annual plan for fiscal year 1980 (272) describes methods to select chemicals for testing: NTP operates under the principle that industry will test chemicals for health and environmental effects as intended and mandated by Congress under legislative authorities. However, some chemicals will not be tested by the private sector, and NTP will select chemicals for its own testing program from the following categories:

1. chemicals found in the environment that are not closely associated with commercial activities;
2. desirable substitutes for existing chemicals, particularly therapeutic agents, that might not be developed or tested without Federal involvement;
3. chemicals that should be tested to improve scientific understanding of structure-activity relationships and thereby assist in defining groups of commercial chemicals that should be tested by industry;
4. certain chemicals tested by industry, or by others, the additional testing of which by the Federal Government is justified to verify the results;
5. previously tested chemicals for which other testing is desirable to cross-compare testing methods;
6. "old chemicals" with the potential for significant human exposure which are of social importance but which generate too little revenue to support an adequate testing program (some of these may be "grandfathered" under FDA laws);
7. two or more chemicals together, when combined human exposure occurs (such testing probably cannot be required of industry if the products of different companies are involved); and
8. in special situations, as determined by the executive committee, marketed chemicals which have potential for large scale and/or intense human exposure, even if it may be possible to require industry to perform the testing.

NTP solicits lists of chemicals from NTP research (NCI, NIEHS, FDA, NIOSH) and regulatory (FDA, OSHA, CPSC, EPA) agencies, other Federal agencies, academia, industry, labor, and the public. All of the chemicals suggested for study are funneled to the NTP Chemical Nominations Group.

The Chemical Nominations Group, composed of representatives from EPA, OSHA, FDA, CPSC, NIH, NCI, NIEHS, and NTP, prepares a dossier describing what is known about the physical properties of each chemical, its production volume, its use, exposures to it, and any toxicological information. Each chemical is judged against the chemical selection principles described above and nominations are forwarded to the NTP Executive Committee which makes final decisions about which chemicals to place on test.

A decision by NTP to test a chemical does not mean necessarily that the chemical will be placed on a bioassay program. It may mean that the chemical will be entered into less expensive, short-term tests first, and depending on the results of those tests, subsequent decisions will be made about whether testing should continue.

The National Center for Toxicological Research

NCTR, a research arm of EPA and FDA was established to develop a better understanding of adverse health effects of potentially toxic chemicals. NCTR's research emphasis is on determination of adverse health effects resulting from long-term, low-level exposure to chemical toxicants (food additives, residues of animal drugs, etc.); determination of the basic biological processes involving chemical toxicants in animals in order to enable better extrapolation of toxicological data from laboratory animals to man; and development of improved methodologies and test protocols for evaluation of the safety of chemical toxicants (good laboratory practices, automated data systems, etc.). NCTR chooses substances for testing from the following categories (271):

1. substances that have no clear industrial sponsorship and for which it is determined that further toxicological data are needed. Usually these are either food contaminants, GRAS (generally recognized as safe food additives) compounds, or cosmetic ingredients.
2. substances that can act as model compounds in a continuing toxicological methods development program.

3. substances for which there is a pressing need to acquire toxicological data above and beyond that which may be supplied by industry.
4. studies as a direct regulatory response to consumer complaints.

Chemical Industry Institute of Toxicology

CIIT was established in 1974 as an independent, nonprofit research laboratory financed by annual contributions from the member companies. Membership in CIIT is open to any corporation or other business entity whose activity consists to a substantial extent of the manufacture, processing, or use of chemicals and any formal association of such entities. CIIT is to provide objective study of toxicological problems problems involved in the manufacture,

handling, use, and disposal of commodity chemicals.

CIIT has developed a set of criteria to select and rank chemicals into priority lists for study. These criteria are:

- volume of production,
- physical and chemical properties,
- estimated human exposure,
- toxicological suspicion and opinion,
- public interest, and
- significance to society.

To date about 40 chemicals have been selected by CIIT for review and study. CIIT's testing showed that formaldehyde caused nasal cancer in rats. Those results have been used by Federal agencies in considering regulations about the chemical.

TIER TESTING

This chapter has so far discussed various test procedures, from quick, low-cost molecular structure analysis through relatively quick, relatively cheap short-term tests to long-term, high-cost bioassays. The fourth category of test, epidemiologic studies, differs from the other three. Detection of a carcinogen because it causes human illness and death can be regarded as a failure in hazard identification, because the other three tests should have or might have predicted the risks before the substance had a chance to inflict harm.

During the last several years, a number of expert committees and panels have discussed an ordered approach to testing—proceeding from quick, cheap tests to longer, more expensive tests. One such "tier testing" plan was developed by an expert group drawn from academic institutions, public-interest organizations, industry and Government agencies (66). A repeated criticism expressed in letters that commented on the plan was the absence of criteria on which to drop a chemical from further testing requirements (66). The point was made that the tier system developed by the Conservation

Foundation was actually a sequential test series, since once a chemical entered the test series it would apparently continue on through every test.

Tier testing has no place in regulations of carcinogens under FIFRA and TSCA, since EPA regulation of substances as a carcinogen requires bioassay or human data (102, 106). To talk of a tier testing system under those regulations is academic, but evidently EPA is considering a role for short-term tests for making decisions about carcinogenicity. In the suit brought by the Natural Resources Defense Council against EPA because of its failure to act on the ITC chemicals, Warren Muir of EPA said: " . . . EPA is in the process of considering what kinds of results from short-term tests suggest the need to require long-term tests for the potential for causing cancer . . . " (243).

An approach to tier testing appears in the 1980 NTP annual plan and is described in figure 20. The close interrelationships between genetic toxicology and carcinogenesis test programs are shown by the lines which connect them. The ab-

Figure 20.—Interrelationships of Major Testing Activities of NTP

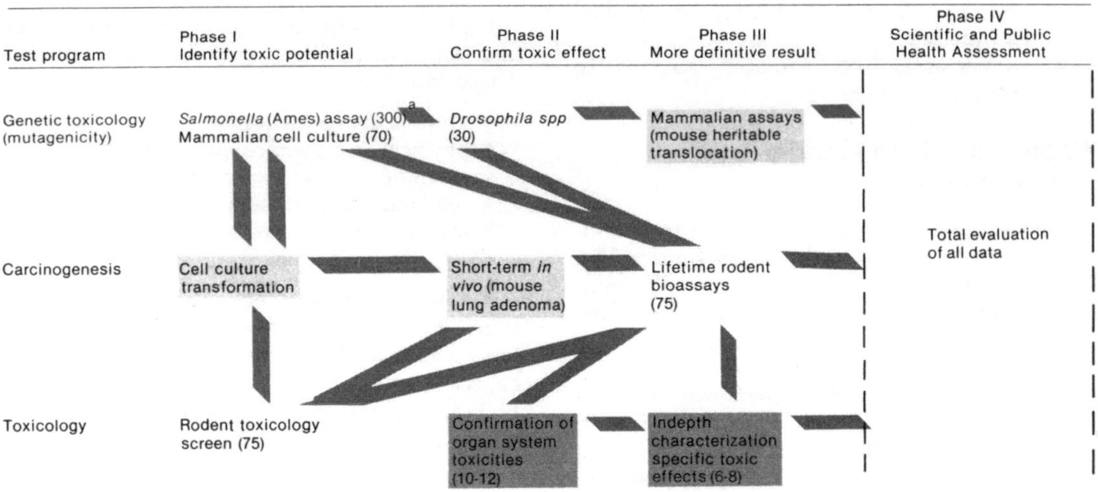

| Test program | Phase I
Identify toxic potential | Phase II
Confirm toxic effect | Phase III
More definitive result | Phase IV
Scientific and Public
Health Assessment |
|---|---|---|---|---|
| Genetic toxicology
(mutagenicity) | *Salmonella* (Ames) assay (300)[a]
Mammalian cell culture (70) | *Drosophila spp*
(30) | Mammalian assays
(mouse heritable
translocation) | |
| Carcinogenesis | Cell culture
transformation | Short-term *in
vivo* (mouse
lung adenoma) | Lifetime rodent
bioassays
(75) | Total evaluation
of all data |
| Toxicology | Rodent toxicology
screen (75) | Confirmation of
organ system
toxicities
(10-12) | Indepth
characterization
specific toxic
effects (6-8) | |

[a]( ) yearly capacity, fiscal year 1980 figures.
SOURCE: Office of Technology Assessment, adapted from NTP (272).

sence of arrowheads on the lines is intentional; according to David Rall, NTP Director (303), there has not yet been enough experience with the scheme to be certain which phase I tests should come first or whether all chemicals should go through all phase I tests.

A critical feature of tier testing is the ability to make decisions about whether or not to continue testing from phase I to II, or from II to III. Guidelines are necessary for making the decision that a chemical is sufficiently without risk and that no further testing is necessary. Rall (303) said that development of decisionmaking guidelines is a priority item for NTP in 1980 and 1981. NTP intends to analyze the testing his-

tories of chemicals that have gone through all three phases (albeit not necessarily under NTP aegis) to determine which test results were most predictive of the ultimate decision about the chemical. NTP will take advantage of the fact that the most expensive and time consuming testing, phase III, has been completed on some chemicals which have not otherwise been tested. Such chemicals will be entered into phase I and II testing to provide additional information about which tests are most predictive. Finally, the NTP decision to continue testing a few chemicals that are negative in phase I tests will provide additional information.

EPIDEMIOLOGY

Lilienfeld (210) defined epidemiology as the study of the distribution of disease in human populations and of the factors that influence disease distribution. Epidemiologic techniques are useful for identifying causative agents and conditions that predispose for cancer. Studies can determine associations in populations between

exposure to carcinogenic agents or between aspects of lifestyle and increased cancer risk.

The earliest association of a factor with cancer was made by Ramazzini in 1713. He found that nuns had a higher rate of breast cancer than other women and, in his Treatie on the Diseases of Tradesman of 1700, he attributed the increase to celibacy (322). That association has been sharpened to include the observation that women who deliver a child at an early age are less likely to develop breast cancer. In addition to identifying cancer risks, epidemiology may play a positive role by pointing out less hazardous diets or agents which are protective against cancer.

For the purpose of this discussion, epidemiologic studies are divided into three general types: 1) experimental, 2) descriptive, and 3) observational. While several basic strategies exist, there are no rigid study designs within any of these categories. Flexibility is important since, unlike laboratory experiments, epidemiology examines groups of unpredictable people living in dynamic environments. The importance of flexibility is underlined by IRLG Guidelines, which state that epidemiologic study design must "be described and justified in relation to the stated objective of the study" (181).

Experimental Epidemiology

The ideal procedure for investigating cause-and-effect hypotheses is through experimental epidemiology. This type of study requires the deliberate application or withholding of a factor and observing the appearance or lack of appearance of any effect. Given the severity of cancer, ethical considerations preclude the administration of suspected carcinogens to people, though it is possible to test agents thought to aid in prevention (292).

Experimental epidemiology studies are difficult to conduct because of the need to secure the cooperation of a large group of people willing to permit an experimenter to intervene in their lives. The investigator must have reason to believe that the proposed intervention, whether a deliberate application or withholding, will be beneficial, but at the same time, he must be somewhat skeptical of the effects. Once sufficient evidence leads to the conclusion that the intervention is or is not beneficial, the experiment must be terminated.

Descriptive Epidemiology

Descriptive epidemiology studies examine the distribution and extent of disease in populations according to basic characteristics—e.g., age, sex, race, etc. The primary purpose of conducting descriptive epidemiologic studies is to provide clues to the etiology of a disease which may then be investigated more thoroughly through more detailed studies. Descriptive studies have focused on international comparisons and comparisons among smaller geographical regions, such as U.S. counties (29).

The identification of high bladder cancer rates in New Jersey males and excess mortality rates from cancer of the mouth and throat, esophagus, colon, rectum, larynx, and bladder in the industrialized Northeast have suggested that occupational factors might be incriminated and have prompted additional investigations. Blot et al. (29) describe NCI's stepwise approach to search for etiological clues. Examination of age-specific rates of disease occurrence or mortality across time (see ch. 2) is another example of descriptive epidemiology.

Observational Epidemiology

Observational epidemiology depends on data derived from observations of individuals or relatively small groups of people. These studies are analyzed using generally accepted statistical methods to determine if an association exists between a factor and a disease and, if so, the strength of the association. Often the hypothesis to be investigated arises from the results of a descriptive study. NCI has embarked on several observational studies based on findings from their county-correlation studies. For example, high rates of lung cancer were found in the Tidewater Virginia area, and a large study was initiated which found elevated risk for lung cancer in shipbuilders and smokers.

Cohort Studies

Two types of observational epidemiology studies, cohort and case-control studies, differ in the selection of the population groups for study.

A cohort study starts with a group of people, a cohort, considered free of the disease under study, and whose disposition regarding the risk factor under consideration is known. Usually the risk factor is an exposure to a suspect carcinogen or a personal attribute or behavior. The group is then studied over time and the health status of the individual members observed. This type of study is sometimes referred to as "prospective" because it looks forward from exposure to development of the disease characteristic (210,225). Cohort studies can be either concurrent or nonconcurrent in design. Concurrent cohort studies depend on events which will occur in the future, while nonconcurrent cohort studies rely on past data or past events.

Case-Control Studies

In a case-control study, individuals with the disease under study (cases) are compared to individuals without the disease (controls) with respect to risk factors which are judged relevant. Some authors label this study design "retrospective" because the presence or absence of the predisposing risk factor is determined for a time in the past (210,225). However, in some cases the presence or absence of the factor and the disease are ascertained simultaneously.

The choice of appropriate controls is rarely without problems. Often, for practical reasons, controls are chosen from hospital records. However, they may not be representative of the population, and they therefore may introduce "selection bias," as discussed by MacMahon and Pugh (218).

In case-control and cohort studies, the groups selected should be comparable in all characteristics except the factor under investigation. In case-control studies, the groups should resemble each other except for the *presence* of the disease, while in cohort studies, the study and comparison groups should be similar except for *exposure* to the suspect factor. Since this rarely is possible in practice, comparability between groups can be improved by either matching individual cases and controls (in case-control

studies) or by standard statistical adjustment procedures (in either case-control or cohort studies). Demographic variables, e.g., age, sex, race, socioeconomic status, are most commonly used for adjustment or matching.

There are advantages and disadvantages with both the case-control and cohort studies (see table 29). Case-control studies tend to be less expensive to conduct, require relatively fewer individuals, and many have been especially useful in studying cancer. The great advantage of cohort studies is that they allow observation of all outcomes, not only those originally anticipated. Bias is somewhat reduced in cohort studies since classification into an exposure category cannot be influenced by prior knowledge that the disease exists. In a concurrent cohort study, it is often necessary to wait many years for the manifestation of enough disease cases to conduct an analysis. The cost and time of the study can be reduced if conducted nonconcurrently. Cohort studies tend to require many more subjects than case-control studies and assignment of individuals to the correct cohort for analysis is difficult.

Causal Associations

A pragmatic view of causality is necessary, particularly when studying complex, multifactorial diseases such as cancer. Analysis of the association between exposure and disease in an epidemiologic study depends on tests of statistical significance. However, finding a positive statistically significant association is not sufficient to conclude a causal relationship. Artifactual and indirect associations must be considered. As MacMahon and Pugh (218) state, " . . . only a minority of statistical associations are causal within the sense of the definition, which requires that change in one party to the association alters the other."

Policy Considerations About Epidemiology

While short-term tests and bioassays are used to evaluate a chemical's carcinogenic potential in the laboratory, the effect on humans is direct-

Table 29.—Advantages and Disadvantages of Case-Control and Cohort Studies

Type of study	Advantages	Disadvantages
Case-control	Relatively inexpensive	Complete information about past exposures often unavailable
	Smaller number of subjects	Biassed recall
	Relatively quick results	Problems of selecting control group and matching variables
	Suitable for rare diseases	Yields only relative risk
Cohort	Lack of bias in ascertainment of risk factor status	Possible bias in ascertainment of disease
	Yields incidence rates as well as relative risk	Large numbers of subjects required
	Can yield associations with other diseases as by-product	Long follow-up period
		Problem of attrition
		Changes over time in criteria and methods
		Very costly
		Difficulties in assigning people to correct cohort

SOURCE: Office of Technology Assessment.

ly assessed by epidemiologic techniques. Well-conducted and properly evaluated epidemiology studies which show a positive association are accepted as the most convincing evidence about human risks.

Negative epidemiologic results show that exposure of a certain number of people to a substance at a specified level did not cause cancer. From such results, it is possible to calculate that human risk is no higher than what the study could have detected. For instance, a study of 1,000 people which showed no excess cancer would be "more negative" than one of 100 people exposed at the same level. Neither study would show that a risk exists, and neither shows that no risk exists, but the larger study shows a lower probability of risk.

The OSHA Generic Cancer Policy (279) proposed that OSHA, after ascertaining the adequacy of the study design, would interpret negative epidemiologic studies as setting an upper limit for human risk. AIHC (8) wants negative human evidence to be considered along with animal data in making decisions about carcinogenicity. The OSHA position, and that of Federal Government regulatory agencies in general (306), is to use epidemiology to estimate limits of risk, but not to weigh negative human evidence against other positive evidence in deciding whether or not a substance is a carcinogen.

The Regulatory Council (306) considers properly designed and conducted epidemiologic studies, which show a significant statistical relationship between human exposure to a substance and increased cancer risk, to provide "good evidence" that a substance is carcinogenic. The Council mentioned some difficulties in epidemiology, e.g., long latency periods, multiplicity of exposures, and cautioned that often "even large increases (which could involve thousands of people) . . . cannot be detected." For these reasons they cite two caveats in using epidemiological studies:

> The failure of an epidemiological study to detect an association between the occurrence of cancer and exposure to a specific substance should not be taken to indicate necessarily that the substance is not carcinogenic.

> Because it is unacceptable to allow exposure to potential carcinogens to continue until human cancer actually occurs, regulatory agencies should not wait for epidemiological evidence before taking action to limit human exposure to chemicals considered to be carcinogenic.

OSTP (281) states that "a positive finding in a well-conducted epidemiologic study can be viewed as strong evidence that a chemical poses a carcinogenic risk to humans." Alternatively, "a negative finding is not nearly so meaningful . . . " and OSTP emphasizes the importance of examining the sensitivity of a negative study, and suggests that the upper limit of risk that might have gone undetected in the study be calculated and presented.

Carcinogens for Which There Is Human Evidence

Through various means, epidemiologic studies have identified several human carcinogens. The first use of epidemiologic principles to relate environmental contaminants to human cancer is credited to Pott in 1775 (322). Pott, a physician in London, suggested that scrotal cancers, which he observed in men who had worked as chimney sweeps when boys, were caused by exposure to soot. Pott is an example of an astute physician recognizing an unusual cluster of cancer cases. A more recent example is vinyl chloride which was identified as a carcinogen after three cases of a rare liver tumor (hepatic angiosarcoma) were diagnosed in workers in a manufacturing plant (71). In the case of vinyl chloride, evidence for its carcinogenicity in laboratory animals was available in advance of the human evidence. In both cases, control action followed the demonstration of occupational risk. The Danish Chimney Sweeps Guild instructed its members about protective clothing and to practice preventive hygiene soon after Pott's report was published, and OSHA regulated vinyl chloride.

IARC bases its evaluation of carcinogenic risk to humans on consideration of both epidemiological and experimental animal evidence. IARC considered human evidence bearing on 60 chemicals and industrial processes and classified 18 as human carcinogens (see table 30). Many of the human data considered by IARC are from studies concerning workplace and medical exposure. This does not necessarily reflect the distribution of carcinogens but more likely the higher exposure and relative ease of performing epidemiologic studies on patients and occupational groups. For instance, the availability of medical records facilitates locating people exposed to a drug and provides information about time of exposure and dose level.

IARC also classified 18 additional compounds as *probably* carcinogenic for humans but there was insufficient evidence to establish causal associations. These 18 were further subdivided according to the degree of evidence, high or low, as displayed in table 30. Insufficient evidence was available to decide about the carcinogenicity of 18 chemicals listed in table 30. Finally, because of time limitations, IARC was unable to evaluate six compounds for which human data exist.

Annual Report on Carcinogens

In an effort to provide information on carcinogens which would be useful to regulatory agencies, Congress passed an amendment to the Community Mental Health Act (Public Law 95-622). It requires the Secretary of DHHS to publish an annual report containing a list of substances which are known to be carcinogens or may reasonably be anticipated to be carcinogens and to which a significant number of persons residing in the United States are exposed. The task was assigned to NTP, and the first report (82) includes the 26 exposures which IARC had determined in 1978 to be human carcinogens (344). Candidates for the 1981 and 1982 list also will be drawn from IARC beginning with chemicals and processes judged "probably carcinogenic for humans." The initial report did not, as required by the statute, list " . . . all substances which either are known . . . or . . . may reasonably be anticipated to be carcinogens . . . . "

One limitation enumerated in the first report was that, "Science and society have not arrived at a final consensus on the definition of carcinogen either in human populations or in experimental animals." The report, by including chemicals and industrial processes already classified by IARC, has sidestepped dealing with the question of what is a carcinogen. A definition for "carcinogen" remains elusive unless it is given in the context of a particular methodology.

Table 30.—Chemicals and Industrial Processes Evaluated for Human Carcinogenicity by the International Agency for Research on Cancer (IARC)

Chemicals and processes judged carcinogenic for humans

	Degree of evidence	
	Humans	Experimental animals
4-aminobiphenyl	Sufficient	Sufficient
Arsenic and certain arsenic compounds	Sufficient	Inadequate
Asbestos	Sufficient	Sufficient
Manufacture of auramine	Sufficient	Not applicable
Benzene	Sufficient	Inadequate
Benzidine	Sufficient	Sufficient
N,N-bis (2-chloroethyl)-2-naphthylamine (chlornaphazine)	Sufficient	Limited
Bis(chloromethyl)ether and technical grade chloromethyl methyl ether	Sufficient	Sufficient
Chromium and certain chromium compounds	Sufficient	Sufficient
Diethylstilboestrol (DES)	Sufficient	Sufficient
Underground hematite mining	Sufficient	Not applicable
Manufacture of isopropyl alcohol by the strong acid process	Sufficient	Not applicable
Melphalan	Sufficient	Sufficient
Mustard gas	Sufficient	Limited
2-naphthylamine	Sufficient	Sufficient
Nickel refining	Sufficient	Not applicable
Soots, tars and mineral oils	Sufficient	Sufficient
Vinyl chloride	Sufficient	Sufficient

Chemicals and processes judged probably carcinogenic for humans
Group A: Chemicals and processes with "higher degrees of evidence."

	Degree of evidence	
	Humans	Experimental animals
Aflatoxins	Limited	Sufficient
Cadmium and certain cadmium compounds	Limited	Sufficient
Chlorambucil	Limited	Sufficient
Cyclophosphamide	Limited	Sufficient
Nickel and certain nickel compounds	Limited	Sufficient
Tris(1-aziridinyl)phosphine sulphide (thiotepa)	Limited	Sufficient

Group B: Chemicals and processes with "lower degrees of evidence."

	Degree of evidence	
	Humans	Experimental animals
Acrylonitrile	Limited	Sufficient
Amitrole (aminotriazole)	Inadequate	Sufficient
Auramine	Limited	Limited
Beryllium and certain beryllium compounds	Limited	Sufficient
Carbon tetrachloride	Inadequate	Sufficient
Dimethylcarbamoyl chloride	Inadequate	Sufficient
Dimethyl sulphate	Inadequate	Sufficient
Ethylene oxide	Limited	Inadequate
Iron dextran	Inadequate	Sufficient
Oxymetholone	Limited	No data
Phenacetin	Limited	Limited
Polychlorinated biphenyls	Inadequate	Sufficient

Chemicals and processes that could not be classified as to their carcinogenicity for humans

	Degree of evidence	
	Humans	Experimental animals
Chloramphenicol	Inadequate	No data
Chlordane/heptachlor	Inadequate	Limited
Chloroprene	Inadequate	Inadequate

Table 30.—Chemicals and Industrial Processes Evaluated for Human Carcinogenicity by the International Agency for Research on Cancer (IARC) (Continued)

Chemicals and processes that could not be classified as to their carcinogenicity for humans—continued	Degree of evidence	
	Humans	Experimental animals
Dichlorodiphenyltrichloroethane (DDT)	Inadequate	Limited
Dieldrin	Inadequate	Limited
Epichlorohydrin	Inadequate	Limited
Hematite	Inadequate	Negative
Hexachlorocyclohexane (technical grade HCH/lindane)	Inadequate	Limited
Isoniazid	Inadequate	Limited
Isopropyl oils	Inadequate	Inadequate
Lead and certain lead compounds	Inadequate	Sufficient (for some soluble salts)
Phenobarbitone	Limited	Limited
N-phenyl-2-naphthylamine	Inadequate	Inadequate
Phenytoin	Limited	Limited
Reserpine	Inadequate	Inadequate
Styrene	Inadequate	Limited
Trichloroethylene	Inadequate	Limited
Tris(aziridinyl)-para-benzoquinone (triaziquone)	Inadequate	Limited

Chemicals and processes for which human data are available, but which were not considered by the IARC Working Group

Ortho- and para-dichlorobenzene
Dichlorobenzidine
Phenylbutazone
2,3,7,8-tetrachlorodibenzo-para-dioxin (TCDD, the "dioxin" of Agent Orange)
Ortho- and para-toluidine
Vinylidene chloride

SOURCE: Office of Technology Assessment, adapted from IARC (185).

SOURCES OF EPIDEMIOLOGICALLY USEFUL DATA

Three major types of information are useful in assessing the carcinogenic risk of a substance: 1) health status of exposed and unexposed populations; 2) exposure data; and 3) physical, chemical, and biological properties of the substance. Information related to each of these categories can come from a variety of sources and can be used in different ways. Testing the substance generates information about its potential hazard, but information about its distribution in the environment and any impacts on human health are necessary to describe its human risk

Health Status Information

DHHS is primarily responsible for administering health data collection, storage, and analysis projects. An overview of existing DHHS programs and other departments' health data collection activities can be found in *Selected Topics in Federal Health Statistics* (283).

National Center for Health Statistics

The National Center for Health Statistics (NCHS), located within the DHHS Office of Health, Research, Statistics, and Technology, was established to collect and disseminate data on the health of Americans. Since 1960, it has played a major role in the development of national health statistics policy and programs. The NCHS Division of Vital Statistics collects information on natality, mortality, marriage, and divorce from the individual States and regions. (See ch. 2 for a discussion of cancer mortality and incidence statistics.) In addition to vital statistics, NCHS conducts several general-purpose surveys that provide statistics about the health status of the U.S. population. Additional information can be obtained from *Data Systems of the National Center for Health Statistics* (253).

Health Interview Survey (HIS).—HIS is the principal source of information on the health of the civilian noninstitutionalized population of the United States. Initiated in 1957, interviews are conducted each week in a probability sample of households to provide data on a range of health measures, including the incidence of illness and accidental injuries, the prevalence of diseases and impairments, the extent of disability, and the use of health care services. Each year, approximately 40,000 households containing about 120,000 persons are sampled.

HIS collects information only about conditions which respondents are willing to report. The basic questionnaires are similar from year to year but supplemental questions may be added. In 1978 and 1979 questions on smoking were added, but these were discontinued in 1980.

The NCHS Study of Costs of Environment-Related Health Effects, mandated by Public Law 95-623, may use HIS as a data source (179).

Health and Nutrition Examination Survey (HANES).—HANES, initiated in 1970, is a modification and expansion of the earlier Health Examination Survey (HES). These surveys collect and use data from interviews and physical examinations to estimate the prevalence of chronic diseases, establish physiological standards for various tests, determine the nutritional status of the population, and assess exposure levels to certain environmental substances. The sampling techniques employed provide representative national data. Two surveys, HANES I (1971-75) and HANES II (1976-79) have been conducted. Both surveys examined approximately 20,000 persons.

HANES is the most extensive national assessment of health and nutritional status of the American people. The nutritional component of HANES includes: information on dietary intake; data from hematologic and biochemical tests; body measurements; and chemical examination for various signs of high risks of nutritional deficiency. Preliminary findings from the HANES II pesticide monitoring program have found an apparent rise in tissue levels of DDT and PCBs. The implications of the observed levels are uncertain.

HANES surveys might become valuable sources of information for cancer epidemiology if sufficient resources were available. Because of its representative nature, aggregate data from the survey can be used to represent "normal" or background levels. For example, white cell count levels determined in HANES I were used for comparative purposes in an epidemiologic study of laboratory workers exposed to suspected toxic chemicals. HANES II contains certain information about dietary intake of substances which have been associated with a lower risk of cancer, vitamins A and C, and substances such as fats which are associated with higher risks.

HANES might be linked with other health data systems, such as the National Death Index (see below) to facilitate assessment of whether particular exposure levels or certain nutritional statuses were associated with cancer mortality. NCHS, with its HANES capabilities, has been asked to participate in studies near Love Canal, and to evaluate the health status of certain high-risk industry groups. It was unable to do so because of limited resources.

The NCHS overall monitoring survey budget for fiscal year 1981 is $28 million. This is a $3 million increase over 1980 and includes $1.1 million for a special HANES study which will focus on Hispanics in selected areas of the United States. The study is designed to describe the health and nutritional status of the Mexican-American, Puerto Rican-American and Cuban-American populations. Studies of specific groups are necessary to acquire data in sufficient detail to describe subgroups of the population which differ from the "average." General national surveys such as HANES I and II produce data about the "average" citizen by sampling groups in proportion to their representation in the total population, and this often results in too small a sample size to be useful for identifiable smaller groups.

As examples of data useful for cancer studies, the HANES Hispanic study will determine:

- name, date of birth, and social security number recorded in machine readable form for subsequent use with the National Death Index;
- history of toxic substance exposure;
- nutritional status including dietary interviews, serum vitamin A levels, prevalence of vitamin C deficiencies; and
- the quantity and frequency of alcohol consumption.

Hospital Discharge Survey.—This survey was established in 1964 to provide representative statistics for the U.S. population discharged from short-term hospitals. The survey collects information on the characteristics of patients, the lengths of stay, diagnosis and surgical operations, and patterns of use of care. Completion of each medical abstract form is estimated to take approximately 5 minutes. Only short-stay hospitals with six or more beds and with an average length of stay of less than 30 days are included in the sample (177).

Vital Statistics Followback Surveys.—NCHS-conducted mortality "followback" surveys have provided information on possible relations between environmental and lifestyle factors and death from cancer. Information is sought about decedents through inquiries addressed to those providing information for the death certificate, such as the medical certifiers, funeral directors, and family members. These surveys are an efficient means to augment the routinely reported information contained in the vital records.

The efficiency of the followback approach for eliciting additional information about deaths is related to the relative rareness of death as an event in the U.S. population. About 1 percent of the population dies annually; and cancer-related deaths are reported for about 20 percent of this 1 percent, or a total of 0.2 percent of the total population. The followback approach permits sampling directly from the file of those death certificates of interest in order to supplement existing information.

Mortality followback surveys were conducted in the United States annually from 1961 through 1968. They have since been discontinued due to inadequate resources, including personnel.

National Death Index (NDI).—Deaths in the United States are registered by the States or other death registration areas (e.g., District of Columbia). The records are transmitted on microfilms or on magnetic tape to NCHS for compilation. Historically, because there was no integration of records for the country as a whole, no mechanism had existed at the national level to determine if a person had died. In 1981, after several years of planning and preparation, the NDI will be placed into operation to serve that purpose. The NDI will code deaths that occurred in 1979 and each year thereafter. Although there has been discussion of coding deaths that occurred before 1979, no plans are now in place to do so.

NDI, administered by NCHS, is designed to provide medical and health researchers with probable fact of death, the death certificate number, and the location of the death certificate, when supplied with a minimum set of identifiers (generally the person's name and social security number or date of birth). The researcher then may contact the registration area where the possible match has occurred to obtain the death certificate or the required information.

NDI will be of immediate use in ongoing long-term studies which include mortality. Beebe (23) described the NDI as the most important recent advance in making vital statistics accessible to researchers. NCI's Surveillance, Epidemiology, and End Results (SEER) program plans to use the NDI to determine deaths of all persons in the SEER registries. This should reduce the number of people lost to followup by SEER and provide better information about survival. Currently, deaths of people who moved or cease to participate are not always recorded by SEER.

National Cancer Institute

NCI, 1 of 11 research organizations of NIH, receives more than one-fifth of all Federal health research funds (283). NCI operates the SEER program, which provides cancer incidence data on approximately 10 percent of the population. Additional information on the SEER program can be found in chapter 2.

Centers for Disease Control

The overall mission of the Centers for Disease Control (CDC) (56) is "to prevent unnecessary illness and death and to enhance the health of the American people." CDC serves as a focus for DHHS efforts in the areas of disease prevention and control, environmental health, health promotion, and health education.

NIOSH, located within CDC, assists OSHA in establishing workplace health standards. Between 1972 and 1974, NIOSH conducted the National Occupational Hazard Survey (NOHS) to provide estimates of the proportion of employees exposed to potential health hazards in various industries. NOHS estimates of exposure are often used in assessing risks from occupational carcinogens. NIOSH periodically conducts studies to identify the health effects of particular industrial processes and to determine the health experience of selected employee populations. The National Surveillance Network, which is operated by NIOSH, collects data from State safety and health inspection programs.

Social Security Administration

The Social Security Administration (SSA) collects information on economic and demographic data in administering the social security system. SSA makes available an annual 1-percent continuous work-history sample (CWHS) to outside users which provides information about employment, migration, and earning status. Six different types of files, all of which contain sex, race, and age data, are available to outside users. For purposes of confidentiality, the employee and employer identification are included in scrambled form. The usefulness of the CWHS for epidemiologic studies is limited by privacy constraints of access and other characteristics, e.g., only wages up to the taxable maximum are reported.

SSA has recently initiated efforts to amass a 10-percent sample of the work force because of the Office of Management and Budget's (OMB)

need for better estimates of intercensal population. This file would constitute the most detailed information on the structure of the labor force so that employment distributions by sex, race, age, wages, and wage changes, work force participation, industry, and regional migration patterns could be analyzed systematically.

The Disability Insurance Fund, managed by SSA, contains information regarding benefit computation and actions related to employee entitlement. SSA routinely prepares reports regarding specific disease entities and has published characteristics of workers disabled by cancer (283).

Exposure Data

The principal data deficiencies for assessing cancer risks are inadequate information about exposures and lifestyle characteristics. Since cancer has a long latent period, relating cancer in today's population to particular exposures might require information from 20 or more years ago. Even when information was collected, records may have been destroyed before they became useful in cancer epidemiology studies.

As the lead agency for regulating chemicals, EPA administers numerous exposure-monitoring programs. Several studies have been critical of EPA's monitoring data collection efforts, and as a result, EPA established a Deputy Assistant Administrators Committee to review and make recommendations regarding agency monitoring and information management activities (113). Three of the major conclusions found by the committee are:

1. A considerable quantity of collected ambient environmental information has not been analyzed or presented to top management.

2. The most serious problem found was the lack of consistent, integrated information on toxic and hazardous pollutants.

3. There is little coordination between EPA offices focusing on the same area. In addition, there is a lack of compatability and sharing of these data.

Exposure data in the workplace are limited even though a number of cancer causing agents have been identified in the occupational environment. NIOSH's National Occupational Hazard Survey collects exposure data in a sample of industries, and OSHA requires monitoring for 6 of the 20 substances regulated because of carcinogenicity.

Death certificates generally include questions on the usual occupation and industry or business of the decedent. However, those questions are not always answered and there is uncertainty about the accuracy of the information that is provided. NCHS, along with NIOSH, is currently assessing the feasibility of using and improving occupational descriptors on death certificates as a surrogate for exposure information. Approximately a dozen States now code the usual occupation of the decedent, and about half of these also code the reported usual industry or business of the decedent. One State, Wisconsin, now publishes such tabulated information in their annual public health report. Other States, with support from NIOSH, have executed special studies on occupational mortality based on data reported on the standard death certificate (45,236).

In England, information reported on the death certificate has been used as a basis for occupational mortality analyses every 10 years since 1851 (with the exception of the war year, 1941). In the United States, a study of this type was conducted in 1950. It involved coding over 300,000 death certificates for the occupation and industry of males aged 20 to 64. The information was used in conjunction with the decennial census information for that year to produce measures of relative mortality risk associated with occupation and industry of decedents (148,149,150,151,196).

The National Human Adipose Tissue Monitoring Program and HIS and HANES, which are described above, are the principal mechanisms for monitoring levels of toxics in the body. This information is used not only to determine normal baseline levels but also to identify populations which may be at high risk.

This assessment did not concentrate on monitoring methods and programs, but the general impression is that data collection efforts are incomplete and that many generate data of limited usefulness. For instance, measurement techniques are not always specified for collected exposure data and ignorance of the sensitivity of the instrument used makes it difficult to compare measurements from different times and sites. Furthermore, a nondetectable measurement does not necessarily indicate that a substance is not present, and may mean only that the instrument was not sufficiently sensitive to measure it. Such negative readings are often not reported, and when they are, they may be misleading. The efforts of organizations such as the EPA Committee (113) mentioned above to improve collection and analysis of monitoring data might be encouraged.

Chemical Information Systems

The lack of toxicological information about many substances and concern over perceived toxic substance problems prompted Congress to enact more than two dozen statutes dealing with toxics. Many of the statutes delegate information-gathering functions to Federal regulatory and research agencies.

Toxic Substances Control Act—TSCA

In 1976, Congress passed TSCA to strengthen the ability of the Federal Government to accumulate information on potentially hazardous chemicals and better enable the Federal Government to protect the public from toxic substances. TSCA required the establishment of several new programs at EPA and a completely new infrastructure had to be organized. This necessitated recruiting an Assistant Administrator and placed a large burden on a small staff. Subsequently, the programs have been slow to get off the ground (141). Recruitment has continually lagged behind authorized staff ceilings which may be inadequate to meet expected program needs. EPA estimated that approximately 1,500 people were needed in fiscal year 1979: 382 permanent positions were authorized, 313 were actually filled.

New Chemicals.—One of TSCA's primary objectives—as stated in the opening paragraph of the Committee on Interstate and Foreign Commerce Report (165), is to provide "for the evaluation of the hazard-causing potential of new chemicals before commercial production begins." TSCA requires manufacturers and importers to notify EPA at least 90 days prior to the manufacture or import of a new chemical substance by submitting a premanufacture notice (PMN). Along with notification, manufacturers are to provide specific information about the new chemical, including any test data which relate to the effects of the substance on human health or the environment. "New" is synonymous with not being listed on the inventory of existing chemicals and subject to TSCA's authority. In May 1979, EPA (105) issued a statement of interim policy covering submission and review of PMNs. Final PMN rules have yet to be issued. In the 2-year period, April 1979 to March 12, 1981, EPA received 488 PMNs, and about 800 are anticipated in fiscal year 1982.

TSCA was not the first Federal law to require a review of new chemicals entering the market. FIFRA and the Food, Drug, and Cosmetics Act, have registration/certification provisions for pesticides and pharmaceuticals respectively. Unlike those laws, TSCA requires neither licensing nor registration, but only notification of intent to manufacture. As mentioned, the PMN must contain any test data available to the submitter, but EPA cannot require testing of a new chemical substance just because it is "new." The act places the burden of proof on EPA to demonstrate that the information available to EPA:

> . . . is insufficient to permit a reasoned evaluation of the health and environmental effects of a chemical substance . . . and . . . [that] in the absence of sufficient information . . . [the substance] may present an unreasonable risk or will be produced in substantial quantities, and there may be significant or substantial exposure.

If such a finding is made, EPA may issue an order under section 5(e) to prohibit or limit the manufacture, processing, distribution, use, or disposal of the chemical. EPA has proposed two such orders and each time the company withdrew its notice and decided not to manufacture.

On two other occasions notices were withdrawn when the companies learned orders to require more information were in preparation.

Lack of regulatory action on a new chemical by EPA does not imply that the substance is "safe" or has been "approved." However, it does grant the manufacturer the right to produce and use the chemical as desired, subject to any other regulations that may be applicable. Under section 5(a)(2) EPA can issue a "significant new use rule" (SNUR) for a chemical when there is concern that a specific use of the substance, other than those proposed in the PMN, may pose an unreasonable risk. Issuance of an SNUR requires that persons must notify EPA 90 days prior to manufacture or processing of a substance for a use subject to a SNUR. Through March 1981, one chemical specific SNUR had been proposed and EPA was considering SNURs on more than 40 chemicals. Once a substance is in production, EPA can require testing under TSCA section 4 and/or submission of human health and environmental monitoring data under a TSCA section 8 rule (see *Existing Chemicals*).

EPA recently published a policy statement describing a recommended list of premanufacture tests for new chemical substances (114). The tests are identical to those under consideration by the Organization for Economic Cooperation and Development (OECD). OECD considers that its base set of tests would generate the minimum amount of information normally sufficient to perform an initial hazard assessment of a chemical (see table 31). EPA is recommending that flexibility be used by manufacturers to tailor this "base set" of tests for the particular chemical substance and intended uses. Use of this base set is voluntary due to EPA's lack of statutory authority to require testing of new chemical substances. The estimated costs of this base set, should all tests be employed, range from $53,000 to $67,850.

EPA has reported that no toxicity data were submitted in 60 percent of the first 199 notices received (141). In fact, 25 percent of the notices contained no data on physical or chemical properties. No chronic test data have yet to be

Table 31.—EPA's Recommended Base Set of Data To Be Included in Premanufacturing Notices

Type of data	Estimated cost
Physical/chemical data	
Data about 11 characteristics........	$ 3,800
Acute toxicity data	
Acute oral toxicity..................	2,000
Acute dermal toxicity	2,800
Acute inhalation toxicity	3,300
Skin irritation......................	700
Skin sensitization	3,200–6,700
Eye irritation (for chemicals showing no skin irritation)..................	450
Repeated dose toxicity data	
14–28 day-repeated dose test(s) using probable route(s) of human exposure..	10,200–12,800
Mutagenicity data	
Gene (point) mutation data	1,350
Chromosomal aberration data	18,000
Ecotoxicity data	
Data about killing of three lower organisms	4,100
Degradation/accumulation data........	3,100–11,850

SOURCE: Office of Technology Assessment, adapted from EPA (114).

presented to EPA in a PMN. In cases where toxicity data are given they are usually limited. The then-Assistant Administrator for Toxic Substances has indicated (192) that the lack of test data:

> . . . has placed an extraordinary burden on EPA's limited resources . . . . Furthermore, we [EPA] believe that our objective will not be achieved until industry assumes more of the burden of generating adequate risk information and assessing the risk of its products.

Unless additional information is received with the notices, EPA's reviews will be "based upon a fundamental lack of information and data. This in turn means that our information will be highly uncertain" (192). In order to evaluate a chemical's carcinogenic potential, EPA staff have had to rely on structure activity relationships and mutagenicity data when available.

Existing Chemicals.—Sections 4 and 8 of TSCA relate directly to the issue of acquiring adequate information for assessing the carcinogenic risk of existing chemicals.

Section 4 grants EPA the authority to require industry testing of a potentially harmful chemical if available information is *insufficient* for a

reasoned evaluation of risk and if the substance: 1) may present an unreasonable risk or 2) result in substantial or significant exposure. TSCA established ITC to recommend chemicals for testing under section 4; ITC and EPA responses to it are described above. To require industry testing, EPA must demonstrate that available information is insufficient to conclude that the substance "presents an unreasonable risk," yet supports the finding that the chemical "may present an unreasonable risk." If available information were sufficient to show that the chemical presents an unreasonable risk, EPA could regulate the substance under section 6 of TSCA. One difficulty EPA faces in using this testing authority is how to define "may present an unreasonable risk."

Section 8 of TSCA required EPA to compile by November 1977 an inventory of chemical substances manufactured in the United States. An initial inventory was published about 2½ years late in June 1979 and updated in July 1980. Information originally requested for the inventory was limited and EPA has proposed rules requiring additional information for certain substances. In February 1980, rules requiring exposure information on approximately 2,300 substances were proposed (108). Additional information-gathering rules are scheduled for proposal in 1981.

Section 8(c) of TSCA also requires manufacturers, processors, and distributors to notify EPA of information which reasonably supports the conclusion that a substance "presents a substantial risk" of injury to health or the environment. In addition, Section 8(c) requires the maintenance of records indicating "significant adverse reactions" alleged to have been caused by a chemical substance. Allegation by employees are to be retained by industry for 30 years and all other allegations for 5 years. These records are to be submitted to EPA upon request, and EPA is investigating means of establishing an automatic reporting system whenever a certain number of allegations are received in a 12-month period for the same substance, process, or discharge (109). Final rules to implement the significant adverse reaction reporting requirement are expected in 1981.

Chemical Substances Information Network (CSIN)

In February 1978, under mandate of TSCA, EPA and CEQ established the Toxic Substances Strategy Committee (TSSC) to facilitate interagency coordination of chemical information collection, dissemination, and classification. The Departments of Health and Human Services, Agriculture, Commerce, Defense, Energy, Interior, State, and Transportation, and OSHA, CPSC, and NSF participate in TSSC. IRLG and the DHHS Committee to Coordinate Environmental and Related Programs are also members. TSSC has formed a number of committees for special tasks, and the data committee recommended the development of a broad-based network of data systems—CSIN. CSIN was adopted by TSSC, and if sufficient resources and personnel are committed, it should go a long way toward the goal of providing convenient access to information about chemicals. Its master file will contain all information collected under TSCA; a subfile, stripped of confidential data about trade secrets, will be available for public use. CSIN will identify about 1 million chemicals and for each one provide selected research and test data, references in the toxicologic and biomedical literature, and information about regulations that pertain to the chemical (345). The system is still in the developmental stages, although some aspects were expected to be operational in 1980 and the entire system is to be completed within a decade.

CSIN will not be a single new system; rather it will incorporate several systems already in use. To facilitate locating information about a single substance in more than one system, EPA is developing an unambiguous identification number system, which was another recommendation of TSSC's data committee. In this way, information about structure, chemical and physical properties, production volume, uses, application, distribution, and toxicity, now stored in different systems, can be linked together. Such systems do not necessarily contain information about human health effects, but they can be used in combination with health information systems.

Collection and Coordination of Exposure and Health Data

Congress has responded to concern about the collection and availability of data for assessing environmental health risks. It has mandated commissions and studies directed at improving data collection, storage, and dissemination.

The Health Services Research, Health Statistics, and Medical Libraries Act of 1974, Public Law 93-353, mandated the U.S. National Committee on Vital and Health Statistics to assist and advise PHS with statistical problems bearing on health and the delivery of health services which are of national interest. A committee recommendation was important to the establishment of the NDI.

The 95th Congress passed two acts which included sections pertaining to data collection for assessing and reducing cancer risks. The Clean Air Act Amendments of 1977 (Public Law 95-95) established the Task Force on Environmental Cancer and Heart and Lung Disease, to focus efforts by EPA and various branches of DHHS on issues relating to these diseases. The task force is composed of representatives from EPA, NCI, NHLBI, NIOSH, NIEHS, NCHS, CDC, and FDA (340). The task force was directed to recommend, among other things (340):

> . . . a comprehensive research program to determine and quantify the relationships between environmental pollution and human cancer . . . [and] . . . recommend research and such other measures as may be appropriate to prevent or reduce the incidence of environmentally related cancer . . . .

Initial efforts were focused on defining problems, categorizing relevant research programs, and exchanging information among member agencies and other appropriate groups. Activities related to prevention and reduction of environmental risks are planned to begin during 1981.

The task force established several project groups to address specific areas of interest. Of particular relevance to this assessment is the Project Group on Exposure and Metabolic

Mechanisms, established in May 1979. The group is examining the interrelationship of exposure to a toxicant and body uptake, metabolism, and affected target organs. It is hoped that this information will increase the ability of researchers to predict a chemical's potential toxicity and establish which symptoms may be associated with trace chemical levels in the body.

The Project Group on Standardization of Measurements and Tests is primarily concerned with obtaining reliable, comparable data on environmental and disease measurements. The group has focused on "potential contributions to the state of the art of environmental and occupational monitoring and testing that would complement, rather than duplicate or overlap, the efforts of individuals or agencies" (340). They identified two problem areas common to task force agencies:

1. There is a need for better resource allocation to optimize the quality of data since agencies and laboratories charged with monitoring activities typically have limited resources.
2. Researchers currently have limited means of assessing the relationship and validity of published environmental monitoring data.

The Project Group on Standardization of Measurements and Tests expects to develop recommendations in these areas.

The Health Services Research, Health Statistics, and Health Care Technology Act of 1978 (Public Law 95-623) mandated the Secretary of DHHS to initiate several efforts relating to the impact of the environment on health. He is to develop a plan for the collection and coordination of statistical and epidemiological data on the effects of the environment on health and prepare guidelines for the collection, compilation, analysis, publication, and distribution of this information. The law also authorized the Secretary of DHHS to "consult with and take into consideration any recommendations of the Task Force" in developing the plan.

NCHS (252) recently published *Environmental Health: A Plan for Collecting and Coordinating Statistical and Epidemiologic Data,* which reviews information currently available from Federal data collection systems. A series of recommendations are made to Congress for correcting gaps and deficiencies in environmental health data systems. These recommendations include the need for priority setting in new data collection efforts, interagency coordination in the environmental data collection process, assurance of the quality of data, and linking data on the environment and health.

NCHS (252) identified 64 ongoing systems in 18 agencies that gather environmental health-related data. At least two-thirds of these collect either information on cancer incidence/mortality or data on cancer risk factors. Most of the data collection systems identified are designed to:

- collect health-related data,
- measure environmental pollutants and individual exposures,
- test specific interrelationships, or
- link data on the environment and health.

Linking systems that collect different kinds of data appear to have the greatest utility for assessing associations of environment and health. For example, the Upgrade system, which is concerned with water quality and health is a joint effort of CEQ, EPA, NIOSH, and NCHS, and integrates data from the Bureau of the Census, mortality data from NCHS, and water quality data from EPA and the U.S. Geological Survey.

OTA encountered an example of the often-voiced complaint that data are not in a form easily accessible and useful to researchers. National mortality data were necessary to carry out the analyses reported in chapter 2, but those data were available in computer readable form only for the years since 1968. OTA had to computerize the data back to 1933 to carry out the analyses. The OTA computer tapes of cancer mortality data will be made available to researchers. These data include deaths by age, race, and sex for selected cancers, for each of the years 1933 through 1978. All of the data on these tapes are consistent with those available on paper from NCHS.

Not all informational systems release data for public use and some that are released are of limited usefulness. Data are often aggregated by geographical regions (e.g., by county or State), which precludes detailed analysis of exposures on health. Individual identifiers are frequently deleted because of privacy and confidentiality constraints. This unfortunately hinders intensive specific epidemiologic investigations which are facilitated by matching an individual's exposures and lifestyle characteristics with health status. Agencies with individually identified records can sometimes conduct followup studies to obtain additional information for investigation, e.g., NCHS recently initiated a followup study, 10 years after the survey, of participants in its HANES I survey. The followup will investigate current health status of participants as it can be related to previously collected data.

Collection of useful epidemiologic information may be indirectly affected by the Paperwork Reduction Act of 1980, which passed during the last days of the 96th Congress. The act is intended to improve use of existing data collection systems and to reduce the Federal paperwork burden placed on individuals, businesses and governments by 25 percent within 3 years. The act empowers the Director of OMB to review and approve Federal agency information collection requests. Various medical and epidemiologic research groups, including NIH, expressed concern that Federal research into disease prevention could be impeded by the Paperwork Reduction Act and advocated the exemption of biomedical and epidemiologic research (64). The Senate Committee on Governmental Affairs decided against this exemption because it determined that the act would not interfere with disease prevention research.

In addition to reducing the paperwork burden, the act directs the sharing of information among agencies to the extent authorized by law and the establishment of a Federal Information Locator System. This system will contain a description of all information collected by the Federal Government, and directions for obtaining the information by all agencies and the public. Successful implementation of this system should enhance the quality of information available for epidemiologic research.

Government Records and Record Linkage

Government records contain a wealth of information about individuals that could be of great value to researchers looking for associations between exposures and disease states. The SSA, Internal Revenue Service (IRS), Veterans' Administration (VA), the Bureau of the Census, and NCHS are organizations with extensive data collections. For the most part, details about individuals are not readily available because of legal and institutional barriers. Most critically, it is difficult to obtain records of the same person from two or more sources. This can be a major obstacle because one record rarely contains all desired information. For example, to do a study relating mortality to occupational exposures, one could extract "occupation" from the IRS record, "employer" and "industry" from information collected by the SSA, and cause of death from the death certificate filed in the State in which the death occurred. The NDI, which is described above, makes it easier to locate death certificates.

Individuals in several Government agencies have been promoting a Linked Administrative Statistical Sample, a project designed to bring together records of IRS, SSA, and NCHS (200). The project planners aim to provide an improved data base for mortality research by compiling statistical information from the participating agencies on a sample of individuals. The starting point will be the 1-percent CWHS (see above). This effort has great importance as a pilot for future projects to study cancer mortality, particularly contributions of occupational exposures.

Records from different agencies have been linked before on an ad hoc basis, e.g., VA has cooperated in several studies (23), but the broader scale now proposed has brought some basic issues to the fore. The most fundamental barrier to researchers acquiring data from more than one file is that which is erected to preserve privacy and confidentiality. Restrictions have been tightened considerably in recent years by the Privacy Act of 1974 and the 1976 amendments to the Internal Revenue Code. Although epidemiologists have not been implicated, well-publicized breaches of confidentiality and privacy have engendered suspicion among legislators and the public, about possible misuse of easily accessible files. MacMahon (217) has summarized the epidemiologist's point of view:

> To determine cancer risks among persons exposed to particular environmental factors, we need to be able to link information relating to the same individual at different times in his life and to determine whether an individual exposed in the past is now dead or alive and in what state of health . . . . Maximum confidentiality means minimum epidemiologic information and minimal effectiveness in identifying new cancer hazards. In my opinion, we are well beyond the point at which concern for confidentiality seriously impairs the extraction of valuable knowledge, even from routinely collected information. Working as an epidemiologist, one comes to recognize the readiness with which most people, patients or nonpatients, will supply even sensitive information if they believe the cause is reasonable. Somehow, the issue of confidentiality becomes more difficult when it is institutionalized or politicized. We must attempt to convince the public's representatives that a reasonable balance can be achieved.

Other linkages, and the means to accomplish them, have been suggested. One current proposal involves drawing a sample of several million individuals from those people who filled out the 1980 long census form for future match-ing to the NDI. This would facilitate matching cause of death with personal characteristics reported in the census. Another proposal has been made to add cause of death information to the SSA's 1-percent CWHS. However, since collection of cause of death data is not part of the mission of SSA, it would presumably require money from outside SSA for implementation.

The cited desirability of making records more available for research purposes runs into conflicts with society's intention of protecting the individual's privacy. The linking of individual records between agencies would allow a person with access to the system to obtain most or all Government-held information about any individual. The potential for abuse is apparent. At the same time, linkage, in the hands of a biomedical researcher, might quickly provide information about behaviors, exposures, and health that could be obtained only with great difficulty in any other system.

The Workgroup on Records and Privacy of the Interagency Task Force on the Health Effects of Ionizing Radiation (182a) has addressed the problems arising from the conflict between access to records for research and the right to privacy. It suggested changes in the Privacy Act, the Tax Reform Act, and commented on pending bills (in 1979) that would have permitted access to records under tightly controlled conditions. The workgroup's report is an excellent starting point for discussion of this complicated subject and provides possible directions for Federal efforts.

SUMMARY

Interest in cancer prevention and acceptance of the idea that some substances cause cancer have spurred developments in methods to determine which substances are associated with cancer.

Epidemiology has played an important role in identifying both carcinogenic substances and exposures which are associated with cancer although the causative agent may not be known.

When available, epidemiologic data about cancer risks are the most convincing. At the same time, identifying a carcinogen on the basis of human disease and death means that other testing methods failed to identify the agent before human illness resulted from it.

The most important laboratory method for determining carcinogencity is the long-term bioassay in laboratory animals, generally rats and mice. The 1960's saw marked increased interest in the test, and NCI has played a major role in designing appropriate test methods. NCI developed a large-scale bioassay program for testing, evaluating, and documenting the carcinogenicity of environmental chemicals. It has also supported the IARC program to review information on environmental carcinogens and publish findings in its authoritative monograph series.

While the bioassay has been improved and is widely accepted as an appropriate method to identify carcinogens, it is expensive (each one costs $400,000 to $1 million) and time-consuming (each takes from a minimum of more than 2 years to a more realistic 5 years). Because of those costs and limited long-term bioassay capacity, other tests are being developed.

The short-term tests measure biological effects other than carcinogenicity (often mutagenicity) in bacteria, yeast, cultured mammalian cells, or in intact lower organisms. Major international efforts have been completed and others are ongoing to validate the ability of these tests to identify correctly carcinogens and noncarcinogens. Some tests perform well in the validation experiments, and it is expected that they will play an increasingly important role in identifying carcinogens.

Deciding to test a chemical in a short-term test or a long-term bioassay involves studying its structure. Some classes of chemicals are more likely to be carcinogenic than others, some are present in high concentrations in the environment, and some are viewed with suspicion for one reason or another. Based on such information a chemical may be selected for testing. NTP is developing a tier-testing scheme which first assays a chemical in a number of short-term tests. The chemicals that appear most risky as a result of short-term tests will be accorded priority for further testing in long-term bioassays. This NTP program promises to improve both the use of information from short-term tests and the usefulness of the bioassay program.

The establishment of NTP, which appears to be moving toward an ordered, careful development of methods for testing and interpretation of results, and IRLG's appearing as a single voice for Federal regulatory procedures and decisions promise further improvements. Additionally, IARC's distinguishing between noncarcinogens and carcinogens and ordering among carcinogens on the basis of test results is an important step in increasing the usefulness of the results.

Not included in testing systems, but discussed here are already useful and potentially more useful data collection systems. Several of these systems were mandated by Congress to collect information about exposures and health status. Currently, inadequate resources and coordination may be hampering the performance of the systems. Another major source of information, the administrative data systems, were not developed as health information resources. However, both SSA and IRS collect some information which might be of great value for epidemiologic studies. Perhaps the most pressing need in adapting the administrative data systems for these uses is more consultation between epidemiologists and the data systems experts.

5.
Extrapolation From Study-Generated Data to Estimates of Human Risk

Contents

LIST OF TABLES

LIST OF FIGURES

5.
Extrapolation From Study-Generated Data to Estimates of Human Risk

INTRODUCTION

Information about carcinogenicity is obtained from exposing animals to measured doses of suspect substances in the laboratory or by studying associations between exposures to suspect carcinogens and development of cancer in humans. In practice, both the animals and certain groups of humans, particularly those exposed in the workplace, are exposed to doses far larger than those encountered by most citizens. A number of "numeric extrapolation" methods have been developed to estimate the effect of exposure to low doses based on observed effects at high doses. When information about carcinogenicity is obtained from animals, "biologic extrapolation" techniques are employed to project from animal results to estimates of human risk. (In this report the word "hazard" is applied to a substance or exposure that harbors a "risk" to people who come in contact with it—i.e., a carcinogenic chemical is itself a hazard. Risk is the probability of cancer developing as a result of a particular exposure to the hazard.)

In most cases, no adequate human data are available for estimating risks, and it is necessary to make both numeric and biologic extrapolation from measured responses in animals to estimate human risk. Less uncertainty attends making numeric extrapolations from observation of human responses at high-exposure levels than extrapolations from animal data. However, such extrapolations are often complicated by poor exposure data.

Extrapolation, like testing, is employed to make regulatory decisions, and as in the case of testing, a number of agencies have made statements about the methods they will employ. These policy statements are necessary to explain, in the absence of agreed-on universal procedures, how the agencies intend to use bioassay and epidemiologic data to estimate risk through the use of extrapolation methods.

NUMERIC EXTRAPOLATION

This discussion describes information that can be obtained from extrapolation, and comments on various extrapolation methods. It is neither rigorous nor inclusive, and the interested (and mathematically sophisticated) reader is referred to Hoel et al. (170), Crump et al. (75) and the Food Safety Council (FSC) (125) for such treatments.

Toxicity testing produces data relating tumor incidence (I) to dosage (D) as shown in figure 21. Generally, a smooth curve drawn between

the experimental points, P_1-P_5, (solid line in figure 21) is sigmoidal, or S-shaped. It can be seen that the incidence of tumor formation decreases with decreasing dosage. The crux of the extrapolation problem is what sort of line best approximates the response in the region for which data are not available. Or, what kind of line should be drawn from point P_1 to lower, unmeasured, response levels.

Graphic representations such as figure 21 do not fully show the difficulties in estimating in-

Figure 21.—A Stylized Dose-Response Curve and Some Extrapolated Curves

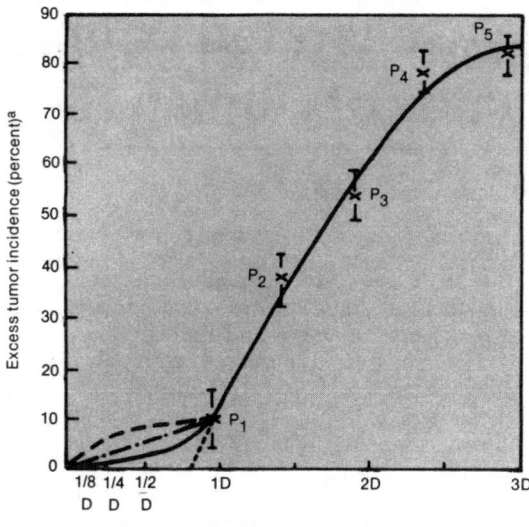

^aExcess tumor incidence (percent) is defined as:

$$\frac{\text{tumors in exposed population}}{\text{number of exposed population}} - \frac{\text{tumors in control population}}{\text{number of exposed population}} \times 100$$

——— a sigmoid dose-response curve; infralinear between O and P₁
—·—·— linear extrapolation
———— supralinear extrapolation
------ line projected to a threshold

SOURCE: Office of Technology Assessment.

cidence at very low doses. The first division on the vertical incidence scale is 10 percent, which means that 1 human or animal out of 10 developed cancer. For many agents, especially those present in air or water, we are interested in knowing what dose is projected to cause an incidence orders of magnitude less, e.g., 1 tumor in 100,000 animals or humans. Such small fractions cannot be seen on the figure, but they can be calculated using any extrapolation method.

The solid curved line drawn from point $\bar{P}_1$ to the origin is a continuation of the curve constructed between the experimentally determined points. It was drawn by eye, and it is representative of a number of smooth, concave upward lines that can connect P_1 and the origin as a continuation of the sigmoidal curve constructed between P_1 and P_5.

The Question of Thresholds

The solid line on figure 21 embodies the premise that there is no threshold. A threshold model would have the curve hit zero incidence at some dose greater than zero, as is shown in figure 21.

The threshold argument contends that there are doses of carcinogens so low that they will not cause cancer, and that no matter how many animals are exposed to doses that low or lower, no tumors will result. The counterargument is that any dose of a carcinogen, no matter how small, has a finite although small, chance of causing a tumor, and, if an experiment were performed with a sufficiently large number of animals, such risk would be detectable.

The concept of a population threshold, which is discussed here, includes the idea that there are exposure levels below which no individual in the population will develop cancer. No solution to the threshold/no threshold argument can be found by doing increasingly larger experiments with more and more animals. If a given dose of chemical causes no excess tumors in 1,000 animals, there is no guarantee that it will not cause an excess when 2,000 are exposed.

Individuals may have thresholds, as suggested by the fact that all heavy cigarette smokers do not develop lung cancer. Possible biologic reasons advanced to explain such differences in susceptibilities include physiologic and genetic variations among people. Another reason for the apparent differences in susceptibility may be chance. Some heavy smokers may be "luckier" than others in that their exposures do not trigger carcinogenesis, and they may not develop cancer, or they may die from some other cause before cancer develops. In any case, it is as yet impossible to predict an individual's threshold for even a single carcinogenic agent and impossible to derive a population's threshold with current knowledge or methods.

In a highly recommended article, Maugh (224) reports on conversations with a number of scientists and administrators from the National

Institutes of Health, private testing laboratories, and industry. The conclusion of the article, apparently shared by the interviewed scientists and administrators, is that resolution of the threshold question is not now available:

> . . . it is extremely unlikely that it would be possible to distinguish between a linear dose-response curve and a highly nonlinear one (threshold), even in a large-scale experiment involving several thousand animals per dose level.

> . . . statistical analysis of standard animal carcinogenicity experiments, Schneiderman [then-Associate Director of the National Cancer Institute (NCI)] concludes, does not now, and probably never will, resolve the threshold question. There are, he says, simply too many "biologically reasonable" mathematical models, both implying and denying the existence of thresholds, that will fit the observed results.

> . . . there is so little data and so many interpretations, Gehring [Dow Chemical Co.] says, arguing about thresholds is an exercise in futility.

The view that thresholds cannot be demonstrated is accepted in publications of the National Research Council (NRC) (262), Interagency Regulatory Liaison Group (IRLG) (180), FSC (125), and, for tumors resulting from somatic mutations, by the American Industrial Health Council (AIHC) (8). Despite the apparent agreement that it is impossible to demonstrate a threshold, many individuals object to the idea that thresholds should not be considered in making decisions about carcinogens.

In particular, some tumors are thought to result from irritation or mechanical injury, and threshold models are postulated for those. An often mentioned example is Clayson's (60) finding that bladder stones are found in conjunction with some bladder tumors. Stone formation may be dependent on intake of large quantities of a chemical; if exposure to the chemical is sufficiently low so that no stones are formed and if stone formation is necessary for carcinogenicity, then a threshold should exist. This and other examples of "epigenetic" tumors can be considered separately from tumors that originate from somatic mutations. Just as thresholds for acute toxic responses differ, thresholds for

stone formation most likely differ among individual animals. Therefore, it may be impossible to determine exactly what dose is necessary to produce a stone and therefore pave the way to a tumor. Nevertheless, if the threshold for stone formation in animals is found to be 100 or 1,000 times greater than human exposure levels, the observation takes on great significance. If stone formation is a necessary precursor to tumor appearance, and no stone formation occurs at human exposure levels, it becomes difficult to maintain the position that human exposure levels present a carcinogenic risk. The difficulties in this argument are the possibility that some humans may produce stones at very much lower doses than animals and that carcinogenicity might not proceed through stone formation in humans. Such caveats seem reasonable to some people; unreasonable to others. Experimentation and more sophisticated models may eventually settle such questions. However, for the present, positions on these issues reflect organizational policy and individual judgment.

Gehring, Watanabe, and Young (139) describe differences between metabolism of chemicals administered at low and high doses. Measurement of these differences is called pharmacokinetics. In general, biochemical mechanisms to detoxify chemicals and to repair damage to DNA are seen as having a better chance of detoxifying and repairing damage at low doses than at high doses. High doses can swamp defense mechanisms resulting in toxic effects; lower doses are seen as presenting little or no risk.

Metabolic differences measured by pharmacokinetics might have important effects on the shape of the dose-response curve. If a metabolite of an ingested substance is the actual carcinogen, and the production of the metabolite increases out of proportion to dose above a certain level, then the dose-response curve might bend upward at that point. Pharmacokinetic data are not always collected, and the standard bioassay which produces data at only two dose levels does not provide sufficient information to see if differences in metabolism might be important in the slope of the dose-response curve.

Biochemistry of a particular compound may be affected by other compounds present in the organism. Cancer is a relatively common disease, and if avoiding cancer involves biochemical detoxification processes, it may be that small doses of many substances can swamp the process as well as large doses of a single substance. If this is correct, the addition of the carcinogens, even at low doses, might be enough to overcome the detoxification mechanism.

Cornfield (67) described quantitative extrapolation models to take into account differences in metabolism at high and low doses. His paper was criticized because it postulated a threshold (see 36,73,229,276,319), and his hope that the paper would lead to discussion of the merit of his models apparently was not realized (68). The difficulty with models which propose detoxification activities for producing thresholds is that the detoxification has to be instantaneous and complete. Otherwise molecules might escape detoxification and initiate a carcinogenic event.

Donald Kennedy, a few months after leaving the post of Commissioner of the Food and Drug Administration (FDA), expressed his opinion that thresholds may exist for some chemicals:

> Dr. Kennedy said that the [Delaney] clause in the FDA's authorizing legislation codifies the hypothesis that there is no threshold concentration below which a chemical does not cause cancer. And although this hypothesis "probably holds most of the time," Dr. Kennedy said that he was "as certain as I can be of any scientific prediction that some day, very soon, some compound will be demonstrated to have a threshold level for cancer causation" . . . (274).

It is difficult, if not impossible, to marshal more evidence on one side of the threshold question than on the other. The ascendancy of the more conservative view, that thresholds cannot be identified for human populations, can be taken as a policy decision made in the interest of protecting the public health. Such a general policy can not exclude the possibility that a threshold may someday be demonstrated.

Numeric Extrapolation To Project Risk at Doses Below Those Tested

The shape of the line in figure 21 depends on the number of tumors observed at points P_1-P_5. No matter what method is used to extend the line below P_1, that extension represents an estimate. Any number of smooth curves can be drawn from point P_1 to the origin; for convenience, the possible lines will be divided into three families: supralinear, linear, and infralinear. A detailed discussion of these models as they relate to radiation and cancer is available in a paper by Sinclair (329).

Supralinear Extrapolation

A supralinear extrapolation is presented on figure 21. It says that some doses less than 1D are relatively more effective in inducing tumors than doses equal to 1D. Conceptually the contention that lower doses are more carcinogenic is easy to address. Further tests at lower doses would resolve the question, but additional tests are costly and time consuming.

Supralinear models are considered for two reasons. In several NCI bioassays, the tumor yield was lower at the high dose than at the low dose (102). In other words, the lower dose was more efficient at producing tumors. The explanation is that the higher dose was so toxic that it killed animals before they developed tumors. The other reason for considering supralinear responses is that some studies of radiation-induced cancer have been interpreted as producing supralinear dose-response curves (e.g., 241), but those interpretations are hotly disputed.

Such responses might result from the presence of a subpopulation of more sensitive individuals. On figure 21, the supralinear response between the origin and P_1 represents the tumors induced in the proposed sensitive fraction of the population; the solid line drawn from the origin to P_5 represents the sensitivity of the remaining members of the population. The difference between the two lines between the origin and P_1

represents the contribution of the sensitive subpopulation to the total response at doses below 1D. It can be seen that the sensitive subpopulation accounts for the majority of tumors that occur below P_1. Clearly, if this model describes risks, reducing doses to $\frac{1}{2}D$ or $\frac{1}{4}D$ would not significantly reduce tumor incidence, and a supralinear dose-response curve would force lowering doses to very small fractions of D to significantly reduce tumor incidence.

Nonartifactual, supralinear dose responses have rarely been observed in bioassays but neither would they be expected. Laboratory animals are highly inbred and each animal should be more nearly equally sensitive than are members of human populations. Supralinear response models have been advanced but do not now receive the acceptance accorded to the other two general models.

Linear Extrapolation

A linear model is shown by the straight line that extends from P_1 to the origin on figure 21. If the true dose-response curve is represented by the solid curved line from P_1 to the origin, then the linear model is "conservative" and overestimates the number of tumors at all doses between P_1 and the origin.

The paper by Crump et al. (75) is an often-cited and important argument for linear dose responses at low doses. The paper points out that 25 percent of the U.S. population will develop cancer as a result of existing carcinogenic influences (see ch.3). Crump et al. (75) propose that any new carcinogenic substance interacts additively with exposures and behaviors already present in the environment. Their mathematical theories predict that regardless of the shape of the dose-response curve at high exposures, at low doses cancer incidence should be proportional (linear) with exposure to the substance under study.

Gaylor and Kodell (137) argue that no risk estimate can be very reliable for doses below that associated with the lowest data point (P_1 in figure 21) because there is no information available below point P_1. They propose the use of "linear interpolation" and the 95-percent upper

confidence level to estimate the *maximum* risk posed by a substance.

Error is associated with any experimental determination, and standard methods can be used to calculate "confidence limits" for each estimate. Usually "95-percent confidence limits" are calculated for carcinogenicity experiments; they are plotted as vertical bars extending from the data points, as shown on the figure. The 95-percent confidence limit says that given the experimentally determined incidence and the size of the experiment, we can be 95-percent certain that the actual incidence represented by the point estimate lies inside the error limits.

In the method of Gaylor and Kodell (137) a line is drawn from the upper limit of the error bar on the lowest data point to the origin. Inspection of figure 21 shows that this method projects a larger risk than does linear interpolation from the point P_1 to the origin. This is not an estimate of risk; it is an estimate of the upper bound of risk.

Objections to including upper confidence levels in extrapolation are frequently voiced. The practice of including them is seen as introducing a "safety factor." Industry spokesmen (9a) and others contend that the best risk estimate should be made and the safety factors added after the estimate is made.

As a practical matter, there is often no alternative to the linear model. The dose-response curve in figure 21 is an outrageous overstatement of the data that are generally available. Bioassays carried out according to NCI's cancer testing guidelines (331) produce only two data points. The Environmental Protection Agency's (EPA) (102) analysis of many such tests showed that tumor incidence was sometimes higher and sometimes only measurable at the lower of the two doses because other toxic effects killed animals at the higher dose. Left with only the response at the lower dose, there is little choice available but to estimate responses at still lower doses on the basis of simple proportionality. Such calculations produce a straight line from the experimental point to the origin.

IRLG (180) did not discuss how to extrapolate when more than one data point is available; it recommends linear extrapolation (proportionality) for making estimates from a single point. IRLG further proposes that the upper confidence level be used as the starting point for extrapolation to achieve "an added degree of protection . . . ."

A linear extrapolation model from the lowest positive data point to zero dose (104) was used by EPA's Carcinogen Assessment Group (CAG) until the summer of 1980. At that time, CAG (48) announced it was going to discontinue use of the linear model and subsequently employ a model developed by Crump. The CAG decision was not made because evidence had shown the linear model was poorer than the new one (48):

> There is no really solid scientific basis for any mathematical extrapolation model which relates carcinogen exposure to cancer risks at the extremely low level of concentration that must be dealt with in evaluating the environmental hazards.

The now-adopted model is linear at low doses, and, in practice, produces estimates of risk at low doses which " . . . are not markedly different from those obtained with the former procedure based on the one-hit [linear] model" (230). However, the new model does allow consideration of data produced above the linear part of the curve (points P_4 and P_5 on figure 21) to influence the slope of the line and the range of error associated with each point.

Infralinear Extrapolation

The curved line between P_1 and the origin on figure 21 or any curved line which remains below the straight line is infralinear. Such models predict lower tumor incidence than the linear model. If it were decided that a certain level of risk were acceptable, higher exposure to the chemical would be allowable under infralinear than under linear models.

A number of such models have been developed and are well described in FSC's (125) report. All of them produce concave upward lines between the origin and the lowest data point (P_1, in figure 21). Different models produce differently shaped lines. It is suggested (e.g., 125) that the model which produces the line that best fits the data points (P_1 to P_5 in figure 21) is the model to use to predict risk between P_1 and the origin. Unfortunately, usually any of the models seems to fit the available data points about equally well (9a,125,138,180). The reasons for the equally good fits are that generally only one, two, or three data points are available and all of them measure incidence above 10 percent. Data points at such relatively high response rates do not often provide enough information to decide what the dose-response curve is at an incidence of 1 percent or less.

QUANTITATIVE EFFECTS OF SELECTING A MODEL

Selection of the appropriate model for estimating risks at low doses would be made easier if some models clearly did not fit the observed data points. As mentioned above, hardly ever is it possible to select the best model or even to reject the worst on the basis of fit to observed data points. The low end of the dose-response curve is most informative for selecting the correct model but it is the part that is most difficult to measure. In practice, incidence rates in animal tests much below 10 percent (5 tumor-bearing animals in a test population of 50) can seldom

be distinguished from the rate of spontaneous tumors.

Table 32, derived from a paper by Brown (35), shows that two infralinear models and the one-hit model, which is essentially linear at doses that cause an incidence of 10 percent or less, are indistinguishable at high doses. For the table, a dose level of one was set as sufficient to cause an incidence of 50 percent. The expected incidence using higher doses or doses as low as one-sixteenth are nearly equal regardless of the

Table 32.—Expected Incidence of Tumors Calculated by Three Models When a Dose of 1.0 Caused Tumors in 50 Percent of the Tested Animals

Dose level	Projected percentage of tumor bearing animals		
	Log-normal model (Infralinear)	Log-logistic model (Infralinear)	Single-hit model (linear at incidence below 10%)
16	98	96	100
4	84	84	94
1	50	50	50
1/4	16	16	16
1/16	2	4	4
1/100	0.05	0.4	0.7
1/1,000	0.00035	0.026	0.07
1/10,000	0.0000001	0.0016	0.007

SOURCE: Adapted from Brown (35).

model. Brown (35) points out that no experiment of practical size could distinguish among the three models at those dose levels.

However, at much lower dose levels of 1/100, 1/1,000, and 1/10,000, the models diverge greatly in their projections of incidence. These greatly lower dose and response levels are often the ones of most interest for estimating human risks, but they cannot be measured. The incidences measured at higher doses do not provide sufficient information to choose the appropriate model. These problems plague all extrapolation efforts.

In general, either a linear or infralinear model is used for extrapolation. The linear model predicts a higher incidence at low doses than does the infralinear model.

Selection of the correct extrapolation model is important for only one of the three possible regulatory strategies for carcinogens. The first strategy is to accept either human or animal evidence as sufficient to identify carcinogens, and once the identification is made, try to eliminate the exposure. This approach requires no quantitative or numeric extrapolation. The second approach uses biologic and numeric extrapolation to rank substances in order from that expected to be most carcinogenic to those that are noncarcinogenic. This relative ranking can be accomplished by consistently applying any model, and the numerical accuracy of the estimated incidence is not critical. The third approach, which includes a quantitative estimate of human risk to be used in risk-benefit computations or to consider levels of acceptable risk requires the most accurate numerical estimate. Clearly, in this case, the selection of models is important because the numbers produced by different models vary across a wide range.

Virtually Safe Doses

A very low risk of cancer, say, one chance in million lifetimes, is sometimes suggested as a virtually safe dose. Any extrapolation model can be used to calculate the dose which will produce such a risk, and different models produce very different estimates for the virtually safe dose (see table 32 and 125,170). As shown on figure 21, infralinear models predict higher virtually safe doses (i.e., lower risks at any dose) than does the linear model.

WHAT QUANTITATIVE PROJECTIONS CAN BE MADE FROM NEGATIVE RESULTS (ZERO EXCESS TUMORS IN A TEST POPULATION)?

No tumors occurring in a test population of 100 animals or no excess tumors among 100 animals as compared with the number of tumors in 100 control animals does not show that zero cancer risk is associated with the chemical. Instead standard statistical calculations based on zero excess tumors in 100 animals show that we can be 95-percent confident that the actual incidence of tumors is no more than 4.5 percent. This estimate of the incidence of tumors that might have gone undetected is called the upper confidence limit. The percentage can be reduced by testing more animals, for instance, finding zero excess tumors in 1,000 animals would mean that we can be 95-percent confident that the actual incidence is no more than 0.45 percent.

Proceeding with the illustration of zero excess tumors in 100 animals, assume that the dose administered to the animals was 1,000 times higher than that to which humans are exposed. Linear extrapolation (proportionality) predicts that exposure of the U.S. population to that chemical at 1/1,000 the level fed to the animals will result in fewer than 10,000 cases of cancer assuming equal sensitivity between man and animals. The estimated risk would be reduced if the experiment on which it is based is more sensitive. For instance, finding zero excess tumors in 1,000 animals (instead of 100) would reduce the estimated risk to fewer than 1,000 cases.

The statistics of the above exercise are not questioned, but they are seldom applied. Although a test cannot show that a substance presents no risk, much less concern is attached to substances that cause no excess of tumors. The risk associated with substances that are negative in bioassays is qualitatively lower, and the consideration of quantitative risk estimates from negative experiments is of minor importance.

OTHER EXTRAPOLATION MODELS

The supralinear, linear, and infralinear models are all dichotomous. They compare the number of tumors or tumor-bearing animals in the exposed population to the number in the controls. In both populations, the analysis depends on the presence or absence of tumors. Other models can be used to make inferences about the times (or ages) at which animals develop tumors in response to exposures.

Two of these models have been used extensively to describe animal and human "time-to-tumor" data. The lognormal model described in Chand and Hoel (57), predicts that the average time-to-tumor is longer at low doses. An important outcome of this model is that at sufficiently low doses, the time necessary for tumor development may exceed the expected lifespan. Such a long latent period would produce a "practical threshold." The Weibull model (also described in 57) predicts that the average time-to-tumor is nearly independent of dose. This prediction means that an increase in dose simply causes more cancers; it does not shift the age distribution at which they occur. The assumptions and predictions of these two models are quite different. Unfortunately both are apt to give adequate fits to any available data set, making it difficult to reject one in favor of the other. IRLG (181) concluded that these models have not received the attention that has been focused on dichotomous dose-incidence relation models, and it recommends more research be directed toward exploring them. The mathematics for these models is sophisticated, and the interested reader is referred to Chand and Hoel (57).

At this time, discussion of other models is more an academic than a policy exercise. Opposing camps are for or against quantitative extrapolation, and among those favoring it, the argument is between those for and against using linear extrapolation (including EPA's new mod-

el). There is no agreement about another single model being offered as an alternative at this time.

EXTRAPOLATION FROM SHORT-TERM TESTS TO HUMAN RISKS

McCann et al. (227) and McCann and Ames (226) showed that about 90 percent of the carcinogens tested in the Ames test were mutagenic (see ch. 4). Meselson and Russell (235) developed a model to compare the mutagenic and carcinogenic potency of tested chemicals. Fourteen chemicals were analyzed because there were sufficient mutagenic and carcinogenic data available to construct dose-response curves for each. The correlation between animal carcinogenicity and bacterial mutagenicity was excellent for 10 of the 14 compounds. The other four compounds (all nitroso-compounds) were more potent as carcinogens than as mutagens.

A spirited exchange of views resulted from the suggestion that quantitative relationships exist between mutagenicity in the Ames test and carcinogenicity in animal tests. Ashby and Styles (18) challenged the idea that such relationships were common, and Ames and Hooper (12) responded that they were.

The International Program for the Evaluation of Short-Term Tests for Carcinogenicity (188) distributed 42 chemicals to each of 12 laboratories for testing in the Ames system: To eliminate bias, none of the laboratories knew the identity of the chemicals. There was excellent agreement among test results obtained in different laboratories and about 80 percent of the carcinogens were scored as mutagens and about 80 percent of the noncarcinogens were scored as nonmutagens. These numbers compare well with those in the literature that describe results from experiments in which the investigators knew before the mutagenicity test was run that the chemicals were or were not car-

cinogenic. Although the 80-percent is lower than the 90-percent accuracy sometimes reported, the program included a number of chemicals that are known to present difficulties for the Ames test. In a qualitative sense, the test performed very well, but mutagenic potency did not correlate with carcinogenic potency. In other words, the results from this program do not support the idea that there is a quantitative relationship between Ames test results and carcinogenicity in animals. Similar results showing good qualitative and poor quantitative agreements between mutagenicity and carcinogenicity were reported by Bartsch et al. (22).

Meselson and Russell (235) reported that sufficient quantitative data were available for two human carcinogens, aflatoxin B and cigarette smoke, to allow comparison of mutagenic potency to carcinogenic potency in humans. Correlation between carcinogenicity in humans and mutagenicity was good for the two compounds, and the Meselson and Russell paper raised the possibility that human cancer risks might be predicted from mutagenicity data. Acceptance of such a procedure is far away and will depend on much more data being available to support the proposed quantitative relationships.

Clearly, controversies now exist about the value of extrapolations made from short-term tests. It seems reasonable that, as use of short-term tests increases, such projections are going to be made, but some initial optimism about the value of quantitative extrapolation from short-term tests to carcinogenicity is apparently fading.

CARCINOGENIC ACTIVITY INDICATORS

The NRC Pesticide Committee (267) recommends calculating potency expressions, "Carcinogenic Activity Indicators" (CAI), for tested chemicals. For each point of a dose response curve (fig. 21), the number of chemical molecules ingested divided by the animal body weight can be related to the excess percentage of tumor-bearing animals in the exposed population.

$$CAI = \frac{\text{excess percentage of subjects in which tumors are observed}}{\text{lifetime dose (molecules/kg of body weight)}} = \frac{\text{tumor incidence}}{\text{dose}}$$

CAIs do not have to be based on total tumors, for instance, site specific tumors may be counted, the analysis may be limited to one sex, only malignant tumors may be counted, or other alterations can be made as wanted. In practice, the number of molecules of different substances, S1, S2, and S3 required to induce the same percentage of excess tumors can be compared to determine which is the most potent carcinogen. CAIs will probably be different for each point on a dose-response curve because the points seldom fall in a straight line, but comparisons can be made at comparable doses.

Using information about exposure levels for human populations, the number of molecules that compare to human exposures can be calculated. Linear extrapolation is then to be used to estimate the animal response at human exposure level. This method is especially appropriate for comparing chemicals with similar uses, and if applied, would assure that the most and least risky ones based on animal data are identified.

The procedure does not make predictions of human cancer risks from animal data and avoids the problems associated with biologic extrapolation. The NRC committee (267) urges that only epidemiologic data be used to estimate human risk; it restricts the use of animal data to making comparisons of carcinogenicity in animals. (Such an approach is especially attractive when deciding about regulating pesticides. Substitutes are often available and CAIs offer a method to decide on the less or least risky one. This suggestion corresponds to the second possible use of extrapolation discussed in *Quantitative Effects of Selecting a Model* above.)

POTENCY

Ames et al. (14) have analyzed more than 1,500 bioassays carried out on some 600 chemicals. For each experiment, they have calculated a potency index, TD_{50}, which is calculated as the total dose of substance necessary to produce tumors in 50 percent of the animals. They expect to compare potency:

1. among multiple tests run on the same substance in the same strain and species;
2. between male and female animals;
3. between different strains of the same animal;
4. between different sites in different animals; and
5. between rodent tests and 26 tests that have been carried out in monkeys.

The results of this massive project is expected to provide much information about biologic extrapolation from species to species and about potencies.

Ames et al. (14) mention that preliminary results show that there is usually less than a tenfold variation in potencies among rodents. This level of agreement was also found by Crouch and Wilson (72) for most of 70 chemicals tested in both rats and mice by NCI. Crouch and Wilson included tumors which were not present at "statistically significant" levels in their analyses. Therefore, some chemicals judged positive in only one species by NCI (146) have potencies that agree within a factor of 10 between rats and mice although one is statistically significant and the other is not. Results showing a substance is much more potent in one species than in another will suggest that metabolism of the chemical differs from species to species. This information will also be important in efforts to improve extrapolation methods.

THE ED$_{01}$ EXPERIMENT AND EXTRAPOLATION MODELS

The National Center for Toxicological Research, a joint FDA/EPA laboratory, tested the known bladder and liver carcinogen 2-acetylaminofluorene (2-AAF) in approximately 24,000 female mice. This experiment was designed to study dose responses down to a 1-percent tumor incidence, i.e., the effective dose for a 1-percent (0.01) response (ED$_{01}$).

Figures 22 and 23 show the results of postmortem examination for liver and bladder tumors in animals exposed to 2-AAF for between 21.5 and 28.5 months. The curve that describes the liver tumors (fig. 22) shows no threshold and increases almost proportionally to dose. The curve that describes the bladder tumors (fig. 23) gives an impression of a "threshold" dose below 60 ppm of 2-AAF. Gaylor (136)

Figure 23.—Proportion (P) of Mice With Bladder Tumors v. Dose (21.5 to 28.5 months)

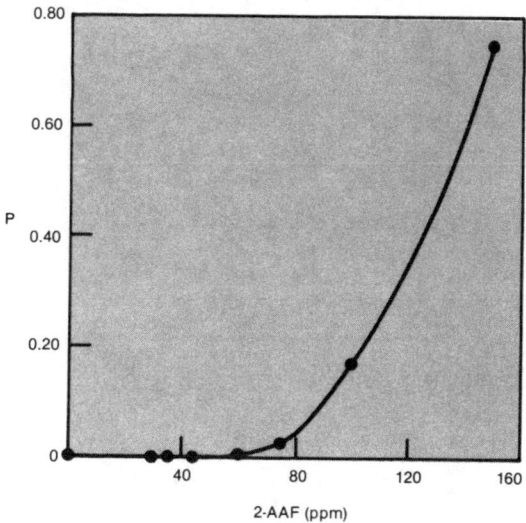

SOURCE: Littlefield, et al. (213).

Figure 22.—Proportion (P) of Mice With Liver Tumors v. Dose (21.5 to 28.5 months)

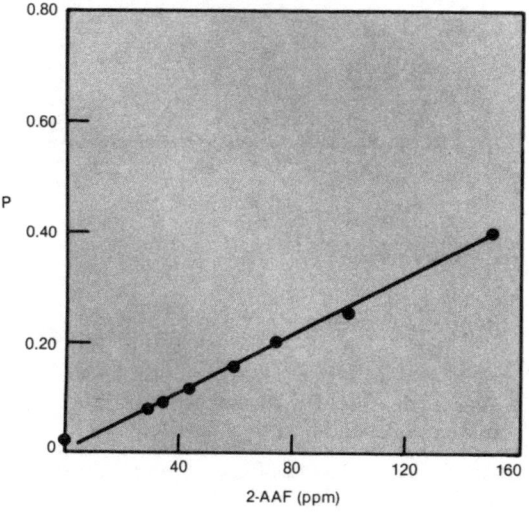

SOURCE: Littlefield, et al. (213).

ascribes the apparent threshold to a lack of resolution of the graph for low tumor rates. He replotted these same data on an enlarged scale (figure 24) to show that the number of bladder tumors increases with dose even at lower doses. This diagram supports the idea that there was no threshold. However, there is a dramatic change in slope of the line between 60 and 75 ppm, and the efficiency of 2-AAF in causing tumors increases greatly at doses above 60 ppm (fig. 24).

Carlborg (50) has also analyzed the data from ED$_{01}$. He does not argue that the bladder cancer data show a threshold, but he does contend that neither the bladder nor the liver data fit a one-hit (linear) model. In addition to trying to fit a one-hit model to the data, he also tried the

Figure 24.—Proportion (P) of Mice With Bladder Tumors v. Dose (21.5 to 28.5 months)

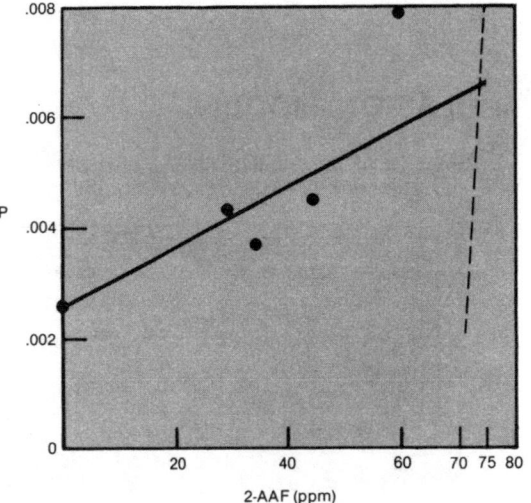

2-AAF (ppm)

NOTE: The vertical scale has been expanded 100 times compared to figure 23.
—— line fitted to data points between 0 and 60 ppm
---- slope of line between 60 and 75 ppm (derived from figure 23)

SOURCE: Gaylor (136) and Office of Technology Assessment.

Figure 25.—Proportion (P) of Mice With Liver Tumors v. Dose (24 months)

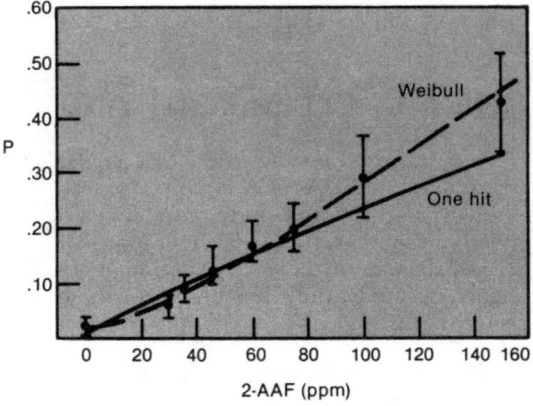

2-AAF (ppm)

SOURCE: Carlborg (50).

Figure 26.—Proportion (P) of Mice With Bladder Tumors v. Dose (24 months)

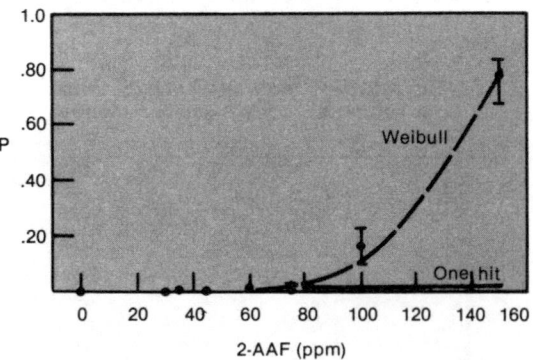

2-AAF (ppm)

SOURCE: Carlborg (50).

Weibull model, a "generalization of the one-hit model." Figures 25 and 26 represent his analysis of the two sets of data, and the "best-fitting one-hit and Weibull models" are plotted in both figures. It can be seen that the Weibull model provides a better fit, especially with the bladder tumor data. Carlborg (50) also states that the one-hit model fits well with only the three lowest dose points from the liver tumor data.

The Weibull model produces a different slope for the line to be drawn from 30 to 0 ppm. Carlborg calculates that a 0.000045 ppm dose of 2-AAF is necessary to produce a one in a million risk of liver cancer using the one-hit model. Using the Weibull model, the calculated dose for a one in a million risk is 100 times higher, 0.0045 ppm. In other words, use of the Weibull model would allow exposures 100 times higher than the linear model if there were agreement that a one in a million risk were acceptable.

Despite the large number of data points from ED_{01}, Gaylor (136) argues that a "best" model cannot be chosen on the basis of fit with the data and that the Weibull model cannot be singled out above all others. Furthermore, he says that several models fit the observed data about equally well, and that they predict very different levels of risk at doses between 0 and 30 ppm 2-AAF (see discussion of different models in 35,49,51,123,170).

Obviously, animal data can be best used quantitatively to estimate potential risks within the same animal species under test conditions. These estimates cannot be used directly to estimate human risks. Other "biologic" assumptions are necessary to extrapolate from animal data to estimates of human risk.

BIOLOGIC EXTRAPOLATION FROM ANIMAL TESTS

Bioassay guidelines call for testing in two species. Qualitative judgments are based on whether a tested substance causes tumors in both, only one, or neither species. Sometimes, a substance is reported positive (causes tumors) in only one species and negative in another. The frequency with which this problem is encountered can be estimated from Griesemer and Cueto's (146) discussion of the results of the NCI bioassay program (see app. A). Of the 98 chemicals for which "very strong" or "sufficient" evidence of carcinogenicity was found in either rats, mice, or both, 54 were positive in only one species. An analysis of test results from 250 substances (300) found 38 percent were carcinogenic in neither rats nor mice, 15 percent were carcinogenic in either the rat or the mouse but not both, and 44 percent were carcinogenic in both. Crouch and Wilson (72) and Ames et al. (14) tend to dismiss these discordant results between rats and mice because tests analyzed by their methods, which consider experimental error and test sensitivity, are in agreement much more often.

In cases in which there are apparent species differences in sensitivity, the positive result is generally accepted as more important. The Office of Science and Technology Policy (281), IRLG (180), the Occupational Safety and Health Administration (279), and American Federation of Labor/Congress of Industrial Organizations (7) all present arguments for following this course. AIHC (8) and Purchase (300) present arguments against deciding that the more sensitive animal is predictive for human response. The disagreement continues, but in Federal programs, extrapolation is based on results from the more sensitive species.

Accepting that experimental animals provide appropriate data for extrapolation to estimates of human risk, a decision has to be made about how to adjust the dose measured in the bioassay to the dose experienced by humans. A mouse or rat, of course, is much smaller than a human, and the dose necessary to cause a carcinogenic response is less than that required in humans. Three "scaling factors" are in general use to make allowance for the different sizes and rates of metabolism between experimental animals and humans. The three are listed below in order from least conservative, that is the one that predicts the lowest human risk, to the most conservative. The fourth scaling factor is less often used, but it is included because it was used for the estimates reported in table 34. For rats and mice, the most commonly used laboratory animals, the relationship between scaling factors and estimated risk in man for the same doses are shown in table 33.

1. Exposures may be adjusted on the basis of relative body weights, milligram of agent/kilogram of body weight/day (mg/kg/day), for animals and humans. This method is most generally used by toxicologists.

2. In cases where the experimental dose is measured as parts per million in food, air, or water and human exposure is through ingestion, the dose of the chemical is expressed as parts per million. This method is generally used by FDA and in some cases by EPA.

3. Exposure may be adjusted on the basis of the relative surface areas of the test animal and humans: milligram of agent/surface area/day, for animals and humans. It is generally expressed as milligram of substance/square meter of surface area/day or $mg/m^2/day$. EPA uses this scaling factor.

Table 33.—Relative Human Risk Depending on How Dose Rate is Scaled From Experimental Animals to Humans

	Risk projected for humans when an identical dose is scaled by different factors			
	Milligram	Parts per million	Milligram	Milligram
Experimental animal	Kilogram body weight/day	In diet	m² body area	Kilogram body weight/lifetime
Mouse	1	6	14	40
Rat	1	3	6	35

SOURCE: Office of Technology Assessment.

4. Exposures may be adjusted on the basis of relative body weight over lifetime, milligrams of agent/kilogram of body weight/lifetime (mg/kg/lifetime).

As can be seen from table 33, the choice of scaling factor can make a difference of up to fortyfold in estimating human risks. The mg/kg/day scaling factor was arbitarily set equal to 1.0. Use of the mg/m²/day factor (for instance) projects that humans would have 14 times the risk of a mouse for equivalent doses measured in mg/kg/day. The information given in table 33 allows a comparison to be made among the scaling factors. However, it is important to remember that great uncertainties surround biologic extrapolation because of possible differences between laboratory animals and man, and no great assurance is attached to any number in table 33.

COMPARING MEASURED HUMAN CANCER INCIDENCE AND MORTALITY TO ESTIMATES MADE USING EXTRAPOLATION

The more troubling and more fundamental problem with biologic extrapolation concerns questions about how closely the test animal resembles humans. This problem is partially related to differences in the greater genetic complexity of human populations. Populations of test animals are highly inbred and are almost genetically identical. Populations of humans are outbred and include greatly differing genotypes. There is no way to deal with the problem of humans that may differ in sensitivities because there is seldom, if ever, a way to associate sensitivities with individuals. The other problem concerns differences in metabolism between test animals and humans. Few are well understood, and many may be unidentified.

Laying these problems aside, a few efforts have been made to compare human cancer incidence or mortality to the levels of incidence or mortality extrapolated from animal studies. The number of such attempts is limited by the few cases for which data are available both from experimental animals and from humans. The Consultative Panel on Health Hazards of Chemical Pesticides of the National Research Council's Study of Pest Control (262), identified six chemicals for which such comparisons could be made. Comparisons were made on the basis of lifetime dosage (expressed as milligram chemical/kilogram body weight/lifetime) in animals and in humans. Table 34 shows those findings. It can be seen that for three chemicals the incidence of human tumors was essentially that predicted from animal studies, and for the other three, extrapolation from animal data overestimated human risk as measured by epidemiology. Crouch and Wilson (72) have made similar comparisons for 13 chemicals (including the 6 in table 34). They reported good agreement between predicted and observed human tumors rates, using a linear nonthreshold extrapolation model. Crouch and Wilson (72) also calculated "scaling factors" from their experiments and concluded that humans are twice as sensitive as mice and between one-third and three times as sensitive as rats to the same dose expressed as mg/kg/day. These values differ

**Table 34.—Comparison of Tumor Rates in Laboratory Test Animals and Humans
Following Lifetime Exposures to Comparable Amounts of Each of Six Agents**
(comparison based on mg agent/kg bodyweight/lifetime)

Chemical	Test animal	Animal tumor site(s)	Human tumor site	Relative tumor rate[a]
Benzidine	Mouse	Liver	Bladder	ca. 1
	Rat	Bladder		
Cigarette smoking	Mouse	Lung	Lung	ca. 1
	Hamster	Larynx		
N,N-bis(2-chloro-ethyl)-2-naphtyl-amine	Mouse	Lung	Bladder	ca. 1
Aflatoxin B₁	Mouse	Liver	Liver	ca. 10
	Rat	Liver		
Diethylstilbestrol (DES)	Mouse	Mammary	Daughters' re-productive tract	ca. 50
	Mouse	Cervix and vagina		
Vinyl chloride	Mouse	Lung	Liver	ca. 500
	Mouse	Mammary		
	Rat	Kidney		
	Rat	Liver		

[a] relative tumor rate = $\dfrac{\text{tumor incidence predicted from most sensitive animal species}}{\text{tumor incidence observed in humans}}$

SOURCE: Adapted from National Research Council (262).

from unity by a factor of 3 or less which is assumed for doses scaled on the basis of mg/kg/day (see table 33).

A decision about whether the reasonably good agreement between extrapolated values and observations (72,262) are of significance, and whether or not these findings mean extrapolation is accurate enough for making quantitative decisions about human risks depends on the observer. The NRC Committee (262) concluded that:

Although there are major uncertainties in extrapolating the results of animal tests to man, this is usually the only available method . . . Despite the uncertainties, enough is known to indicate what dependencies on dose and time may operate and to provide rough predictions of induced cancer rates in human populations.

Regulating Pesticides, a report prepared by the National Academy of Science's Committee on Prototype Explicit Analyses for Pesticides (267), says that seven previous National Re-

search Council reports have recommended extrapolating from animal data to projected human risk. The Committee (267) took a different position and recommended that only epidemiologic data be used to estimate human risk:

OPP [Office of Pesticide Programs, EPA] should abandon its attempts to produce numerical estimates of the effects of the use of pesticides on human mortality and morbidity except when reliable human epidemiological data are available. In the usual case, in which major reliance has to be placed on the results of bioassays, those results should be used to construct indicators of the relative pathological activity of the pesticide under review in comparison with other pesticides and compounds.

Documented differences between the metabolism of a chemical in test animals and in humans would be very useful in any attempt at biologic extrapolation. Poor understanding of comparative biochemistry hampers research in the basic biology of cancer. As research continues, knowledge of metabolic differences between animals and humans may provide clearer direction, but such information will always be limited by strong constraints on studying metabolism of carcinogens in humans.

SUMMARY

Animal tests or epidemiologic studies yield data that relate cancer (or tumor) incidence to exposure levels (dosage) of the substance under study. The accuracy of the relation between exposure and incidence is always limited. Practical restraints on the number of animals that can be tested means that the data are always subject to significant experimental error; it also means that only relatively high incidences, almost always greater than 10 percent, can be measured in the experiments. Epidemiologic studies may be limited by small numbers of people available for study, or by unknown or uncertain exposure levels. In all cases, deficiencies in experimental design and execution may further limit the accuracy of relating incidence to dose.

Quantitative extrapolation begins with the experimentally determined relationship between incidence and exposure and may use one of several methods to derive an estimate of incidence at exposure levels likely to be encountered in the environment. When animal data are used for extrapolation one of four scaling factors can be used to extrapolate from animal results to expected human response. The scaling factors vary some fortyfold in the risk they project for humans, and agreement has not been reached about which one is most appropriate.

There is also no agreement about which mathematical models best extrapolate from the exposure levels measured in studies to those encountered in the environment. Linear models, which assume that incidence is proportional to exposure at low-exposure levels, are used by Federal agencies. Some other organizations favor nonlinear models in which estimates of incidence decrease faster than dose decreases. A special feature of some models is the incorporation of a threshold, a low, but nonzero exposure level at which the estimated incidence is zero. Nonthreshold models, which are used by Federal agencies, associate some positive estimate of incidence with all doses above zero.

Suggestions are frequently made that careful inspection of available data and testing various extrapolation models against them will allow selection of the best model. Unfortunately data are not sufficient to make such judgments. Another method to decide which model is appropriate is to make projections from animal data and compare those to observed incidence in humans. The cases where human data are available to make comparisons are few, but the conceptually simple, linear, nonthreshold model is reported to estimate human incidence reasonably well.

The increasing importance of short-term tests has led to efforts to extrapolate from them to estimates of carcinogenic risks in humans or animals. Qualitatively short-term tests perform well in predicting whether a substance will be carcinogenic or noncarcinogenic in an animal test. Quantitative agreement between mutagenic potency in short-term tests and carcinogenic potency in animal tests for carcinogenicity is not nearly so good.

6.
Approaches to
Regulating Carcinogens

Contents

LIST OF TABLES AND FIGURES

6.

Approaches to Regulating Carcinogens

PUBLIC PERCEPTION ABOUT CANCER AND THE LEGISLATIVE RESPONSE

The importance of cancer in U.S. policies about disease is illustrated by the attention focused on cancer research. The first institute of the U.S. Public Health Service to be devoted to a single disease was the National Cancer Institute (NCI), established in 1937. Initially a freestanding institute, it was incorporated into the National Institutes of Health (NIH) which was organized in the 1940's. Thirty-four years after NCI's establishment, a nearly successful effort was mounted in Congress, in 1971, to separate NCI from NIH and to establish a National Cancer Authority, that would have set cancer further apart from other biomedical research activities. While the National Cancer Act of 1971 was unsuccessful in establishing a new authority, it elevated NCI to bureau status, a higher organizational level than all other institutes at NIH until the National Heart, Lung, and Blood Institute was also made a bureau. The 1971 legislation established a three-person cancer panel, appointed by and responsible to the President; no other disease has been singled out in such a way. The attention bestowed on cancer research reflects the importance of the disease to the public. It is the number two killer in the United States, the number one disease killer among people younger than 55, and it is the most dreaded disease (307).

In the 1960's and 1970's, public and congressional interest in cancer prevention was spurred by associations being drawn between environmental exposures and cancer. Congressional testimony mentioned associations between the environment and cancer, and several laws were enacted to provide Federal agencies with regulatory mechanisms to reduce exposures to carcinogens.

Public fear and dread of cancer is not likely to decrease, and despite the current antiregulatory mood, Americans still favor health and environmental regulations. A survey of 2,000 people, commissioned by Union Carbide in 1979, found continued public support of Government efforts "to protect individual health and safety and the environment." Seventy percent of those surveyed favored stronger measures to protect workers from cancer; 65 percent favored stronger measures to protect consumers from cancer (352).

Concern about cancer is likely to provide impetus for continued efforts to reduce its incidence and to improve its treatment. Efforts to improve treatment are seen as highly desirable and excite little controversy, but efforts to reduce cancer incidence by regulatory intervention generate great passion about whether the expected benefits from the regulations justify their costs. As is pointed out in the earlier chapters of this report, some uncertainty is associated with estimates made of the cancer risk posed by particular exposures. Part of the controversy about regulatory intervention, whether it is worth it or not, flows from those uncertainties, but controversy also stems from the fact that the regulations bring two societal goals into conflict. The majority of people want protection from carcinogenic risks, and at the same time want to reduce regulatory costs and burdens. Choosing between these two goals or reaching compromises between them will remain an important point of contention in policies about the control of cancer.

Several Federal agencies administer regulatory programs for the control of carcinogenic and other health risks to humans from chemical substances. These programs differ in their objectives and regulatory authority. Some were designed by Congress to deal with several different types of risks, including carcinogenic risks, in the workplace or in consumer products. Others were designed to protect humans and the environment through control of toxic substances in air, water, and food.

Regulatory decisionmaking for control of cancer risks to humans is guided by specific legal mandates and administrative procedures and depends on technical determinations con-cerning the existence and magnitude of risk. This chapter first discusses statutory mandates related to carcinogen regulation, then moves to an examination of risk assessment issues. A concluding section focuses on the process of making regulatory decisions for controlling carcinogens.

STATUTORY MANDATES

Regulations of carcinogenic substances are designed to reduce health risks. The laws that require such regulations differ in whether they direct regulators to consider only health risks or to consider both health risks and other factors. The other factors to be considered may include the costs of reducing the exposure and the costs of foregone benefits from reduced availability of the substance.

Table 35 lists 10 laws under which some action has been or may be taken to reduce exposure to carcinogens. Of the applicable statutes, the Federal Food, Drug, and Cosmetic Act (FDCA), the Clean Water Act (CWA) of 1977, and the Toxic Substances Control Act (TSCA) specifically mention carcinogens. The remaining statutes provide for regulating all toxics, and carcinogens are included in the more general term. The list includes the laws most often discussed in relation to carcinogens but not all laws under which carcinogens might be regulated. For instance, laws governing transport of hazardous substances might be used to regulate carcinogens, and the U.S. Department of Agriculture regulates carcinogens in poultry and meat.

The earliest laws reflecting congressional concern about toxics centered on the food supply. Those laws, enacted around the turn of the century, established the Food and Drug Administration (FDA). In line with the importance society attaches to a safe food supply, the first law to apply directly to carcinogens was aimed at carcinogenic food additives. The Delaney clause, incorporated into the Food Additives Amendment of 1958, forbids the incorporation into food of any additive shown to induce cancer in humans or other animals.

The late 1960's and the 1970's saw the identification of carcinogens in various parts of the environment, and Congress provided legislative authority to regulatory agencies to reduce such exposures. The number and diversity of laws produces a "balkanized" Federal regulatory effort. Whether or not carcinogen regulation would be better accomplished under fewer, broader laws is a question worthy of consideration, but it is beyond the scope of the present assessment.

Bases for the Laws

Although many of the laws deal with other toxics in addition to carcinogens, the discussion here will focus on carcinogens to the exclusion of other health and environmental risks. The existence of the laws clearly states that Congress has seen cancer risks as deserving Government attention. At the same time, despite the fact that some of the laws are attacked as proposing an unobtainable risk-free society, Congress has recognized that cancer-risk management can sometimes involve balancing and comparing of risks against other societal goals. The 10 laws in table 35 can be divided into "risk-based laws" (or zero-risk laws) which allow no balancing of health risks against other factors, "balancing laws" which require balancing of risks against benefits of the substance, and "technology-based laws" which direct regulatory agencies to impose specified levels of control (306).

Risk-Based Laws

For this discussion, "risk-based" refers to legislation that provides for regulations to reduce risks to zero without considering other factors. The primary example is the Delaney clause which specifies that carcinogenic food additives are to be eliminated from the food supply. Section 112 of the Clean Air Act (CAA) and section 307(a)(4) of CWA call for the reduction of exposures to levels which allow an "ample margin of safety." Because Federal agencies do not accept threshold levels below which carcinogens pose no risk, strict interpretation of "ample margin of safety" would also require reductions to zero exposures. The Resource Conservation and Recovery Act (RCRA) is also risk-based, but no regulation about carcinogens has yet been issued under it.

When it enacted the Delaney clause, Congress was aware that over 1,000 substances were present as additives in the U.S. food supply. Many of those substances had been poorly tested (if at all) for acute toxicity and hardly any had been tested for chronic toxicity. Congress recognized that some of the additives might pose health problems, and the Delaney clause reflects its conclusion that no benefit could militate against banning a carcinogenic additive.

The most recent application of the Delaney clause was the proposed removal of saccharin from the "generally recognized as safe" (GRAS) list of food additives. This action, based on the finding that saccharin causes bladder cancer in rats, would then have resulted in the ban of saccharin from use as a food additive (282). Few people question that saccharin is a rat carcinogen, and the Delaney clause is clear: Saccharin should be removed from the market on the basis of the animal study. Peter Hutt, former General Counsel of FDA, points out that a zero-risk approach, such as the Delaney clause, may work reasonably well so long as there are substitutes. When no substitute is available, controversy flares. It flamed in the case of saccharin.

Because FDA had banned cyclamates on the basis of animal tests in 1969, the banning of saccharin would have meant that there would be no nonnutritive sweetener on the market. No one could have the pleasure of sweetness without the cost of calories. Citizens who objected to the ban, aided by postage-paid postcards inserted into cartons of saccharin-sweetened soft drinks, deluged Congress with mail. Congress delayed the imposition of the saccharin ban and called for more studies. In 1980, it continued the delay.

At the request of Congress, both OTA (282) and the National Research Council (NRC) (269) reviewed the scientific data and conclusions about saccharin and agreed with the FDA decision that saccharin is a carcinogen. The congressional decision to forestall action on saccharin can be viewed as the Congress reopening discussion about its earlier decision that benefits of carcinogenic food additives could not be weighed against their risks. It is aware of the evidence of risks (from animal studies) and benefits (from public outcry), and by delaying the ban, it is giving weight to the benefits.

Whether the saccharin moratorium presages an eventual voiding of the Delaney clause is an open question. Congress may retain the Delaney clause but, from time to time, exercise its prerogative to overrule agency decisions when it decides that benefits, whether measured or not, outweigh risks.

Comments are sometimes heard that the Delaney clause was appropriate for the state of knowledge in 1957 when it was enacted, but that times have changed. It is said that at that time there was general agreement that few substances were carcinogenic and that those few could be eliminated from commerce with little difficulty. However, more and more substances, including many useful and some apparently essential ones, have been identified as carcinogens. Some people make a connection between these discoveries and the apparent turning away from risk-based laws such as the Delaney clause.

Despite the fact that some of the laws written in the 1970's were technology-based or balancing (see below), section 112 of CAA, 1970, and RCRA, 1976, are risk-based. They direct that risks to health be reduced or eliminated without specifically calling for consideration of other factors. An important consideration in these

Table 35.—Public Laws Providing for the Regulation of Exposures to Carcinogens

Legislation (Agency)	Definition of toxics or hazards used for regulation of carcinogens	Degree of protection	Agents regulated as carcinogens (or proposed for regulation)	Basis of the legislation	Remarks
Federal Food, Drug and Cosmetic Act: (FDA)					
Food	Carcinogenicity for *additive* defined by Delaney Clause	No risk permitted, ban of additive	21 food additives and colors	Risk	
	Contaminants	"necessary for the protection of public health..." sec. 406 (346)	Three substances—aflatoxin, PCBs, nitrosamines	Balancing	
Drugs	Carcinogenicity is defined as a risk	Risks and benefits of drug are balanced.	Not determined	Balancing	
Cosmetics	"substance injurious under conditions of use prescribed."	Action taken on the basis that cosmetic is adulterated.	Not determined	Risk. No health claims are allowed for "cosmetics." If claims are made, cosmetic becomes a "drug."	
Occupational Safety and Health Act (OSHA)	Not defined in Act (but OSHA Generic Cancer Policy defines carcinogens on basis of animal test results or epidemiology.)	"adequately assures to the extent feasible that no employee will suffer material impairment of health or functional capacity..." sec. 6(b) (5)	20 substances	Technology (or balancing)	
Clean Air Act (EPA)					
Sec. 112 (stationary sources)	"an air pollutant...which ...may cause, or contribute to, an increase in mortality or an increase in serious irreversible, or incapacitating reversible, illness." sec. 112(a) (1)	"an ample margin of safety to protect the public health..." sec. 112(b) (1) (B)	Asbestos, beryllium, mercury, vinyl chloride, benzene, radionuclides, and arsenic (an additional 24 substances are being considered)	Risk	Basis of the Airborne Carcinogen Policy
Sec. 202 (vehicles)	"air pollutant from any ...new motor vehicles... or engine, which...cause, or contribute to, air pollution which may reasonably be anticipated to endanger public health or welfare." sec. 202A(a) (1)	"standards which reflect the greatest degree of emission reduction achievable through...technology ...available..." sec. 202(b) (3)(a) (1)	Diesel particulates standard	Technology Sec. 202(b) (4) (B) includes a risk-risk test for deciding between pollutant that might result from control attempts.	Sec. 202(b) (4) (A) specifies that no pollution control device, system, or element shall be allowed if it presents an unreasonable risk to health, welfare or safety.
Sec. 211 (fuel additives)	Same as above (211(c) (1)).	Same as above (211(c) (2) (a)).	—	Balancing. Technology-based with consideration of costs, but health-based in requirement that standards provide ample margin of safety.	A cost-benefit comparison of competing control technologies is required.
Clean Water Act (EPA) Sec. 307	Toxic pollutants listed in Committee Report 95-30 of House Committee on Public Works and Transportation. List from consent decree between EDF, NRDC, Citizens for Better Environment and EPA.	Defined by applying BAT economically achieveable (sec. 307(a) (2)), but effluent levels are to "provide(s) an ample margin of safety." (sec. 307(a) (4))	49 substances listed as carcinogens by CAG.	Technology	
Federal Insecticide, Fungicide, and Rodenticide Act and the Federal Environmental Pesticide Control Act (EPA)	One which results in "unreasonable adverse effects on the environment or will involve unreasonable hazard to the survival of a species declared endangered..."	Not specified.	14 rebuttable presumptions against registrations either initiated or completed; nine pesticides voluntarily withdrawn from market.	Sec. 2(bb) Balancing: "unreasonable adverse effects..."	"Unreasonable adverse effects" means "unreasonable risk to man or the environment taking into account the economic, social, and environmental costs and benefits..."

Table 35.—Public Laws Providing for the Regulation of Exposures to Carcinogens (Continued)

Legislation (Agency)	Definition of toxics or hazards used for regulation of carcinogens	Degree of protection	Agents regulated as carcinogens (or proposed for regulation)	Basis of the legislation	Remarks
Resource Conservation and Recovery Act (EPA)	One which "may cause, or significantly contribute to an increase in mortality or an increase in serious irreversible, or incapacitating reversible, illness; or, pose a...hazard to human health or the environment..." sec. 1004(5) (A) (B)	"that necessary to protect human health and the environment..." sec. 3002-04	74 substances proposed for listing as hazardous wastes	Risk. The Administrator can order monitoring and set standards for sites.	
Safe Drinking Water Act (EPA)	"contaminant(s) which...may have an adverse effect on the health of persons." sec. 1401(1) (B)	"to the extent feasible...(taking costs into consideration)..." sec. 1412(a) (2)	Trihalomethanes, chemicals formed by reactions between chlorine used as disinfectant and organic chemicals. Two pesticides and 2 metals classified as carcinogens by CAG, but regulated because of other toxicities.	Balancing	
Toxic Substances Control Act (EPA)					
Sec. 4 (to require testing)	substances which "may present an unreasonable risk of injury to health or the environment." sec. 4(a) (1) (A) (i)	Not specified.	Six chemicals used to make plastics pliable.	Balancing: "unreasonable risk"	
Sec. 6 (to regulate)	substances which "present(s) or will present an unreasonable risk of injury to health or the environment." sec. 6(a)	"to protect adequately against such risk using the least burdensome requirement" sec. 6(a)	PCBs regulated as directed by the law.	Balancing: "unreasonable risk."	
Sec. 7 (to commence civil action against imminent hazards)	"imminently hazardous chemical substance or mixture means a...substance or mixture which presents an imminent and unreasonable risk of serious or widespread injury to health or the environment."	Based on degree of protection in sec. 6			
Federal Hazardous Substances Act (CPSC)	"any substance (other than a radioactive substance) which has the capacity to produce personal injury or illness..." 15 USC sec.	"establish such reasonable variations or additional label requirements...necessary for the protection of public health and safety..." 15 USC sec.		Risk	"Highly toxic" defined as capacity to cause death, thus toxicity may be limited to acute toxicity.
Consumer Product Safety Act (CPSC)	"products which present unreasonable risks of injury...in commerce," and "'risk of injury' means a risk of death, personal injury or serious or frequent injury." 15 USC sec. 2051 "imminently hazardous consumer product' means consumer product which presents imminent and unreasonable risk of death, serious illness or severe personal injury." 15 USC sec. 2061	"standard shall be reasonably necessary to prevent or reduce an unreasonable risk of injury." 15 USC sec. 2056	Five substances: asbestos, benzene, benzidine (and benzidine-based dyes and pigments), vinyl chloride, "tris"	Balancing: "unreasonable"	Standards are to be expressed, wherever feasible, as performance requirements.

SOURCE: Office of Technology Assessment.

two laws is that they deal with pollutants. Pollutants benefit no one, and their reduction or elimination improves the environment and public health.

A problem arises because eliminating the pollutants costs money. Furthermore, in the case of carcinogens, the evidence that a substance poses a risk is not always accepted by everyone. As a result, the cost of reducing exposure to a pollutant is often offered as an argument against the projected health benefits expected from regulation, and suggestions are made that the costs be considered against the benefits before regulation, even in cases where the law does not call for such considerations.

Balancing Laws

The "balancing laws," such as the Consumer Product Safety Act (CPSA), the Federal Insecticide, Fungicide, and Rodenticide Act (FIFRA), and TSCA, put a qualifying word, such as "unreasonable" in front of the word "risk." This construction implies that some risks are to be tolerated, and, in practice, means risks from a substance are to be weighed against other factors in the process of deciding whether and how to regulate. TSCA requires that "the benefits . . . for various uses, . . . the economic consequences of the rule, . . . the effect on the national economy, small business, technological innovation, the environment, and public health" [TSCA sec. 6(c)(D)] be considered in deciding whether a substance does or does not pose an unreasonable risk.

Balancing is equated with some kind of comparison of benefits and costs, but none of the laws explicitly requires formal benefit-cost analysis. For instance, the Committee on Interstate and Foreign Commerce Report (65) on TSCA says that, "a formal benefit-cost analysis under which a monetary value is assigned to the risks" is not required. And a court decision about an action taken under CPSA declared that the Consumer Product Safety Commission "does not have to conduct an 'elaborate cost-benefit analysis' to conclude that 'unreasonable risk' exists" (145).

All of the laws provide for the regulation of carcinogens which threaten human health. In the case of the balancing laws Congress requires that other considerations be balanced against the health risk. In practice health risk signals an agency that it should consider regulation; the stringency of that regulation is at least partially determined by balancing.

Technology-Based Laws

CWA and CAA are, in general, technology based. For instance, CAA directs the Administrator of the Environmental Protection Agency (EPA) to reduce particulate emissions to some percentage of existing levels. The regulations may be "technology-forcing" because new techniques may be required to achieve the reduction. In other cases, the laws specify that pollution control is to be achieved by using "best practical technology" (BPT) or "best available technology" (BAT). Such regulations do not force new technology, but bring all control efforts up to standards established by existing control technologies.

An important consideration of the technology-based laws is that EPA has not yet been required to produce studies to show that the imposition of new standards will improve public health. Imposition of the standards reduces exposures, and in the case of carcinogens, given a nonthreshold approach to carcinogenic risks, it follows that reducing exposures should improve public health.

The Occupational Safety and Health Act (OSH Act) requires:

> The Secretary, in promulgating standards . . . shall set the standard which most adequately assures, to the extent feasible, on the basis of the best available evidence, that no employee will suffer material impairment of health or functional capacity . . . . In addition to the attainment of the highest degree of health and safety protection for the employee, other considerations shall be . . . the feasibility of the standards . . . (OSHA; sec. 6(b)(5))

In the sense that feasible has a technological meaning, the OSH Act can be considered as a technology-based law. However, the Supreme Court may issue a decision in a case involving an OSH Act standard for exposure to cotton dust, that will determine whether or not benefits and costs have to be calculated to justify the standard. That case may not be heard since the Occupational Safety and Health Administration (OSHA) has withdrawn its proposed standard.

Freeman (131) has argued that the "technology-based" laws require balancing, pointing out that BPT implies balancing. How else can "practical" be defined? Likewise, deciding what is BAT involves balancing costs of the technology against the expected gains.

Doniger (95) cites a significant difference between technology-based and balancing laws. He suggests that once a hazard is identified under a technology-based law, the next step is to determine the best means to control it and then decide if there are any compelling reasons to back off from the best means. Under a balancing law, he says, once a hazard is identified, the next step is to quantify the risks it presents in order to balance those against costs of control.

The tripartite division of the laws—risk, balancing, technology—while useful, does not neatly describe all the laws when subjected to closer inspection. Complex laws contain sections that have different bases, and carcinogen regulations are generally developed under risk-based or balancing sections of the those laws.

An Example of Balancing

FDA can balance costs and benefits in regulating carcinogens in food except when the carcinogen is a food additive. An example of that balancing is the FDA (124) regulation of polychlorinated biphenyls (PCBs) in fish. FDA considered three possible levels for PCBs in fish from the Great Lakes (see table 36). Fish that contain PCBs up to the FDA-established tolerance level can be sold; those having more PCBs cannot be sold.

Few (perhaps no) people dispute that PCBs are a human health hazard. The acceptance of that fact is amply demonstrated by TSCA (sec. 6(e)) directing that PCBs be regulated. The in-

Table 36.—An Example of Balancing Cancer Risk v. Revenue Loss. The FDA's Setting a Tolerance for PCBs in Fish

Proposed tolerance ppm	Projected cancer cases/year	Estimated loss of revenue
5	46.8	$ 0.6 million
2	34.3	5.7 million
1	21.0	$16.0 million

formation in table 36 may illustrate that once a risk is accepted as real, i.e., worthy of regulatory attention, the stringency of the regulation is set by economic or other factors. It is reasonable to assume that more cancer would result from PCBs at 5 ppm than at 1 ppm, but given the uncertainties of quantitative risk assessment, it is difficult or impossible to accept that the projected number of cases is accurate. Nevertheless, FDA decided that "the balance between public health protection and loss of food is properly struck by a 2-ppm tolerance."

The Precautionary Nature of the Definitions of Toxic Risks in the Laws

Reduction of exposures to carcinogens are intended to prevent cancer. Given the long latent period between exposure and overt disease symptoms, prevention must depend on the identification of carcinogens in test systems. The alternative, waiting for human evidence of carcinogenicity exposes some portion of the population to a carcinogen. Even if the substance is then withdrawn completely, the legacy of the exposure would be a continuing number of cases as some of the exposed people develop cancer. Reflecting these concerns, the definitions of toxic substances under which carcinogens are regulated do not require evidence of human disease. In accepting evidence from other sources, each of the laws is precautionary.

The Delaney clause is most direct; it accepts evidence of animal carcinogenicity as sufficient to ban a food additive. Section 112 of CAA calls for regulation of pollutants that "may cause . . . [an] increase in mortality;" RCRA and the Safe Drinking Water Act also use a "may" construction in defining toxics. TSCA directs EPA to require testing of new chemicals which "may present an unreasonable risk" (sec. 5), but has a more stringent, but still precautionary phrase, "presents or will present an unreasonable risk" in section 6 which authorizes regulating a toxic substance already present in commerce.

Regulatory Definitions of Carcinogens

The Delaney clause contains an operational definition for carcinogens:

> . . . no additive shall be deemed safe if it is found, after tests which are appropriate for the evaluation of food additives, to induce cancer in man or animal.

Although the other laws do not define what properties of a substance make it a carcinogen, a number of Federal documents (e.g., 180,279) specify what technical results agencies will consider in deciding about carcinogenicity.

In most cases, animal data are the only basis for decisions about carcinogenicity. Seemingly endless arguments can be mounted about test results: that the tested animal may not be a surrogate for humans, that the dose was too high, that lesions in animals may not parallel human disease states. Given the current state of knowledge, those argument cannot be answered to everyone's satisfaction. In the absence of agreement among all concerned parties, agency statements about methods to be used in making decisions about carcinogenicity represent the Federal Government's position. It can only be expected that the methods will remain disputed until basic science provides more information about carcinogenic mechanisms and human response to carcinogens.

Degree of Protection

A balance between health and other considerations is struck by defining the degree of protection in each law. The Delaney clause, in which the balance is on the side of health, requires banning and the maximum degree of protection.

The other definitions of degree of protection in table 35 are not so clear, and at least one posed a difficult task for a regulatory agency. Section 112 of CAA is the basis for EPA's (111) proposed airborne carcinogen policy. It directs:

> The Administrator shall establish any such standard at the level which in his judgment provides an ample margin of safety to protect the public health from such hazardous pollutant [CAA sec. 112(b)(1)(B)].

The proposed airborne carcinogen policy (111) states that EPA has, "as a matter of prudent health policy, taken the position that in the absence of identifiable effect thresholds, carcinogens pose some risk of cancer at any exposure above zero." The position that no threshold can be assumed for carcinogenicity makes it impossible to achieve an "ample margin of safety" unless zero emissions are imposed. However, EPA also decided that zero emissions for some substances would impose a too heavy economic burden, and that such controls were not what Congress had in mind. EPA solved this problem by proposing that BAT controls will be imposed, and if they leave an unreasonable residual risk, further controls will be considered (111):

> Final standards for source categories presenting significant risks to public health would, as a minimum, require such sources to use best available technology to reduce emissions. If, however, the risk remaining after the application of best available technology is determined to be unreasonable, further control is required.

A striking contrast in the use of the words "ample margin of safety" is seen in comparing CAA (sec. 112) and CWA (sec. 307). Under CWA, the first level of regulation is to be BAT which is also the language chosen for the proposed airborne carcinogen policy, after it had been concluded that an "ample margin of safety," the language of section 112, was unattainable. If after BAT has been applied, residual risk remains, "effluent standards" may be written to reduce effluents to achieve "an ample margin of safety" (see table 37).

Table 37.—Ample Margin of Safety as Used in Two Laws

	Clean Air Act	Clean Water Act
Level of protection	Sec. 112(b) (1) (B) "*ample margin of safety* to protect the public health..."	Sec. 307(a) (2) in accordance with sections 301(b) (2) (A) and 304(b) (2) sets "effluent limitations" according to BAT[a].
Regulatory language	No threshold level is assumed for carcinogens and an *ample margin of safety* is unattainable therefore BAT[a] is imposed.	
What happens if BAT[a] is judged inadequate?	Stricter measures can be employed to control residual unreasonable risk.	Sec. 307(a) (4) an "effluent standard" can be promulgated to provide "an *ample margin of safety.*"

[a]Best available technology.

AGENCY ADMINISTRATIVE PROCEDURES FOR CARCINOGEN REGULATION

The Administrative Procedures Act of 1946

The executive branch of Government administers hundreds of different laws. Agency procedures for carcinogen regulation as well as other subject areas are substantially dictated by the Administrative Procedures Act of 1946, specific formulas mandated by Congress within certain enabling statutes, and, in certain cases, by Executive orders. To varying degrees these formulas aim to safeguard individual rights and due process, while balancing potentially conflicting national goals and policies.

The Administrative Procedures Act (APA) was passed in 1946 after more than 10 years of painstaking study and drafting. Since then, there has been no major reform of regulatory procedures. According to Senator McCarran (228), who supported and explained the bill before the Senate, its purpose is to:

. . . improve the administration of justice by prescribing fair administrative procedure . . . . [it] is a bill of rights for the hundreds of thousands of Americans whose affairs are controlled or regulated in some way or another by agencies of the Federal Government. It is designed to provide guaranties of due process in administrative procedures.

APA is generally applicable to all regulatory agencies and sets forth required procedures for agencies to follow when they engage in rulemaking (e.g., rules which set standards) and adjudication (e.g., licensing). The procedures involved may range from those which allow informal, mostly written, decisions without prior hearings, to those which require formal adjudicatory hearings complete with the right to cross-examination. While APA contains no specific guidance on informal decisionmaking requirements, different levels of procedural detail have developed depending on the kinds of issues involved. As has been noted:

In terms of ordering the procedural values, one might organize (categories of administrative decisions) on a scale of maximum to minimum procedures. At the top of the scale, the hearing procedures employed may come close to the full adjudicative model, since the issues at stake resemble those decided in the civil or criminal process. Toward the bottom of the scale (e.g., planning and policy making) there may be few, if any, procedural requirements . . . . Even in these categories, however, certain procedural ingredients appear; in effect, notice and reasons requirements approximate a minimum procedural model (355).

Most of the agencies discussed in this study use "informal rulemaking" to make regulatory decisions. Therefore, the minimal procedural requirements apply of providing public notice of proposed and final rules, and an opportunity for affected interests to comment. However, specific procedural requirements are imposed by some enabling statutes. TSCA, for instance, provides an opportunity for an informal hearing with cross-examination as a part of the rulemaking process. It goes beyond the more simplified APA informal rulemaking, but does not go as far as to require APA formal rulemaking procedures.

Judicial Review

APA and some enabling statutes provide for judicial review of the process by which agency decisions are made. In the case of informal rulemaking, the tendency is to require that agency performance not be, "arbitrary, capricious, an abuse of discretion, or otherwise not in accordance with law" (5 U.S.C. sec. 706). Judicial review then examines the agency record to see whether the agency has provided notice, responded to comments, and given reasons for its actions to the public.

A more stringent judicial review is applied to formal rulemaking. In those cases, the court may "set aside agency action, findings, and conclusions found to be . . . unsupported by substantial evidence" (5 U.S.C. sec. 706). The court must decide whether or not the agency record contains substantial evidence to support the proposed action, but there is the presumption that the court will defer to agency expertise on technical matters contained in the record.

There is a tendency for judicial review of informal rules under the "arbitrary and capricious" standard to be increasingly stringent to the degree that it is converging on the "substantial evidence" standard prescribed by APA for judicial review of adjudicatory and formal rulemaking decisions (20). The reasonable conclusion is that both standards are coming to mean the same thing in terms of agency accountability when subjected to judicial review. As recently noted by Judge McGowan (231):

If you're raising the question of the difference between arbitrary and capricious review and substantial evidence in the record, I think the judiciary is finally having to accept the fact that, because Congress has used them so loosely and so interchangeably, we have to assure ourselves that there is very little difference, if any, between them.

The practical effect of this merging of judicial review standards is to require closer judicial scrutiny of agency records and evidence in all reviewable actions. Some argue that agency flexibility and innovation, even to the extent allowed by APA, to meet the particular situation of each case has been almost eliminated by the threat of more critical judicial review. There is some concern that these developments have caused confusion in the courts and agencies, as well as worked considerable mischief on procedural regularity and the unifying function that APA was originally designed to perform for all branches of government and the public (355).

As the subject matter of regulation becomes increasingly complex, agencies are required to work more and more with incomplete or approximate data. Scientific uncertainty, compounded by the need to balance and value often conflicting goals, has raised questions about the continued workability of the present regulatory framework.

Regulatory Reform

The following remarks reflect some of the frustrations with the present system which are feeding the calls for reform. In a paper presented before the National Conference on Federal Regulation, September 1979, Richard Neustadt, then-Assistant Director of the White House Domestic Policy Staff, observed (275):

[The 1946 Administrative Procedures Act] predated most of the health and safety programs, concentrated on issues of procedural fairness, and took little account of the problems of economic impact and inconsistent policies.

Cutler (76), in expressing the views of the American Bar Association Commission on Law and Economy, has charged:

[W]e have a regulatory system in which . . . the buck stops nowhere. We pursue each of our numerous and conflicting and competing goals with single-minded devotion regardless of the effect of one upon another.

Numerous regulatory reform proposals have been generated during the past few years, creating a widespread attack on the existing Federal regulatory system. The lack of effective balancing mechanisms in light of present economic and other national goals and policies has been raised with increasing frequency as a major failing. Furthermore, as observed by Costle (69), the concern for reform extends to cancer regulation:

> There is no question about the need for better management of the regulatory process. For example, I will be announcing in the next several days a national policy on the regulation of carcinogens [306]. There are 21 statutes on the books that authorize the regulation of carcinogens. Thus, the necessity of having a consistent national policy is self-evident.

> But the issue of regulating carcinogens also illustrates a larger point, which is that we have not had a national road map of the cumulative effect of regulation, nor of where that regulation is taking us in terms of conflicting national goals . . . [We] have lacked a systematic way of tracking, effectively and intelligently, the multitude of regulatory activities that are ongoing every day.

Many of the recent regulatory reform proposals have called for substantive change through deregulation or severely restricted regulation.

Procedural Reforms

One category of reform proposals focuses on procedural improvements within the existing regulatory framework to make regulation more efficient, effective, and responsive to public needs. Through various means these efforts aim to improve agency administrative procedures, agency analytic and management capability, and public input for better regulatory decisionmaking. The executive branch, in the present and in previous administrations, has acted to improve the procedure through Executive or-

ders. Legislative reforms are proposed in Congress.

Executive Order No. 12044 (Under President Carter) and No. 12291 (Under President Reagan)

In a major step toward regulatory reform at the executive level, President Carter issued Executive Order No. 12044 in March 1978. It directed each executive branch agency to publish a semiannual agenda of significant regulations under review or development, to provide greater opportunity for public participation, and to prepare regulatory analyses on all proposed regulations that may have major economic consequences (an annual economic effect of $100 million or more). To assist individual agencies in meeting the goals of this order, President Carter established the Regulatory Analysis Review Group, to prepare reports on particularly important proposed rules, and the Regulatory Council, to prepare a biannual regulatory calendar and deal with areas of overlapping and conflicting regulations.

This order had a significant and controversial impact on agencies charged by Congress with regulating risks to health, safety, and the environment. Office of Management and Budget (OMB) guidance encouraged the use of cost-benefit and other economic analyses to resolve health, safety, and environmental problems. However, there was no uniform policy or guidance for dealing with the methodological limitations of cost-benefit analysis—use of discount rates, how to value health and environmental benefits, how to allocate costs and benefits to different societal groups, etc. (20). In spite of the order's alleged faults and deficiencies, the Administrator and others at EPA, one of the agencies most experienced with this order, defended it as an encouraging beginning to resolving regulatory conflicts and shaping agency decisions in a manner that reflects overall policy objectives (69).

President Reagan issued Executive Order No. 12291 in February 1981. It preserved many features of the earlier order and provides for an increased role of OMB and cost-benefit analyses in deciding about regulations.

A conflict that arose under the old order is expected to continue. Some segments of society want to know the contents of a proposed draft regulation both when it leaves the agency and when it returns from OMB. Presently no public record is required of such drafts, and, in fact, such materials cannot be disclosed under the Freedom of Information Act. Protection of such documents is seen as necessary for the smooth functioning of the agencies and to allow regulators and decisionmakers to explore ideas and positions before going to the public with them. Resolution of the conflict between the public's right to information and the Government's desire for confidentiality may be reached in the courts.

Legislation

In 1979, the administration transmitted to Congress a bill that would have strengthened the reforms enacted by Executive Order No. 12044, made them permanent, and applied them to all regulatory agencies, including the independent regulatory commissions (S. 755). It also would have overhauled key parts of the Administrative Procedures Act. Other bills of the 96th Congress proposed procedural changes, some of which paralleled portions of the administration's bill (e.g., S. 262, S. 755, S. 1291, S. 2147, and H.R. 3263).

Several proposals require an agency regulatory impact analysis before issuance of major rules. Many require that the agencies set deadlines for rulemaking and a schedule for review of significant existing rules. There are new provisions for agency rulemaking and adjudication, appointment of administrative law judges, and greater involvement of the Administrative Conference. Measures to increase public input include establishment of a Government-wide program of assistance to public intervenors.

The Regulatory Flexibility Act of 1980 (Public Law 96-354) was enacted to lessen the impact of Federal regulation on small businesses and small Government units. This law requires, where there is a likelihood that agency rules may have a "significant economic impact on a substantial number of small entities," that the agency prepare annual agendas for such rules and a flexibility analysis of each proposed rule. This analysis is for the purpose of explaining the rationale for agency action, considering flexible regulatory proposals, and examining alternatives which might minimize economic impact. While the scope of this law is somewhat limited, determined movement toward procedural reform is clear.

Structural Reforms Through Shifts in Oversight

Another category of reform proposals offers a more far-reaching approach by shifting existing regulatory authority to Congress, the courts, or the executive branch. The proposals call for structural reform in the sense that regulatory authority and, ultimately, political power are redistributed. They challenge the fundamental role of administrative agencies as they now exist, by imposing new outside oversight and review controls. Examples of these proposals include the legislative veto, the presidential veto, and the Bumpers amendment.

The Legislative Veto

A major study on Federal regulation by the Senate Committee on Governmental Affairs during the 95th Congress recommended that Congress substantially change its agency oversight processes to improve evaluation, coordination, and systematic review of agency programs. However, when it came to the legislative veto, it concluded that although this approach "may be appropriate in limited situations, the Congress should reject use of the legislative veto for regulatory agency rules . . . [and] should also refrain from routinely adding a legislative veto provision to regulatory agency statutes" (63).

Nevertheless, a number of reform proposals would enact various forms of the legislative veto. Depending on the bill, the approach would subject some or all agency proposed and existing rules to congressional scrutiny, with either House having authority to veto the rule within a specified time (e.g., H.R. 1033, 96th Cong.; H.R. 460, H.R. 495, H.R. 532, H.R. 1858, and S. 1463, 95th Cong.).

Serious questions have been raised about the efficiency of such an all-encompassing approach, particularly in complex areas of regulation, such as those dealing with carcinogens. The legislative veto option could conceivably result in technical decisionmaking being transferred from expert agencies to generalists in Congress. There may be some constitutional problems as well, concerning the separation of powers, congressional delegation of authority, the role of the President, and bicameralism where only a one-House veto is required.

Increased Presidential Authority: The Presidential Veto

Another structural reform proposal with far-reaching consequences would give the President increased authority over regulatory decisions. Again, there are a variety of forms to this proposal. One generating ongoing debate was developed by the American Bar Association (4). It would authorize the President to direct an agency to take up or reconsider and modify certain critical kinds of regulation, require cost-benefit regulatory analysis, and subject the President's actions to limited congressional review. While an agency would continue its normal rulemaking procedure, the President would have, in effect, final rulemaking authority over critical areas, since he could direct the agency to reconsider, modify, or reverse its decision.

As with the legislative veto proposals, a fundamental impetus for this kind of approach is the perceived loss of Government accountability resulting from overly broad delegations of authority to the agencies. Because of the many often conflicting national goals, to which the President must be responsive, and the narrower responsibility of single-mission agencies, greater Presidential authority is seen as needed for an effective balancing process and more responsible and accountable Government.

Questions similar to those raised with the legislative veto are again raised here. Constitu-

tional and political issues related to overly broad delegation of legislative authority; Presidential efficacy, particularly when overseeing technical agencies; further delay and bureaucratic overload; and maintaining procedural safeguards are all concerns which must be examined with this approach to regulatory reform. Additionally, the shift in decisionmaking from the agencies, which have technical expertise, to individuals in the Office of the President who may lack technical expertise, can be viewed as inappropriate.

A Greater Role for the Courts: The Bumpers Amendment

Some structural reform proposals would shift power to the courts. A major example, which continues to spark interest is the Bumpers amendment, adopted by the Senate as a floor amendment in September 1979 (S. 111, 96th Cong., 1st sess., 1979). The amendment would do two things. First, it would remove the presumption of validity that accompanies a regulation when it is challenged in court. Second, it would require an agency to support the validity of a rule by preponderance of the evidence, a higher standard than either "arbitrary or capricious" or "substantial evidence."

The amendment is seen as an attempt to curb problems associated with overregulation, and the courts would play a greater role and have greater influence. The role of the courts would extend to both overregulation and underregulation, since the courts also would be the forum for challenges that an agency is not regulating vigorously enough.

Levin (206) says that application of the amendment raises many ambiguities and difficulties of interpretation. While agencies could still be expected to conduct normal rulemaking activities, it appears that the proposal would require the courts to give little or no weight to an agency's decision. If so, the very reason for administrative agencies to retain expertise may be undercut. The likely outcome would be more litigation and challenge of regulations. Some observers have expressed doubts about the amendment's ability to facilitate more effective and efficient regulatory programs, especially in light of the increased workloads to come to the Federal courts. Others are of the opinion that agencies, knowing of the judicial review to come, would develop stronger cases.

Substantive Change: Deregulation

Some of the most drastic regulatory reform proposals call for deregulation or severely restricted regulation. These proposals raise a presumption against an agency's continued existence and legislative renewal except where there is explicit action to reauthorize.

One of the most popular concepts involved has been labeled "sunset"—in other words, an agency or function will expire by a certain date unless there is enacted in the meantime a statute reauthorizing the activity in question. Various versions of regulatory sunset proposals have been put forth for a number of years (e.g., S. 2 and S. 445, 96th Cong.). Some would require that every regulatory program covered by a sunset requirement be reviewed at a minimum once every 10 years. The most drastic would call for termination of the program, with no provisions to safeguard against termination by inaction, if not authorized by Congress within this review period. Intermediate versions would require systematic review and reexamination of existing programs and legislation by the authorizing committees, with no automatic termination.

The most extreme regulatory reform is outright deregulation. In such areas as airline operations and natural gas production, this course has been taken. Apparently, the fundamental consideration underlying deregulation must be whether the objectives for which regulation was initiated can be accomplished by self-regulation in the marketplace. While most people view this approach as inappropriate for health, safety, and environmental matters, commentators have written about movement in this direction (59). For the present, the conclusions of the Senate study (63) of Federal regulation cited above provide insight into the question of marketplace possibilities for self-regulation:

> Generally speaking, "free market" solutions are not, in the environmental area, a viable option. The activities of a single polluter affect thousands and even millions of other firms and individuals, with whom there usually are no ongoing market relationships. Such relationships do not exist, in large part because neither firms nor individuals have clear property rights to environmental resources.

ESTIMATES OF RISK AND REDUCTION OF CARCINOGENIC EXPOSURES

Risk Assessment

Recent years have seen a proliferation of organizations devoted to the study of risk. As examples, the National Academy of Sciences (NAS) recently formed the "Committee on Risk and Decision Making" that will consider how society and its institutions might better assess, compare, and manage health, safety and environmental risks. The National Science Foundation has an active "Risk Analysis Program" in its Division of Policy Research and Analysis, and several universities sponsor institutes for risk analysis.

A number of different terms—risk assessment, risk analysis, and risk evaluation—are used to describe the process of associating a specific risk with a substance. Figure 27 is an example of a three-step process for making an estimate of carcinogenic risk and a fourth step which lists other factors that may be considered in making a decision about reducing risk. The figure shows where the methods described in this assessment are used.

The first step, hazard identification, is necessary to separate carcinogens from other substances. Some laws, the Delaney clause as dis-

Figure 27.—Assessing Carcinogenic Risks and Considering Other Factors in Making a Decision about Risk Management

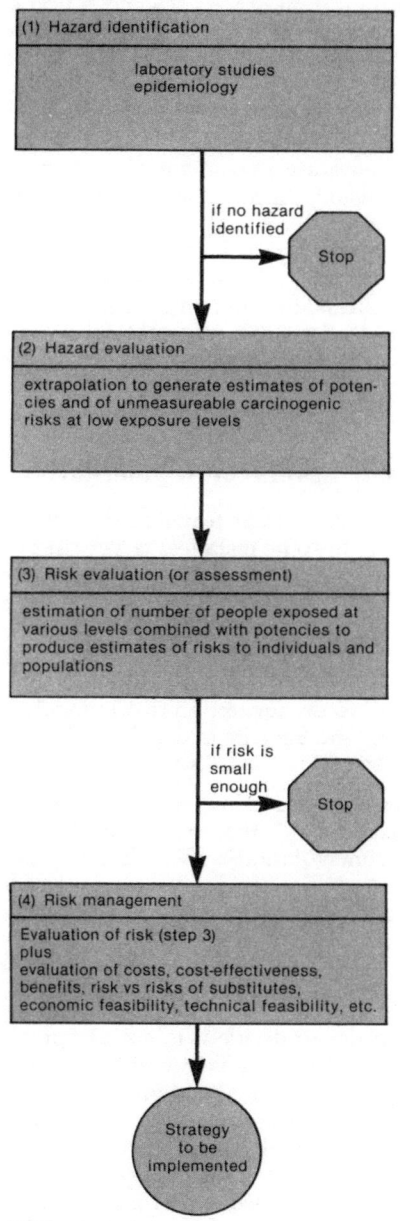

SOURCE: Diesler (81)

cussed above, require only this step to make a regulatory decision. The second step, risk evaluation, produces qualitative and quantitative expressions of the hazard associated with the substance. The quantitative expressions allow a rough ordering of hazards.

The third step, risk assessment, which can produce a quantitative estimate of the potential effect of the substance on humans, is limited by all the uncertainties involved in hazard identification and evaluation. Additionally, in this step, other uncertainties are introduced along with the estimates of the number of people exposed and the levels of their exposure. Some observers object to the third step because of these many uncertainties. However, uncertainties do not make it impossible to attempt to quantify risk asessments; they do affect the form the assessment takes and the form in which the result is presented.

The third step is necessary before quantitative comparisons can be made between risks and other factors. Such comparisons are shown in step 4.

The critical function of step 3 is quantitative risk assessment. The generally good agreement that epidemiology and laboratory tests can identify carcinogens does not extend to agreement that currently available data and risk assessment techniques can accurately predict the level of human risk, and the usefulness of quantitative risk assessment is argued.

Some observers view quantitative risk assessment efforts, especially when applied to chronic health problems, including cancer, as premature. They see the techniques as uncertain, the results they produce as potentially misleading, and express concern that the users of the results do not appreciate the reservations attached to the numbers generated in quantitative risk assessments.

The advocates of quantitative risk assessment say that the methods are necessary to decide which of the many identified carcinogens present intolerable risks and which do not. To counter the argument that the techniques are imperfect, they cite the great amount of interest in risk assessment and say that the methods are being improved.

Quantitative risk assessment is likely to take on increasing importance in Federal decision making about carcinogens. For instance, the requirement for benefit-cost analysis under Executive Order No. 12291 will result in greater demands for quantitative risk assessment. Additionally, the Supreme Court decision about workplace exposure to benzene (337) apparently requires that OSHA make some estimate of risk to support regulations. The fact that benzene is a carcinogen was not disputed in the case, but the court returned the proposed standard to the agency for reconsideration because OSHA had not found,

> . . . that the toxic substance [benzene at the level currently encountered in the workplace] . . . poses a significant health risk in the workplace and that a new lower standard is . . . "reasonably necessary or appropriate to provide safe or healthful employment"(20).

The requirement to show a "significant health risk" will surely result in greater pressure on OSHA to estimate the number of workers likely to suffer ill-effects from exposures. The pressures for use of risk assessment will probably increase, and opponents will continue to voice concern about its uncertainties.

Limits to Quantitative Risk Assessment

Rowe (316) draws attention to limits that he sees surrounding the accuracy of quantitative risk assessment. In particular he cites problems with choosing an extrapolation model, the widely variant estimates produced by the use of different models (see ch. 5), and the problems inherent in animal tests because of the relatively small numbers of animals that can be tested (see ch. 4). Rowe suggests that results of testing particular substances in short-term tests and bioassays be established as benchmarks. Then, as other substances are tested, they can be classified as less hazardous, equally hazardous, or more hazardous than the benchmark substances. At the same time, data about use and exposure can be obtained, so that the number of

people at risk, along with potency, can be considered in deciding what next to do.

Importantly, in Rowe's scheme, a next step is to consider whether or not additional testing might change the conclusion reached on presently available data. To facilitate making that decision, Rowe developed a statistic to allow consideration of the probability that a test will provide information that might alter a previously made decision. Application of the statistic estimates the limits of knowledge that are attainable. Considering the limits of tests and extrapolation models will allow decisionmakers to select additional testing only when the tests will yield more definitive information. When that condition does not prevail, the decisionmaker can choose to do nothing or to consider various methods to restrict exposures.

"Trigger" Levels for Regulation

Individuals in their private lives accept nonzero risks. In some instances larger risks are accepted, presumably, because the benefits associated with the risk-taking are also large. In other situations, smaller risks are avoided, again presumably, because the benefits are seen as not worth even the small risk. Such observations lead to the suggestion that individuals balance risks and benefits in deciding which voluntarily assumed risks are "acceptable."

Exposures to carcinogens in air, water, the workplace, and other environments are different from voluntary risks. In few cases is it possible for an individual to know the identity and magnitude of the risk. In many cases, the individual has no choice but to bear the unknown risk because contact cannot be avoided.

It is not necessary, in all cases, to quantify a risk in order to decide it is not acceptable. An example of such an unacceptable, unreasonable risk is the use of thalidomide by pregnant women. The association of that drug with children suffering multiple anatomic abnormalities led to a suspension of its use. A more recent example was the association of a particular brand of tampon with toxic shock syndrome. Before a quantitative evaluation of the lifetime risk of toxic shock syndrome was published, the manufacturer recalled the product. In these two cases, substitute products were readily available, and the cost of avoiding the risk was largely restricted to the lost sales of the manufacturers.

Regulatory agencies identify and quantify risks, and the ability to quantify risks has produced suggestions for managing risks based on their size. A small chance of risk can be set as a "floor," and substances presenting a risk less than the floor might be considered acceptable. Risks above the floor level would be divided into two groups. Intermediate risks would be considered for reduction, and benefits and risks would be balanced in making a regulatory decision. Above a still higher level of risk, no balancing would be necessary, and any substance presenting a risk of that magnitude or higher would have to be regulated (3).

Products of a quantitative risk assessment (see fig. 27, step 3) can be estimates of the lifetime risk of cancer to: 1) members of the general population; and 2) to members of highly exposed populations. These risks are expressed in scientific notation as 10^{-4}, 10^{-5}, 10^{-6} (or as fractions, 1 chance in 10,000, 1 in 100,000, and 1 in 1,000,000, respectively). Carcinogens differ a millionfold in potency as measured in laboratory animals, and more potent ones are associated with higher risks (10^{-3}) and less potent ones with lower risks (10^{-7}).

Albert (3) and others have suggested that substances associated with individual lifetime risks of 10^{-5} might be considered as presenting risks so low that they require no action to reduce them further. Such low, negligible risks would represent a "floor" on risks. An idea of the magnitude of this risk is furnished by recalling that a 10^{-5} lifetime risk means that one person of 100,000 exposed at that level is expected to develop cancer from that exposure. Currently, about 20,000 of every 100,000 Americans die of cancer. Exposure of 100,000 people to a substance that increases risk by 10^{-5} could increase the number of cancer deaths to 20,001. Whether or not this number seems reasonable, it may be important to consider that a lifetime risk of 10^{-5} for the U.S. population (220 million people) is equal to 2,200 cancer cases in those people's life-

spans. The annual number of cancer deaths from exposing the U.S. population to a 10^{-5} risk would be about 30, assuming a lifespan of 70 years.

A fundamental objection to the idea that some fraction of the population might be allowed to die because of exposure to a risk that is viewed as acceptable is expressed in an argument called "the murder of the statistical person." If the identity of the 30 people who died annually as a result of a 10^{-5} risk were known, there is little doubt that much greater effort would be expanded to reduce the risk. Objections to the idea of society deciding that some risks are negligible are raised by those who consider that statistical people as well as identified people deserve protection.

It is apparently more difficult to suggest a level of risk so high that it demands regulatory action than it is to suggest a level so low that it requires none. Nevertheless, toward the high end of the risk scale, agreement might be reached that an exposure that produced a lifetime risk of cancer of 10^{-2} (1 in 100) is so high that the Government should regulate it as a health risk with little or no regard for other considerations. The magnitude of this risk may be compared to the tenfold higher chance (10^{-1} lifetime risk) of cancer that is voluntarily borne by lifelong smokers (362).

Another consideration is that the low-level risks, those of 10^{-5} or less, add up. If there are ten 10^{-5} risks and the risks are additive, their total risk is 10^{-4}. (Of course, if synergism exists among any of the 10, the combined risk from both might greatly exceed 10^{-4}). What is to be done about the next identified 10^{-5} risk? Should it be regulated, or should small risks, even if there are 100 or 1,000 or more of them go unregulated?

If agreement could be reached on such limits, risks above a certain level (10^{-3} to 10^{-2}) might be declared unreasonable no matter what, and risks below a certain level (10^{-5}) might be declared reasonable or acceptable or negligible. In between, the risks that range from 10^{-5} up to 10^{-3} or 10^{-2} would require balancing of the risks and benefits to decide whether or not to regulate.

The inaccuracy of the risk estimates alarms many people. Crouch and Wilson (72) find "good correlations" between cancer rates measured in animals and those detected in humans due to exposure to the same chemicals. The number of chemicals for which data are available is small (fewer than 20) and the "good correlation" is good within a factor of 10 or 100. In other words, an estimated risk of 10^{-5} might be as high as 10^{-3} or as low as 10^{-7}.

Deisler (80) has approached the problem of the existence of many small risks by suggesting that a ceiling be placed on total risk in "exposure situations." He cites industrial exposure as one situation and discusses a maximum allowable amount of cancer that might be set as tolerable for workplace exposures. As was pointed out earlier, estimates for occupational contributions to cancer vary from less than 5 percent to about 40 percent, and Deisler (80) suggests:

> . . . the first interim goal should be . . . to assure that industrially related cancer becomes *less* than a truly small fraction of today's total cancer incidence in the United States . . .

As an example of a possible interim goal, he suggests that workplace exposures be set so that they account for 1.5 percent of the total cancer burden. The 1.5 percent is only an example, and Deisler suggests that the selection of a goal might be negotiated in a public forum, possibly through a congressional commission.

When a ceiling is established, the risks within the exposure situation would be inventoried. If total risk exceeds the ceiling, the risk would be reduced by addressing one or more individual exposures. This appears to be a cost-effective system because the easiest-to-control, least costly-to-control exposures would be attacked first. If the inventory of risks totaled less than the ceiling, the ceiling could be reduced. The individual exposures in the inventory are expected to interact additively, but allowances could be made for synergisms if they occur. The ceiling also provides a method to deal with the identification of previously unrecognized carcinogens in an exposure situation. Such a carcinogen would be, as a first step, controlled to the point that the ceiling is not exceeded.

Despite the demonstrated existence of unacceptable, unreasonable (and generally unquantitated) risks, it has been impossible to assign "trigger" risk levels. Deciding on the "trigger," 10^{-3} or 10^{-2} on the high side, 10^{-5} or 10^{-6} on the low side would be difficult, and problems with the accuracy of the estimates and equity in that those who most directly bear risks may not most directly benefit are problems to be solved. Currently, quantitative risk assessment does not provide a tidy fix for the dilemma of deciding if and when to regulate. At the same time the fact that "acceptable" and "reasonable" risks are discussed implies that not all risks are equal and that society has the task to decide which are to be regulated and which are not.

LOCATIONS OF FEDERAL CARCINOGENIC RISK ASSESSMENT ACTIVITIES

Carcinogenic risk assessment involves a group of people considering the available evidence, drawing conclusions from the data, and, using methods they accept, deciding whether or not the substance is carcinogenic and, in some cases, estimating carcinogenic potency or human risk. Groups which have prepared statements about methods to be used in evaluating data differ in their interests and responsibilities, and their statements reflect the differences. In addition, there is much discussion about who should consider the data, apply the methods, and make the decisions.

Scientists in each regulatory agency now evaluate data about carcinogenicity of substances that may be regulated by their own agency. They may consider advice from expert committees in their decisions. The decision is then forwarded to the individual named in the appropriate law who announces the decision and his intentions to act on it.

The Office of Science and Technology Policy (OSTP) (281) proposed a change from agency-by-agency decisionmaking. It suggested that all carcinogenic risk determinations be made in a single governmental body. Representative Wampler proposed such a body in a bill he introduced; the American Industrial Health Council (AIHC) (10) and Markey (222) have also suggested central locations for making technical decisions for regulatory purposes. These proposals differ from each other, but all have in common a central panel of technical experts.

Panel proposals are all directed at decisions made by or for regulatory agencies. At the research agency level, the National Toxicology Program (NTP) has established a Peer-Review Panel of Experts to review draft reports from its bioassay program. The panel is to assure (273):

. . . carcinogenesis bioassays have been carried out using the prevailing scientific state-of-the-knowledge and that the interpretations and conclusions reflect a logical and accurate analysis of the collected experimental data.

The panel can either approve draft reports or return them to NTP for revision. If panel members disagree about whether a report and its conclusions should be approved, a majority and minority report can be filed. The panel is composed of 14 experts from academe, environmental groups, and industry and began meeting in late 1980.

The issuance of the Interagency Regulatory Liaison Group (IRLG) guidelines (180) provides some uniformity to governmental decisions because all agencies are to use similar methods for evaluating risks. Agencies appreciate that consideration by nonagency scientists may improve their decisionmaking and may call upon experts to aid them. For instance, the proposed OSHA Generic Cancer Policy (279) allowed the Secretary of Labor to assemble a panel of Government experts to cooperate in making decisions about carcinogens. Such interagency workgroups are a common response of the Federal

Government to complex and sensitive technical issues.

Some legislation requires that agency decisions be discussed with advisory groups of non-Federal experts. Under FIFRA, EPA is required to refer any decisions to initiate a pesticide cancellation to EPA's Scientific Advisory Board (SAB). SAB review comes at a point in time after EPA has made a decision about whether or not the pesticide presents a toxic hazard, and it is an example of an advisory panel functioning in a review capacity.

FDA has made extensive use of technical advisory panels. In 1962, FDA was required for the first time to screen drugs for efficacy. Thousands of drugs were involved, and the task was immense. FDA asked that NAS assemble technical panels for different types of drugs and that the panels advise FDA about which drugs were not efficacious. The panels were quite successful and since then, FDA has added technical panels to advise about drugs, medical devices, and food additives.

The augmentation of agency expertise can be accomplished through calling on Government or non-Government scientists. There is now no legal requirement for such consultation in decisions about carcinogenicity, and advice can be rejected by the agency. Seeking or requiring advice from scientists outside the agencies is the least radical proposal for changing the current decisionmaking system. A number of other proposals would move some parts of decisionmaking about carcinogenicity out of the agencies altogether.

Three dimensions can be considered in setting up a decisionmaking apparatus. The first is *personnel*, whether the technical experts are to be from the Federal Government, the private sector, or both. Each of the proposals to be discussed below is specific about the organizational association of the experts. The *procedure* that might be used by the panel ranges from collegial to adversarial. The proposals tend toward the former pole; each provides the technical panel with a staff to develop information for the panel's consideration. The *power* of the panel can range from advisory to decisionmaking to review. Most expert panels are now advisory, and the SAB is a reviewing panel. Some of the proposals call for the technical panel to make the decision for the agencies, others to review contested decisions.

OSTP Proposal for Decisionmaking

OSTP (281) divided Federal decisionmaking about carcinogens into two phases. Phase I is the identification and quantitative characterization of risks and encompasses steps 1 and 2 and part of 3 in figure 27. Phase II is making the regulatory decision to control the identified and characterized risk. OSTP proposes that phase I activities for all agencies be brought together and located within NTP.

The current responsibilities of NTP do not include phase I judgments for regulatory decisions. However, OSTP argues that just as NTP has a centralized coordination role in toxicological research so should it have a central role in interpretation of data.

Gilbert Omenn, an author of the OSTP paper (281), insists that decisionmaking about carcinogenicity should remain the responsibility of Federal officials. He makes the point that laws dealing with carcinogens are designed to protect public health and that Federal officials are entrusted with responsibility for administering the laws.

Having a panel of Federal officials decide about carcinogenicity is a major difference between the OSTP proposal and the proposals from AIHC and Representative Wampler. The latter two proposals centralize decisionmaking, but they would delegate carcinogen decisionmaking authority to new non-governmental organizations which would include non-Federal experts.

The American Industrial Health Council Science Panel Proposal

The AIHC (10) proposal for a science panel draws a distinction between scientific ("Phase I") and regulatory ("Phase II") decisionmaking as does the OSTP proposal. The science panel would be composed of "the best scientists available" and located centrally within Government or elsewhere. The panel would review existing data and not conduct or control research. Briefly, when a regulatory agency reached the point of considering regulatory action against a chemical, it would bring its data and conclusions about carcinogenicity to the panel. The panel would solicit additional data from industry, public interest groups, and other Government agencies and review all such data. It would assess the evidence and communicate its conclusions to the agency about whether or not the substance was a carcinogen. If sufficient exposure information and dose-response data were available, the panel would also evaluate the human hazard and risk posed by the carcinogen.

In the AIHC proposal, the panel would have to reach a decision within a certain time limit which would assure that it worked to a schedule. The panel would consider only scientific questions and its findings would not be binding. An agency could reject the panel's conclusions by explaining its reasons for rejection.

AIHC recommends that Congress establish a science panel consisting of 15 members who would assemble from time to time to consider data. It could appoint ad hoc members to workgroups to consider particular cases, and it would be provided with full-time professional staff to manage its workload.

Representative Wampler's National Science Council Proposal

Representative Wampler's bill to establish a National Science Council (NSC) was introduced on February 13, 1980 (H.R. 6521) and reintroduced as H.R. 638 on January 5, 1981. It would establish a 15-member council to review decisions concerning chemical toxicity. A company or individual who objected to an agency's assessment of toxicity during the agency's adjudication could request NSC review of the agency decision. Subjects of meetings of NSC would be announced in the Federal Register and open to the public except when trade secrets or confidential information were discussed. The bill offers amendments to CPSA, FDCA, the

Federal Meat Inspection Act, the Poultry Products Inspection Act, the OSH Act, and TSCA. The amendments would make the decisions of NSC final with respect to scientific fact under those laws.

Mr. Wampler's proposal stipulates that NSC members would be appointed by the President to full-time Federal posts for 2 years and have appropriate staff support. This full-time service differs from AIHC's proposal. The AIHC Science Panel would convene "periodically to assess materials," but its members would maintain their usual employment while serving.

Judge Markey's Proposal for Legislative Branch Review of Risk Decisions

Each proposal so far discussed—convening of Federal committees, non-Federal advisory groups, or creation of scientific boards within or outside of the Government—seeks to improve decisionmaking before regulations are written. A strikingly different idea has been advanced by Judge Howard Markey of the U.S. Court of Customs and Patent Appeals.

Markey (222) proposes no change in the way agencies make decisions about carcinogenicity and regulations. However, he does propose that OTA, as an agency of Congress, review agency decisions about risks. The review would be initiated if a regulated industry or a public interest group objected in court to a regulation on the basis that the agency had made a mistake in science.

Markey goes on to say that if OTA or some other agency designated by Congress cannot reach an agreement about the correctness of the agency decision about risk, "OTA would turn to Congress, where the final decision on acceptable risk could be made by the people through their representatives."

Summary Comments About Technical Panels and Study of Their Feasibility

The number of proposals for risk determination panels almost guarantees that the panels will remain an issue in Federal policy about car-

cinogens. Establishment of such a panel would represent a significant change in the process used by the Federal Government to make decisions about health risks.

Proponents of panels claim they would improve the efficiency of the regulatory process. A panel would make technical decisions for all the agencies, which is seen as assuring consistent scientific findings. Secondly, a time limit imposed on panel deliberations would ensure that it complete its work quickly. Finally, a regulatory agency could initiate the panel review of data about a suspect substance, and therefore the review could take place when it best fits the agency schedule.

Public interest, labor, environmental organizations, and the Federal regulatory agencies oppose these suggestions. They see regulatory agencies as the appropriate and lawful locations for making decisions about risk. In general they see a science panel as another layer of bureaucracy that might hinder regulatory activities, and worry that a single panel might be more sensitive to pressure from interested parties. Furthermore, they see the division between "science" and "policy" in decisions about cancer as illusionary. They argue that such a panel might have the power to delay decisions by imposing a higher standard of proof that a substance was a carcinogen than is required by law. This would stymie preventive "precautionary" governmental action which they view as necessary to protect lives and health when certainty cannot be achieved.

Congress has appropriated $500,000 to FDA to place a contract to investigate the feasibility of a centralized science panel, and a report is expected in 1982. The results of that study should answer questions about how the panel might function and how, or if, scientific and technical decisions can be made separately from policy or regulatory decisions. The FDA-sponsored study may also reveal whether difficulties associated with chemical regulations have hinged on scientific or on regulatory controversies. If the study shows that scientific errors have seldom resulted from processes used by the Government or that the errors have been of little importance, changes in the process of making scientific decisions would seem to have little merit. Conversely, if many examples of incorrect scientific decisions are found, changes might be appropriate.

MAKING REGULATORY DECISIONS

Possible Decisionmaking Frameworks

Each environmental health law seeks to reduce risks to the public health. Lave (204) discusses "frameworks" under which regulatory decisions can be made, and his categorizations are the basis for this section. He arrays the frameworks from that requiring the least information and analysis—the no-risk framework—to that requiring the most information and analysis—the benefit-cost framework. Some are familiar, describing the way in which decisions are made today; some suggest possible future directions.

1. The Delaney clause is most frequently mentioned as an example of the *no-risk framework*. It is a statement that Congress, concerned about the safety of food additives, has done the balancing of risks and benefits and has decided no benefits of food additives can outweigh a demonstrated cancer risk. FDA, the agency that administers Delaney, must show a risk before it bans an additive; it does not have to identify and measure benefits. Even if other organizations identify and measure benefits, FDA cannot balance benefits against risk.

2. The *risk-risk framework* requires a comparison of the risks associated with continued use of a substance to any risks generated by its use being controlled or discontinued. Generated risks would include those inherent in substitutes that might be employed in place of the substance. The best and most direct example of risk-risk analysis is the use of dangerous drugs to treat life threatening diseases. The risk from use of the drug can be compared with the risk of death if it is not used. A regulatory risk-risk determination is required under section 202 of CAA. As an example, a control device that reduced particulate emissions might, at the same time, produce chemical emissions. The risks from allowing continued particulate emissions would be compared to the risks from the chemical emissions.

Direct risk-risk analysis could also have been applied to nitrites added to food if the Federal Government had sustained its case that nitrites were carcinogenic and deserving of regulation. Eliminating or reducing use of nitrites as a preservative would have increased the risk of botulism (severe food poisoning). Its continued use might be associated with a cancer risk. Under the risk-risk framework, a decision to ban, to reduce use, or to allow curent use patterns might have been made by comparing expected deaths from botulism and from cancer under the different levels of regulation.

3. *General balancing of risks against benefits* differs from the first two frameworks and parallels all others in that it allows consideration of effects other than health. Lave says that the framework is purposefully loose and vague; it requires enumeration of all effects, but weighing and balancing them, as well as deciding which to quantify, is left to the regulator. He includes determination of "feasibility" under the OSH Act and regulations of air and water pollution which require BPT and BAT under this framework. In reality there is no best available technology. It can always be made better, (e.g., by placing two control devices in series) but at some point costs are judged to be prohibitive. The hallmark of this framework is balancing of risks and benefits without quantification and analysis. Because of deficiencies in available and attainable information a general balancing approach is probably used in most decisionmaking.

4. *Cost effectiveness* compares the costs of different ways to reach the same goal. (*The Implications of Cost-Effectiveness Analysis on Medical Technology* (285) discusses this

method and its application to medical practice.) In general, the framework assumes a fixed budget and produces an allocation of resources (money) among different programs which share a common objective. Programs selected for funding are those that go farthest toward reaching the goal, in this case, reduced cancer incidence and mortality, at the least cost.

The expenditure of public funds is required to develop, promulgate, and enforce regulations. Private funds are expended to argue against regulations and to buy and maintain control devices. Cost-effectiveness techniques can be used to compare the total cost of a regulation, i.e., agency costs, industry costs, and costs passed onto consumers to the benefits of the regulation. Alternatively, cost-effectiveness analysis can compare benefits to either public or private costs separately.

Regulations that are expected to prevent the most cancers at the lowest cost would be identified in a cost-effectiveness framework. The difficulties of evaluating costs and benefits make it unlikely that the technique can distinguish between regulations of near equal benefits and costs, but distinctions should be possible between the most and least cost-effective.

Informal discussions with officials at EPA and OSHA suggest that Government costs are about the same for every regulation because each regulation is likely to be challenged in court, and each one requires about the same amount of staff time, whether its impact is large or small. Although this opinion was commonly expressed, no attempt was made to verify it. If it is true, an agency can select its goals by concentrating on those that will produce the biggest health benefit.

The regulatory budget strategy applies cost effectiveness to non-Government costs. Under it each agency might be granted an amount of private sector costs that its regulations could generate. Working within that amount, the agency would then propose regulations that it intends to promulgate and submit them for executive approval. This approach considers only costs to be borne by the private sector and could set an upper limit on those costs. OMB (280) reported that difficulties in estimating such costs make this approach infeasible.

5. *Benefit-cost or cost-benefit analysis* is similar to general balancing of risks against benefits but is more formal and quantitative. In this framework, all costs and benefits are expressed in dollars, and this analysis requires placing a monetary value on human life. After all items under consideration are converted to dollar terms, the benefits and costs are compared and if the benefits of the regulation exceed the costs, the decision is weighted toward making the regulation. Placing a dollar value on human life is one of the most controversial aspects of this method, and it is simply repugnant to many people.

Lave claims the benefits of this framework are that it is the most flexible, requires the most information and analysis, and drives qualification where possible. Formal benefit-cost analysis is not now required by any carcinogen regulating law, but it is required by Executive Order No. 12291 where legislation does not forbid it, and it is frequently mentioned in plans for regulatory reform. A hearing of the Subcommittee on Oversight and Investigations (334) of the then House Committee on Interstate and Foreign Commerce provides a juxtaposition of opposing views of the applicability of the technique to regulatory decisionmaking.

Feasibility and Limits of Benefit-Cost Analysis

Traditional benefit-cost analysis is an economic tool that requires listing of all benefits and costs and assigning a dollar value to each. Carcinogen regulations involve the ultimate considerations—life and death—and opinions differ about whether or not a monetary value can be placed on life. In what ever way that controversy is settled, certain comments can be made about the usefulness of benefit-cost analysis.

In the case of a carcinogen regulation, expected benefits include the health gains from reducing exposure to the agent, and uncertainty is attached to the calculation of these gains. Presenting the expected health gain as a number does not add certainty to the estimate, but it adds to the estimate's importance. A frequent observation is that caveats and reservations attached to the numbers in the analysis are lost. The number of premature deaths to be averted ("lives saved") as well as the number of dollars to be spent to achieve the benefit take on lives of their own and are unencumbered by statistical reservations about accuracy. In this way, with no more information behind them, the numbers become more certain in the public's and the decisionmakers' minds. Too much reliance on imprecise numbers becomes a special problem in benefit-cost analysis which reduces the benefits and costs to dollar figures. This problem is commonly acknowledged but a practical solution is not readily apparent.

Many criticisms are directed at benefit-cost analysis. Lave (204) claims that a well-done analysis will always favor the status quo; change costs money. Change can be produced by going either from regulation to no regulation or from no regulation to regulation. Lave goes on to say that it would be surprising if the present state is truly the pinnacle of social evolution. If such a tilt toward the status quo exists when all measurements and calculations are accurately done, it is easy to imagine how a bias on the part of the analyst could affect the analysis. Not all economists agree with Lave's statement that benefit-cost analysis will always favor the status quo, and Freeman (132) cites the NAS 1974 study, *Air Quality and Automobile Emissions Control,* as an example of cost-benefit analysis which favored tighter controls.

Two other criticisms are directed at benefit-cost analysis. Equity considerations are not a part of benefit-cost analysis. For instance, the health benefits from a regulation accrue to those individuals whose risks are decreased; the cost of reducing the risks is borne by those who pay for the control devices or procedure. However, the situation before the control is implemented has the exposed people bearing a health risk which spares anyone in society from having to pay to reduce the exposure. The technique of cost-benefit analysis is silent about whether either case is just.

Another difficulty encountered with benefit-cost analysis is its inability to consider intergenerational effects. As a specific example, many substances are both carcinogens and mutagens. Such a substance may cause cancer in people exposed to it and mutations in their germ cells. The mutations are expressed in the next generation. Quantifying genetic damage is at least as difficult as expressing the value of a life in dollars.

A quite different problem in dealing with the future is economic. The discount rate chosen to project monetary costs and benefits is very important to these analyses, but there is no agreement about the appropriate rate, especially in inflationary times.

A response to objections about valuing lives in dollar terms is seen in the suggestion of the Conservation Foundation (78) that different types of analyses can be carried out under the benefit-cost rubric. It suggests use of the term "single-value analysis" to describe benefit-cost analyses which express all items in dollar terms and "two-value analysis" for analysis that compare "lives saved" to "dollars cost."

The Conservation Foundation found "two-value" analysis appropriate for carcinogens when the major concern is death. It is less easily applied when additional considerations, such as damage to an ecosystem, are involved. "Multi-value analysis" is suggested as a method to consider three or more irreducible elements. It enables tradeoffs to be made, e.g., human health risk v. costs of reducing exposure, and ecosystem risk v. costs, but the analysis becomes more difficult. The claimed advantage of benefit-cost analysis (that it forces a detailing of what is being considered) is equally applicable to the one-, two-, and multi-value methods. The two- and multi-value methods involve balancing of health risk against other factors, and fit within Lave's third framework of general balancing of risks and benefits.

While two-value or multivalue benefit cost analysis may be attractive because of its rigor and its not placing a dollar value on life, it is not, strictly speaking, benefit-cost analysis. A benefit-cost analysis drives toward a single number, the quotient obtained when benefits are divided by costs. If the quotient exceeds 1.0, the benefits are greater than the costs, and the project should, on an economic basis, proceed. If it is less than 1.0 it should not. Two-value and multivalue benefit-cost analyses produce no such quotient. Instead they compare the benefits in one term (i.e., lives) v. costs (in dollars). The comparison is useful in a cost-effectiveness approach, where various approaches to a common goal can be ranked, but it does not produce a number that indicates "yes" or "no."

A working panel of the NAS Committee on Principles of Decision Making for Regulating Chemicals in the Environment (263) concluded that:

> The systematic application of the tools of decision analysis and benefit-cost analysis can provide the decision maker with a useful framework and language for describing and discussing trade-offs, noncommensurability, and uncertainty. This framework should help to clarify the existence of alternatives, decision points, gaps in information, and value judgments concerning trade-offs.

Decision analysis, as described in the NAS report, is a careful detailing of regulatory options, expected outcomes and uncertainties of risks, benefits, and costs. Its "main contribution . . . is to organize information for the decisionmaker to assist him in his unavoidable balancing task."

The NRC committee (263) endorsed the use of benefit-cost analysis and concluded that the technique is useful in making decisions, but that it should not be the only consideration in the decision. Furthermore it did not recommend continued research to improve the techniques because "highly formalized methods of benefit-cost analysis can seldom be used for making decisions about regulating chemicals in the environment."

If market prices and shadow prices are fully utilized to value economic efficiency effects, the initial list of noncommensurate effects of the decision will have been reduced to:

- fully commensurate economic efficiency benefits and costs measured in dollars; and
- noncommensurate effects, described and quantified in other units, of which the most significant are likely to be hazards to health and life, damages to the environment and ecosystems, and the distribution of benefits, costs, and hazards among individuals and groups.

The NRC definition of benefit-cost analysis does not require that all costs and benefits be expressed in a common unit (dollars), and it too would fit in Lave's third framework.

This assessment, which deals with the science and policy of making decisions about carcinogens, has emphasized uncertainties in determining risk. The Conservation Foundation (78) and NRC (263) also draw attention to uncertainties in projecting costs of regulations. Both sides of the benefit-cost analysis are difficult, subject to human error, and encumbered by uncertainties. Nevertheless, this method, whether one-, or two- or multi-value has its advocates, and it is increasingly mentioned as at least a tool to be used by decisionmakers.

An Alternative to Benefit-Cost Analysis for Making Regulatory Decisions

Sometimes the world seems divided between economists and lawyers. Economists favor decision frameworks that rely on quantitation and, in benefit-cost approaches, on converting all values into dollars. Lawyers are more comfortable with qualitative concepts as developed on a case-by-case basis under common law. In making decisions about risks under common law, courts rely on concepts of reasonableness of behavior, of duties and responsibilities to learn and to inform, of assumptions of risk that are made by different parties, and of contributory behavior. Application of these concepts is constrained by common law precedents, procedural rules, and rules about admissibility of competent evidence. Quantitative considerations of costs and benefits play a minor role (20).

Regulatory law differs from the common law. Its history is shorter, and it is constrained and governed by many specific and varied enabling statutes, the Administrative Procedures Act, the Regulatory Flexibility Act, and Executive Order 12291. However, more importantly, the regulatory agencies rely heavily on semiquantitative and quantitative risk assessment techniques, on experts, and, increasingly on a benefit-cost framework for decisionmaking. Agency emphasis on quantitation, which "invites . . . playing with the numbers" to reach certain analytical outcomes is producing a "lack of credibility or acceptance in the public and the regulated industries" according to Baram (20).

Offered against these criticisms of benefit-cost analysis are "the rational approach to decision-making that it allegedly fosters" and that "it emphasizes economic considerations, it retards excessively zealous regulations, it ensures that in general only incremental controls will be promulgated."

This has now become the central controversy for the regulatory agencies: How to implement their mandates to control carcinogenic risk in a fair, objective and accountable manner by using a "rational" framework (e.g., cost-benefit) which emphasizes economic cost factors, when the health and environmental benefits at stake are generally considered as being unmeasurable in economic terms (20).

Baram offers a decision framework that considers costs, but which also relies on qualitative considerations for regulatory agency consideration. His framework has six steps. The first two are common to any such decisionmaking scheme—hazard identification and risk measurement—but beyond those steps, he considers risk management options that he says are now overlooked.

1. *Hazard identification.*—This step involves the technologies discussed in this report and is initiated when a test shows a substance is a carcinogen. The development of the initial finding of hazard can be accomplished by Government or non-Government testing, because of a governmental rule requiring a test by private industry, or by presentation of a petition for rulemaking to an agency.

2. *Risk measurement.*—This step, too, involves some technologies discussed here. Baram emphasizes that agencies can improve their performance at this step.

Since agencies can use evidence in their rulemaking which would not be considered competent for admission in a trial in court, there are few legal protocols governing the quality of the evidence . . . [used] . . . in rulemaking. Clearly, there is a need for the agencies to establish such admissibility of evidence protocols and to bind themselves to the protocols if the competency and probative quality of the evidence used is to be improved and the confidence of the public and regulatees in agency findings is to be increased. Costs will be a major factor in establishing such protocols . . . . Thus, it is imperative that agencies jointly address how to manage their resources for risk measurement collectively in the most efficient manner, and to establish collectively the costs to be imposed on industry for risk measurement when the measurement task is mandated for industry by law (20).

3. *Risk management options selection.*— This step is absent from current regulatory programs. It would identify and roughly assess the efficacy of regulatory and nonregulatory approaches to risk management. Regulatory options include both a) setting new standards and b) enforcing in-place standards. Nonregulatory approaches include a) recourse to common law, b) voluntary industrial standard setting, c) restrictions on future Federal procurement from sources of risk, and d) education or public disclosure programs.

4. *Economic and technical feasibility analyses.*—These analyses are required by some enabling statutes, Executive Order No. 12291, and the Regulatory Flexibility Act. They would focus on the management options identified in step 3.

The second, third, and fourth stages of measuring risk, assessing options, and costing options should ideally be kept separate and independent to ensure that risk measurement and option identification results are objectively arrived at on the basis of the best data and analytic methods for risk estimation. This accords with the findings of many critics of the regulatory management of risk who have found a breakdown in risk measurement objectivity when it is influenced by cost considerations. This important reform need not be Congressionally mandated, but can be accomplished by the responsible exercise of agency discretion under existing statutes. It permits each agency then to conduct its fourth stage of economic and technical analysis in a structured fashion—as cost-effectiveness analyses of each option separately and in certain combinations (20).

5. *Ordering of risk management initiatives.—*

Having identified and measured risks and selected the most efficacious and cost-effective management options which are technically feasible, each agency separately (and in conjunction if several find the same carcinogen falling within their regulatory jurisdiction) should then . . . [order] . . . risks it will choose to manage on the basis of the carcinogenic risk reduction benefits to be achieved.

For instance, EPA might decide that the benefits of managing the carcinogenic risks of asbestos alone far outweigh the benefits of managing the risks of many chemical substances, and thereby would be in a position to allot rationally a proportionate amount of its resources to asbestos (20).

6. *Deployment of risk management options— regulatory and nonregulatory—for selected priority chemicals.—*

Finally, an agency is at the point where it can proceed to engage in rulemaking and other regulatory efforts, and foster the use of available alternatives to regulation, for reducing the risks from exposure to the selected priority chemicals. The use of alternatives in conjunction with regulation can be particularly appropriate in those cases where the number of exposed persons is relatively small (as determined in step 2); the alternatives are promising in terms of their efficacy for reducing the risk (as determined in step 3); regulatory approaches do not appear to be cost-effective or technically feasible (as determined in step 4); or the agency has determined that an optional allocation of its resources on the basis of its selected priority chemicals militates against pro-

mulgating and enforcing regulations (as determined in step 5). Thus, although the rational approach to risk management precludes regulating such chemicals, the agency assumes the continuing responsibility of fostering alternative approaches to manage such risks in keeping with societal values which support the protection of individuals from the dangerous acts of others. Following these actions, the agency has the responsibility to monitor results and take necessary corrective steps—e.g., in the case when the use of alternatives has failed, the agency may renew its efforts to foster the use of alternatives or decide to regulate (20).

Agencies can adopt either this specific risk management approach or some other approach, without congressional intervention or mandate. Baram proposes that agencies publish two rules to govern their use of the framework in order to guard against ad hoc or case-by-case subjective determinations. The first would describe the procedures it will follow; the second, any agency assumptions about subjective elements of its analyses.

This scheme shares drawbacks with any that involves ordering of regulatory goals. The decision that a risk is number one may be challenged, and concern about the accuracy with which the actual number one is identified may prolong the ordering process. Also, the publication of a number one risk, say, asbestos in step 5 above, might be accompanied with a list of "also-rans." Whether such risks would go unchecked because it is clear that agency resources would never reach them or whether voluntary risk reductions would flow from the publication is a ponderable question.

Baram's step 3 may be the most critical difference between what is now done and what might be done. Considering alternatives, discussing and comparing them, would better ensure the public and the regulated industry that the most efficacious approach was being selected. It also incorporates the cost-effectiveness framework to choose between alternatives. The scheme enjoys a powerful attractiveness in that it considers nonregulatory management of risks while reserving the regulatory "club" if it is necessary.

Making an Unreasonable Risk Decision

"Unreasonable risk," the operational term in TSCA and CPSA, was of special interest to this assessment. It is a balancing term, and Congress decided not to define it, either in the laws or in the legislative history.

The House version of CPSA attempted a definition of "unreasonable risk" which involved comparing the severity and frequency of potential injury to the utility of the product, but the definition was deleted in the conference committee (145). In TSCA, the term was left undefined to allow maximum latitude to the EPA Administrator in making decisions. However, the House Interstate and Foreign Commerce Committee report accompanying TSCA states that unreasonable risk determinations involve (65):

> . . . balancing the probabilities that harm will occur and the magnitude and severity of that harm against the effect of proposed regulatory action on the availability to society of the benefits of the substance or mixture, taking into account the availability of substitutes for the substance or mixture which do not require regulation, and other adverse effects which such proposed action may have on society.

OTA undertook two efforts to learn about the term "unreasonable risk" and how it might be applied in regulatory efforts. The first effort was a letter of inquiry to knowledgeable people and the second was a workshop held by the New York Academy of Sciences. They are described in appendix B.

Some responses to the letter viewed any risk of cancer as unreasonable in itself. Other respondents favored balancing the risk of cancer against benefits of the substance in question. These two groups of responses parallel two approaches to regulatory law that were discussed earlier. Another suggestion was that consumers should make their own unreasonable risk decision about consumer products. The Government would tell them of the risk; they would decide whether or not to accept the risk.

The same division between risk-based and balancing approaches to regulating carcinogens was reflected in discussions at the workshop. The workshop heard a number of talks and discussions favoring cost effectiveness as a method for deciding on regulatory approaches.

Unreasonable risk has been used as the basis of regulatory action in a limited number of cases. To date, EPA has promulgated three regulations under TSCA to limit unreasonable risks from substances in the environment. TSCA required that EPA regulate PCBs; EPA regulated fully halogenated chlorofluoroalkanes, which threaten the ozone layer in the atmosphere, and it prohibited a company from disposing of 2,3,7,8-tetrachlorodibenzo-para-dioxin ("dioxin") at a particular facility. The few regulatory actions so far undertaken do not provide a coherent picture of how EPA will make unreasonable risk decisions. It is noteworthy that each of these actions dealt with a substance associated with cancer.

In response to a General Accounting Office (141) report, EPA stated that it had not developed "decision criteria" to make unreasonable risk decisions in the course of premanufacture review under section 5 of TSCA. The agency has considered drawing up such criteria, but found that the amount and variety of information to be weighed in such decisions precluded their developing criteria. Premanufacturing notices (PMNs) (see ch. 4) are considered on a case-by-case basis, and EPA considers that approach satisfactory at this time.

EPA assembles health and economic data about a substance considered for regulation and, in different offices, carries out a risk assessment and an economic assessment. These two assessments are then used to reach a decision about unreasonable risk. EPA guidelines (101) for making judgments about carcinogenicity, govern risk assessments. EPA has not yet published information about how it will carry out economic assessments (20). Each assessment carries with it some uncertainties and the quality of the data that go into the assessments varies, but eventually the results of the assessments go to the Administrator (78):

> The last stages of determining unreasonable risk (under TSCA) involve the Administrator of EPA, the Assistant Administrator for Toxic Substances, and perhaps one or two other high-level

officials evaluating the evidence and analysis, sorting through their own personal values, perhaps testing the political winds, and then coming to a conclusion. It is definitely not a process that can be subjected to tidy rules or guidelines.

The Administrator, who is appointed by the President, makes and publishes the decision. He is responsible for the decision made, and if it is shown to be incorrect, he can be removed from his position.

Not "Unreasonable Risks" and What To Do About Them

It seems likely that testing of chemicals will reveal a substantial number that present "limited" but not "sufficient" evidence for carcinogenicity. The words "limited" and "sufficient" are borrowed from the International Agency for Research on Cancer's (IARC) classification (see ch. 4 and app. A). In the case of "limited," the available evidence supports the idea that the substance is a carcinogen, but it is less than "sufficient" to force a conclusion.

A regulator might consider a substance for which only "limited" evidence exists as deserv-ing of regulation. He might come to this decision because many people or very sensitive people, such as young children, were exposed or because a substitute was readily available.

Whatever his reasons for considering regulation, economic assessment of most chemicals in commerce will probably show that significant costs would attend any regulatory scheme. In other words, often there may be a small risk and large costs. With those assessment results, it is likely that further analysis will not result in an answer that says "regulate" under the formal, rigorous balancing mechanisms discussed here.

A regulator who sees his first responsibility to be the protection of public health might be uncomfortable with that decision, and the producer of the substance, although not wanting to be regulated, might be uncomfortable also with continuing exposure at current levels. Methods to deal with these situations through discussion and incentives might reduce the antagonism between regulators and the private sector and promote public health (19, 20).

RESPONSIBILITY FOR MAKING DECISIONS

Quantification of risks and benefits is never likely to be so precise that estimates of these variables can be plugged into a formula to produce a number that dictates a decision. Instead, after all the analyses, a decision about whether a risk is acceptable or unacceptable and reasonable or unreasonable will be made by a few individuals. Those judgments reflect societal values and would, ideally, be made by citizens as a whole. In our form of Government, elected representatives are responsible for expressing societal values, and this responsibility is sometimes delegated by elected representatives to executive or judicial branch officials.

Executive Branch Decisions

The size and complexities of Government have resulted in elected representatives del-egating authority to make judgments about acceptable risk to executive branch agencies. A number of commentors, including Markey (222), point out that many executive branch officials are civil servants with almost lifetime tenure. While high-level appointees, such as the EPA Administrator, are at some risk if they make poor decisions, tenured civil servants are not. Citizens who feel aggrieved as a result of executive branch decisions have little opportunity for redress (222).

Field (120) cites a number of legal scholars who contend that "vague mandates" such as TSCA's directions to reduce or eliminate "unreasonable risks" give too much discretion to agencies:

> If regulatory decisions are to be broadly acceptable, the governing statutes must do more

than provide for decisions about what is safe or what is an unreasonable risk. They must also do more than merely list factors to be considered. The legislative process must make the basic value judgments and tell the agencies how to make the necessary trade-offs. . . .

Insofar as statutes do not effectively dictate agency actions, individual autonomy is vulnerable to the imposition of sanctions at the unruled will of executive officials, major questions of social and economic policy are determined by officials who are not formally accountable to the electorate, and both the checking and validating functions of the traditional model are impaired (120).

Baram (19) draws attention to the frequent absence of congressional direction about what factors agencies are to consider in reducing risk. Absence of that direction, he says, causes the agencies to face extensive litigation.

Judiciary Branch Decisions

Markey (222) expresses concern about the judiciary becoming too involved in making decisions about acceptable risk. He sees such decisions as best made in the political arena by officials responsible to the electorate. Judges, he points out, often enjoy lifetime tenure and are more removed from the electoral process than are executive branch officials.

Vague definitions such as "unreasonable risk" that occur in the balancing laws are seen as inviting legal challenge and judicial involvement in risk decisions. The courts have generally given great weight to "agency procedural safeguards, substantiality of evidence, and consistency" (120), but two recent developments may alter such preference. As discussed above, the Bumpers amendment would erase the judicial preference shown to agency expertise, and the courts would entertain challenges to agency expertise. Judicial involvement is also increased because of industry challenges to agency rules and consumer, environmental, and labor organization challenges to agencies for not regulating. Whatever the source of challenge, judicial reviews have an impact on what level of risk will be acceptable. Should a court modify an agency-decided risk level, it is reasonable to

assume that the agency, in making its next decision, will consider the courts' decree.

Directions From Congress

Congressional attention to details about what to balance and how to balance are seen as solutions to some of the problems of the regulatory agencies. Interestingly, regulatory agency attorneys interviewed by Field (120) generally favored balancing laws. They see their agencies well able to do an adequate job of balancing risks and benefits and evidently do not share the concerns about vague mandates.

Attorneys for four environmental interest groups were also interviewed (120). Three were opposed to balancing laws and favored that the Congress impose clearer mandates for regulatory action. Vague, balancing laws were seen as favoring industry because of its greater resources for influencing decisions in the agencies and in the courts. The fourth environmental attorney suggested that lack of money hampered public interest group representation and that Federal funding for preparation of their cases would ease their difficulties.

Clearly, different laws impose different standards, and the balancing laws are not specific about what is to be balanced. Litigation results from these characteristics of the laws. Congressional intervention to define standards and to detail what to balance should reduce litigation from those sources.

However, there is no guarantee that clearer directions from Congress will eliminate litigation—e.g., FDA's banning of the artificial sweetener, cyclamate, begun in 1969, was contested until 1980 (and may be reopened). Of all the carcinogen laws, the Delaney clause, which was the basis of the cyclamate ban, provides the clearest definition of a carcinogen, and it is the simplest in the sense that it allows no balancing. Nevertheless, administrative law hearings contesting the quality of the evidence about carcinogenicity were held off-and-on for a decade. The FDA decision was upheld.

Congress cannot engage in the day-to-day business of agencies; it does not have the time. It must delegate authority to the agencies. If it shares the opinions of some observers that it does not provide sufficient direction to the agencies about acceptable risk and balancing, it might provide the direction or it might more often exercise its right to intervene in regulatory activities.

Some risks are inherent in either remedy. Overly strict directions, which provide many points for judicial review might so encumber the agencies that no preventive regulatory action is possible. On the other hand, Congress cannot intervene too often in regulatory matters without hobbling its capacity to deal with other issues.

Regulations are seen as too burdensome by some and too weak by others, but the regulations are required by law. The laws are congressional expressions that public policy requires a certain level of protection for public health.

REGULATED CARCINOGENS

Table 38 lists 102 substances and categories of substances regulated under the laws discussed above. In every case, some evidence existed to indicate that the substance is a carcinogen. In many cases, evidence about the substance was generated in the NCI bioassay program (146) and/or evaluated by IARC (185,186). The left-hand columns of the table describe what conclusions were drawn about the human and animal substances by NCI and IARC.

IARC has classified 18 substances or processes as human carcinogens and another 18 as probable human carcinogens. The data in table 38 show that 20 of those chemicals are regulated. Each of those 20 is identified by a "C," carcinogen or "PC" probable carcinogen, in the "H," human evidence, column under IARC.

About one-third of the chemicals tested by NCI or reviewed by IARC present "sufficient" evidence to conclude that they are carcinogens in animals and they can therefore be assumed to present a carcinogenic risk for humans (see, e.g., 185). Chemicals from those classes are indicated with an "S" on the table in the "A," animal evidence, column; the "I" classification means the available evidence is limited but presents a strong warning of carcinogenicity.

About half of the chemicals reviewed by IARC and/or tested by NCI presented neither sufficient nor limited evidence of carcinogenicity. Only one chemical for which there is only inadequate (I) evidence of carcinogenicity appears in table 38. It is not possible to decide from the data in the table that risky chemicals are being regulated at the proper pace, but the data do lead to the conclusion that nonrisky chemicals (as judged by IARC and NCI) are not often regulated. The conclusion then suggests that regulations are not so haphazardly drawn as to regulate large numbers of chemicals that present no or very little risk.

The absence of an entry under "NCI" or "IARC" does not necessarily mean that there is poor or limited evidence about carcinogenicity. For instance, although the first substance, 2-acetylaminofluorene, does not occur on either the NCI or the IARC list, it is an accepted animal carcinogen (see ch. 5). Furthermore, other chemicals have been reviewed since the IARC (186) publication, but the results of the reviews are not yet available.

Some complexities of regulating carcinogens are demonstrated by the table. Some substances present a risk in locations covered by different laws, and separate regulations are necessary for each exposure. Under CAA, EPA has proposed regulation for, or regulated, 6 carcinogens and is considering an additional 24. Section 311 of CWA deals with oil and hazardous spills, and is not focused on regulating carcinogens, but "hazardous discharge reporting levels" have been promulgated for the listed chemicals, and carcinogenicity was considered in setting those levels. The 49 substances for which regulation is required under section 307 of CWA were included in the law in 1977. Standards have been set for trihalomethanes, including chloroform, under the Safe Drinking Water Act. A few

Table 38.—Substances Regulated as Carcinogens Under Various Acts

NCI A	IARC H	A	Chemical	CAA	CWA §307	CWA §311	SDWA	FIFRA	OSHA	FDCA	CPSA
—	—	—	2-acetylaminofluorene (2-AAF)	—	—	—	—	—	OSHA	—	—
—	PC	S	Acrylonitrile	C	RR	L	—	V	R	—	—
—	PC	S	Aflatoxin	—	—	—	—	—	—	R	—
L	—	L	Aldrin	—	RR	L	—	V	—	—	—
—	C	S	4-aminobiphenyl	—	—	—	—	—	R	—	—
—	—	S	Aramite	—	—	—	—	V	—	—	—
—	C	I	Arsenic	P	RR	—	R^a	R	R	—	—
—	C	I	Arsenic compounds	—	RR	L	—	R	—	—	—
—	C	S	Asbestos	R	RR	—	—	—	R^a	—	R
—	—	S	Benz(a)anthracene	—	RR	—	—	—	—	—	—
—	C	I	Benzene	P	RR	L	—	—	R	—	R
—	C	S	Benzidine	—	RR	L	—	—	R	—	R
—	—	S	Benzo(b)fluoranthene	—	RR	—	—	—	—	—	—
—	—	S	Benzo(a)pyrene	C	RR	—	—	—	—	—	—
—	PC	S	Beryllium	R	RR	—	—	—	—	—	—
—	PC	S	Beryllium compounds	—	RR	L	—	—	—	—	—
—	—	L	Bis(2-chloroethyl)ether (BCEE)	—	RR	L	—	—	—	—	—
—	C	S	Bis(chloromethyl)ether (BCME)	—	RR	—	—	—	R	—	—
—	PC	S	Cadmium	C	RR	—	R^a	R	—	—	—
—	I	S	Cadmium compounds	—	RR	L	—	R	—	—	—
—	I	S	Carbon tetrachloride	C	RR	L	—	—	—	—	—
S	I	L	Chlordane	—	RR	L	—	R	—	—	—
S	—	L	Chlorobenzilate	—	—	—	—	R	—	—	—
S	—	S	Chloroform (a trihalomethane, THM)	C	RR	L	R	—	—	—	—
—	C	S	Chloromethyl ether	—	—	—	—	—	R	—	—
—	C	S	Chromium compounds (hexavalent)	—	RR	L	—	—	—	—	—
—	C	S	Coal tar and soot	—	—	—	—	R	—	—	—
—	—	N	Coke oven emissions (polycyclic organic matter; "POM")	C	—	—	—	—	R	—	—
—	—	N	Creosote	—	—	—	—	R	—	—	—
—	—	N	Cyclamates	—	—	—	—	—	—	R	—
—	—	N	D&C Blue No. 6	—	—	—	—	—	—	R	—
—	—	N	D&C Red No. 10	—	—	—	—	—	—	R	—
—	—	N	D&C Red No. 11	—	—	—	—	—	—	R	—
—	—	N	D&C Red No. 12	—	—	—	—	—	—	R	—
—	—	N	D&C Red No. 13	—	—	—	—	—	—	R	—
—	—	N	D&C Yellow No. 1	—	—	—	—	—	—	R	—
—	—	N	D&C Yellow No. 9	—	—	—	—	—	—	R	—
—	—	N	D&C Yellow No. 10	—	—	—	—	—	—	R	—
—	I	L	DDT (dichlorodiphenyltrichloroethane)	—	RR	L	—	R	—	—	—
—	—	S	Dibenz(a,h)anthracene	—	RR	—	—	—	—	—	—
S	—	S	1,2-dibromo-3-chloropropane	—	—	—	—	R^a	R	—	—
—	—	N	1,2 dibromoethane	C	—	L	—	R	—	—	—
—	—	S	3,3'-dichlorobenzidine	—	RR	L	—	—	R	—	—
S	—	S	1,2-dichloroethane	C	RR	L	—	—	—	—	—
I	I	L	Dieldrin	—	RR	L	—	R	—	—	—
—	—	N	Diethylpyrocarbonate	—	—	—	—	—	—	R	—
—	C	S	Diethylstilbestrol (DES)	—	—	—	—	—	—	R	—
—	—	S	4-dimethylaminoazobenzene	—	—	—	—	—	R	—	—
L	—	N	2,4-dinitrotoluene	—	RR	L	—	—	—	—	—
S	—	S	1,4-dioxane	C	—	—	—	—	—	—	—
—	—	N	1,2-diphenylhydrazine	—	RR	L	—	—	—	—	—
—	—	L	Dulcin	—	—	—	—	—	—	R	—
—	I	L	Epichlorohydrin	C	—	L	—	—	—	—	—
—	—	N	Ethylene bis dithiocarbamate	—	—	—	—	R	—	—	—
—	PC	I	Ethylene oxide	C	—	—	—	R	—	—	—
—	—	N	FD&C Red No. 2	—	—	—	—	—	—	R	—
—	—	N	FD&C Violet No. 1	—	—	—	—	—	—	R	—
—	—	N	Formaldehyde	C	—	L	—	—	—	—	—
—	—	N	Graphite	—	—	—	—	—	—	R	—
(S)	—	L	Heptachlor	—	RR	L	—	R	—	—	—
—	—	S	Hexachlorobenzene	—	RR	L	—	—	—	—	—
—	—	N	Hexachlorobutadiene	—	RR	L	—	—	—	—	—

Table 38.—Substances Regulated as Carcinogens Under Various Acts (Continued)

Evaluation by NCI A	IARC H	IARC A	Chemical	CAA	CWA §307	CWA §311	SDWA	FIFRA	OSHA	FDCA	CPSA
—	I	L	Hexachlorocyclohexane	—		L	—	—	—	—	—
—	—	N	α-hexachlorocyclohexane	—	RR	L	—	—	—	—	—
—	—	N	β-hexachlorocyclohexane	—	RR	L	—	—	—	—	—
(S)	—	N	Hexachloroethane	—	RR	L	—	—	—	—	—
—	—	S	Ideno(1,2,3-cd)pyrene	—	RR	—	—	—	—	—	—
S	—	S	Kepone (chlordecone)	—	—	L	—	V	—	—	—
—	—	L	Lindane	—	RR	L	R^a	R	—	—	—
—	—	N	Mercaptoimidazoline	—	—	—	—	—	—	R	—
—	—	S	4,4' methylene bis (2-chloroaniline)	—	—	—	—	—	R	R	—
—	—	L	α-naphthylamine	—	—	—	—	—	R	—	—
—	C	S	2-naphthylamine	C	—	—	—	—	R	—	—
—	PC	S	Nickel	C	RR	—	—	—	—	—	—
—	PC	S	Nickel compounds	—	RR	L	—	—	—	—	—
—	—	N	Nitrosamines	—	—	—	—	—	—	R	—
—	—	L	4-nitrobiphenyl	—	—	—	—	—	R	—	—
—	—	S	N-nitrosodi-n-butylamine	—	—	L	—	—	—	—	—
—	—	S	N-nitrosodiethylamine (DENA)	—	—	L	—	—	—	—	—
—	—	S	N-nitrosodimethylamine (DMNA)	C	RR	L	—	—	R	—	—
—	—	S	N-nitrosodi-n-propylamine	—	RR	—	—	—	—	—	—
—	—	S	N-nitroso-N-ethylurea (NEU)	C	—	—	—	—	—	—	—
—	—	S	N-nitroso-N-methylurea (NMU)	C	—	—	—	—	—	—	—
—	—	N	Oil of calamus	—	—	—	—	—	—	R	—
—	—	N	P-4000	—	—	—	—	—	—	R	—
I	—	N	Pentachloronitrobenzene (PCNB)	—	—	—	—	R	—	—	—
—	I	S	Polychlorinated biphenyls (PCBs; Toxic Substances Control Act-RR)	C	RR	L	—	—	—	R	—
—	—	S	β-propiolactone	—	—	—	—	—	R	—	—
—	—	S	Safrole	—	—	—	—	V	—	R	—
—	—	N	2,3,7,8-tetrachlorodibenzo-p-dioxin (TCDD, "dioxin")	C	RR	—	—	—	—	—	—
(S)	—	N	1,1,2,2-tetrachlorethane	C	RR	L	—	—	—	—	—
(S)	—	N	Tetrachloroethylene (perchloroethylene)	C	RR	L	—	—	—	—	—
—	—	S	Thiourea	—	—	—	—	—	—	R	—
S	—	S	Toxaphene	—	RR	L	R^a	R	—	—	—
(S)	—	N	1,1,2-trichloroethane	—	RR	L	—	—	—	—	—
(S)	I	L	Trichloroethylene	C	RR	L	—	—	—	—	—
S	—	N	2,4,6-trichlorophenol	—	RR	—	—	—	—	—	—
—	—	N	Trihalomethanes (THM)	—	—	—	R	—	—	—	—
—	—	N	"Tris" (flame retardant)	—	—	—	—	—	—	—	R
—	C	S	Vinyl chloride	R	RR	—	—	—	R	—	R
—	—	N	Vinylidene chloride	C	RR	L	—	—	—	—	—
—	—	—	Radionuclides	R	—	—	—	—	—	—	—

Abbreviations

NCI — National Cancer Institute data (146)
IARC — International Agency for Research on Cancer evaluation (185, 186)

A = animal evidence
S = sufficient evidence for carcinogenicity (for more description see Chapter 4, Appendix A)
(S) = Class 3 of NCI; very strong evidence is 1 species; no evidence in 2nd species
L = limited evidence for carcinogenicity
I = inadequate evidence for carcinogenicity
H = human evidence
C = identified as a carcinogen from human studies
PC = identified as a probable carcinogen from human studies
I = inadequate evidence to reach a conclusion about carcinogenicity from human studies
N = not evaluated

CAA — Clean Air Act
CWA 307 — Clean Water Act §307
CWA 311 — Clean Water Act §311
SDWA — Safe Drinking Water Act
FIFRA — Federal Insecticide, Fungicide, and Rodenticide Act
OSHA — Occupational Safety and Health Act
FDCA — Food, Drug, and Cosmetic Act
CPSA — Consumer Product Safety Act

C = being considered for regulation
P = regulation proposed
R = regulated
RR = regulation required by Act
L = discharge levels restricted
V = voluntarily withdrawn from market

[a]Regulation based on non-carcinogenic toxicity (in addition to those indicated, many other listed substances encountered in the workplace are regulated because of toxicities other than carcinogenicity).

metals and pesticides which are identified as carcinogens are regulated under the same act but because of other toxic properties. Implementation of FIFRA has resulted in voluntary withdrawal of pesticides before regulations were promulgated as well as regulations restricting or forbidding use.

OSHA has regulated the substances shown because of carcinogenicity and many other substances on the list are regulated in the workplace because of other toxicities. FDA regulation of carcinogenic food additives and colors has eliminated most of the listed colors and sweeteners from the food supply. The Consumer Product Safety Commission has regulated five chemicals and benzidine-containing dyes.

The table does not discriminate between regulations that set a permissible limit, such as the OSHA standards, and those that ban a substance, such as FDA regulations of food colors. The entry "R" indicates only that some regulation is in effect.

The laws are designed to reduce exposure to carcinogens. They may regulate too many or too few chemicals, but chemicals are being regulated. Furthermore, apparently, few nonrisky chemicals have been regulated under the current system.

Appendixes

Contents

Appendix A.—A Comparison of the National Cancer Institute's and the International Agency for Research on Cancer's Evaluation of Bioassay Results

A working group assembled by the International Agency for Research on Cancer (IARC) reevaluated data about 354 chemicals previously evaluated and described in the first 20 IARC monographs (185,186). The working group developed the following criteria for grading evidence about carcinogenicity. The first three categories are essentially the same as those used in earlier IARC compilations (344), and two new categories were added:

Sufficient evidence of carcinogenicity indicates that there is an increased incidence of malignant tumours: (a) in multiple species or strains; (b) in multiple experiments (preferably with different routes of administration or using different dose levels); (c) to an unusual degree with regard to incidence, site or type of tumour, or age at onset. Additional evidence may be provided by data concerning dose-response effects, as well as information on mutagenicity or chemical structure.

Limited evidence of carcinogenicity means that the data suggest a carcinogenic effect but are limited because: (a) the studies involve a single species, strain, or experiment, or (b) the experiments are restricted by inadequate dosage levels, inadequate duration of exposure to the agent, inadequate period of follow-up, poor survival, too few animals, or inadequate reporting, or (c) the neoplasms produced often occur spontaneously or are difficult to classify as malignant by histological criteria alone (e.g., lung and liver tumours in mice).

Inadequate evidence indicates that because of major qualitative or quantitative limitations, the studies cannot be interpreted as showing either the presence or absence of a carcinogenic effect.

Negative evidence means that within the limits of the tests used, the chemical is not carcinogenic. The number of negative studies is small, since in general, studies that show no effect are less likely to be published than those suggesting carcinogenicity.

No data indicates that data were not available to the working group (185).

IARC (185) made the following statement about the value of bioassay results:

. . . in the absence of adequate data in humans it is reasonable, for practical purposes, to regard chemicals for which there is *sufficient evidence* of carcinogenicity (i.e., a causal association) in animals *as if they presented a carcinogenic risk for humans.* The use of the expressions "for practical purposes" and "as if they presented a carcinogenic risk" indicates that at the present time a correlation between carcinogenicity in animals and possible human risk cannot be made on a scientific basis, but rather only pragmatically, with the intent of helping regulatory agencies in mak-

ing decisions related to the primary prevention of cancer. (Emphasis in original.)

The largest single testing effort is the National Cancer Institute's (NCI)'s Carcinogenesis Testing Program (now a part of the National Toxicology Program (NTP)). Griesemer and Cueto (146) analyzed the results of NCI's testing 190 chemicals and placed each tested chemical into one of nine classifications (see table A-1). Ninety-eight of the 190 were judged to be carcinogenic (classifications 1 through 5); 28 were equivocal (classification 6); and 64 were noncarcinogenic (classifications 7 through 9). The NCI results had earlier been reviewed by a panel of governmental and nongovernmental experts and Griesemer and Cueto drew on that review in their compilation.

A significant difference between the data analyzed by Griesemer and Cueto (hereafter referred to as the "NCI list") and by IARC is that all the NCI experiments were carried out according to a standard protocol (331). The IARC evaluations consider experiments carried out under a variety of protocols including those done by NCI.

Thirty-three chemicals appearing on the IARC list of 354 also appear in the NCI list. In table 39, such chemicals are listed in the class to which they were assigned by Griesemer and Cueto. For instance, the chemical chloroform appears in the NCI class 1, and it is also present on the IARC list. Following each listed chemical is an S, L, or I. The letters indicate IARC's classifications of sufficient, limited, or inadequate evidence for carcinogenicity. In some cases, additional data that became available between the compilation of the 1978 (185) and 1979 (344) IARC lists changed a chemical from I or L to S; these changes are reflected in the table.

Comparisons between the NCI and IARC lists are not direct because different criteria were used, but the following scheme may be useful.

Evidence	IARC classification	NCI classification
Strongly positive	Sufficient evidence (S)	Classes 1, 2
Positive	Limited evidence (L)	Classes 3, 4, 5
Not Positive	Inadequate evidence (I)	Classes 6, 7, 8, 9

Agreement is good about the strongly positive chemicals. Seven of the 12 NCI class 1 chemicals were found to have "sufficient evidence" for carcinogenicity by IARC. Of the remaining five, some are likely to be reevaluated by IARC. For instance, reserpine was classified in the "inadequate evidence" group by IARC before the results of the NCI bioassay

Table A-1.—National Cancer Institute (NCI Analysis of the Results of Testing 190 Chemicals[a] and the International Agency for Research on Cancer (IARC) Analysis of Chemicals[b c] That Appear on the NCI List

NCI Group A: Five categories of results showing increased tumor incidence, ordered with most convincing category being number 1.

Very strong evidence in 2 species.
31 chemicals

Chemicals among the 31 that appear on the IARC lists	Evidence for carcinogenicity, IARC 1979[c]	1978[b]
Chlorodecone (kepone)	S[d]	—
Chloroform	S	I
2,4-diaminoanisole	—	I
2,4-diaminotoluene	S	L
Dibromochloropropane (DBCP)	S	S
1,2-dichloroethane	S	—
1,4-dioxane	S	S
5-nitroacenaphthene	S	S
Phenoxybenzamine hydrochloride	—	L
Reserpine	I[e]	I
Selenium sulfide (IARC entry is selenium compounds)	—	I
Ortho-toluidine hydrochloride	—[e]	I

Very strong evidence in 1 species,
sufficient evidence in 2d species.
9 chemicals

None of the 9 chemicals appears on the IARC lists.

Very strong evidence in 1 species,
no evidence in 2d species.
35 chemicals

Chemicals among the 35 that appear on the IARC lists		
4-amino-2-nitrophenol	—	I
Aniline hydrochloride (IARC entry is aniline)	—	I
Azobenzene	—	L
Chlordane	L	—
Chlorobenzilate	—	L
Cinnamyl anthranilate	—	I
Heptachlor	L	I
Lasiocarpine	S	S
Oestradiol mustard (IARC entry is estradiol mustard)	—	L
Trichloroethylene	—	L
Toxaphene	S	—
4-chloro-ortho-toluidine hydrochloride (IARC entry is parachloro-ortho-toluidine hydrochloride)	—	I

Sufficient evidence in 2 species.
4 chemicals

None of the 4 chemicals appears on the IARC lists.

Sufficient evidence in 1 species,
no evidence in 2d species.
19 chemicals

Chemicals among the 19 that appear on the IARC lists		
Aldrin	—	I
Ethyl tellurac	—	I

NCI Group B: One category showing insufficient evidence to lead to a conclusion about carcinogenicity.

Table A-1.—National Cancer Institute (NCI) Analysis of the Results of Testing 190 Chemicals[a] and the International Agency for Research on Cancer (IARC) Analysis of Chemicals[b] [c] That Appear on the NCI List (Continued)

	Evidence for carcinogenicity, IARC	
	1979[c]	1978[b]
Equivocal evidence in 1 or 2 species.		
28 chemicals		
Chemicals among the 28 that appear on the IARC lists		
Phenacetin (tested by itself by IARC; tested in combination with aspirin and caffeine, APC, by NCI)	L	—
Styrene	L	—
NCI Group C: Three categories showing no evidence of carcinogenicity.		
No evidence in limited experiments.		
51 chemicals		
Chemicals among the 51 that appear on the IARC lists		
Dieldrin.....................................	L	L
Endrin..	—	I
Ethionamide	—	I
Lindane	—	L
Methoxychlor.................................	—	I
No evidence in 1 species.		
10 chemicals		
1 chemical among the 10 appears on the IARC lists		
Anthranilic acid...............................	—	I
No evidence in 2 species.		
3 chemicals		
None of the 3 chemicals appears on the IARC lists.		

[a]Griesemer and Cueto, 1979.
[b]Tomatis, et al., 1978; Tomatis, 1979.
[c]IARC, 1979; IARC, 1980.
[d]S indicates "sufficient evidence of carcinogenicity."
 L indicates "limited evidence of carcinogenicity."
 I indicates "inadequate evidence of carcinogenicity."
[e]See text.

of that drug were available, and ortho-toluidine hydrochloride is being reevaluated by IARC. Both NCI and IARC found that phenoxybenzamine hydrochloride is carcinogenic. Therefore the lists may only differ significantly over two chemicals, and those differences, too, may disappear as more data become available.

Agreement is not as good about chemicals that are less positive. NCI's classes 3, 4, and 5 roughly correspond to IARC's L group, but 5 of the 11 NCI class 3 compounds common to both lists were put in the "inadequate evidence" category by IARC. Additionally, NCI found no evidence for carcinogenicity for any chemical in classes 6 through 9, but IARC found "limited evidence" for carcinogenicity for five of the eight chemicals that it reviewed in those classes.

As was mentioned, the data considered by IARC and NCI are not independent of each other; IARC considers NCI results in addition to all others. The differences in classification may result from the different criteria used by the two organizations, as well as from IARC considering other results.

Comparison of the 1978 and 1979 IARC listings shows that the evidence for the carcinogenicity of some chemicals became more positive. The progression to more-significant-evidence classes may be important to the contention that repeated testing increases the chances that a chemical will be determined to be a carcinogen.

Neither the IARC nor the NCI list include reviews of all chemicals of interest. For instance, neither saccharin nor sodium nitrite appears on either list, but both compounds have been much discussed by regulators and potentially regulated industries.

The last sentences of the Griesemer and Cueto (146) paper draw attention to the importance attached to positive results.

> Those compounds for which evidence for carcinogenicity was not found. . . cannot necessarily be considered as noncarcinogens since the tests were conducted under a limited set of circumstances. It is possible that evidence for carcinogenicity might be found if, for example, a different strain of animal or a different route of exposure were used.

The quote illustrates the impossibility of proving a negative, and in a more immediate sense, it also shows that rules are not established to allow classifying a chemical as safe. A workable approach to allow making a decision that a chemical should be regarded as safe rather than as a potential risk may be necessary to separate important problems from minor and nonexistent ones. In fact, Griesmer and Cueto's group C which includes four grades of negative evidence shows that conclusions can be drawn that chemicals were found not to be risky under conditions of the tests.

To learn more about the concept of "unreasonable risk," the assessment made inquiries of a group of experts and cosponsored a workshop about the subject. The inquiry was directed to 36 individuals, selected by the Assessment Advisory Panel and OTA Staff, and the workshop was held in March 1980 at the New York Academy of Sciences (NYAS).

Responses to Letter Inquiries About Unreasonable Risk

Informed individuals were asked to comment on unreasonable risk. Each individual received the letter and attachments shown in figure B-1. The 22 who responded are acknowledged in table B-1.

Responses ranged from telephone calls or notes, to reprints of papers and speeches, to discursive letters. No attribution of a particular opinion to a specific individual is made in the description of responses that follows. The inquiry letter was couched in reference to the Toxic Substances Control Act (TSCA), but it did not specify that discussions of "unreasonable risk" were to be restricted to a balancing approach to controlling carcinogens. Both zero-risk and balancing approaches were mentioned in the responses, but no response mentioned a technology-based approach to regulation.

Zero-Risk Approaches to Unreasonable Risk

A number of respondents treated cancer, especially workplace-related cancer, as an unreasonable risk, regardless of the number of people affected. Proponents of a purely health-based reading of unreasonable risk contend that workers should suffer no impairment of health as a result of workplace exposures.

These responses did not reflect a naive position that all workplace exposures can be eliminated immediately. Instead, it represented a starting position for regulatory efforts. A respondent said that, "currently when a carcinogen is identified, the first step is to estimate how much of it can be tolerated." He would favor instead that the first step be to set as a goal the elimination of exposure. If that is impossible, each "essential" exposure could be considered in turn to construct a pattern of allowed exposures above zero. Every effort should then be made to reduce the allowed exposure.

Another respondent likened the present workplace situation to Thomas More's Utopian caste system, in which laborers may be sacrificed for the greater societal good:

Not accepting the caste system, only *necessary* risks would be taken and a standard would be promulgated acceptable to labor, but not to management . . . [Workers] want standards set so there will be no increased risk of getting cancer as a result of their exposure to chemicals in the working environment.

Recognizing that zero exposure levels will not be possible in all situations, limiting exposure to low levels is seen as an intermediate goal to be accomplished by imposing every available control measure. There is no balancing in this approach and the respondent objected to "the entire process of weighing dollar costs to employers against the value of a human life."

Another respondent advocated applying all available controls for workplace exposures to known carcinogens and specifically concludes that the time for quantitative risk assessment has not yet arrived. He cited the continued presence of such obvious and indisputable hazards as asbestos, benzidine dyes, and aluminum-reduction pot-room carcinogens as examples of risks which need immediate attention. He stated that even when control techniques are available, they are not required or applied to the fullest extent.

Interestingly, an alternative health-based approach to unreasonable risk involves a very different methodology and leads to different actions. Quantitative risk assessment would be used to estimate human risk for each identified hazardous substance. All estimates would be expressed as the risk that a person might develop cancer during his lifetime as a result of exposure to the substance at the level now encountered. The risks would be expressed as 1/10, 1/100, 1/1,000, etc. Some value for the risk factor, would be designated as a critical value. Risks less than that value would be tolerated; risks greater than that value would be declared unreasonable and candidates for regulation. Costs of regulation would not intrude into the decision to regulate.

Balancing Approaches to Unreasonable Risk

The majority of respondents indicated a preference for a form of balancing some combination of risks, costs and benefits. The spectrum within this ideological grouping however, ranges from suggesting very subjective, case-by-case determinations, to the use of formal quantitative calculations that could be applied to all cases. Individuals who place little faith in quantitative risk assessment and economic analysis of costs and benefits cluster around the "subjective and qualitative" position. The "objective and quantitative" position is occupied by people who are more

Figure B-1.

Dear   :

We would like your help in attacking a particularly vexing problem as part of the ongoing Assessment of Technologies for Determining Cancer Risks from the Environment. For your information, a one page description of the Office of Technology Assessment, a one page description of the assessment, and a list of the members of the Assessment Advisory Panel are included.

In order to move against a substance under the Toxic Substance Control Act, the Administrator of the Environmental Protection Agency must determine that the substance poses an "unreasonable risk." The legislative history of TSCA states that Congress decided not to attempt a definition of the term, and intended that its use as an operational term would allow the administrator flexibility in dealing with toxics.

We are asking a number of individuals and organizations (list enclosed) to comment on their impressions and thoughts about unreasonable risk as a concept and an operational term. The enclosed list of questions may be useful to you. If you like, you may, of course, answer each one, or you can use them as a general guide, or ignore them.

We will acknowledge all people and organizations that respond to this request in the assessment report to be published in November, 1980. We will not attribute your comments and ideas to you unless you ask us to do so.

I know that you are busy, and on behalf of the Assessment Advisory Panel and OTA staff, I thank you in advance for your time and consideration.

Sincerely yours,

Michael Gough

1. Unreasonable risk, most probably, represents estimating the projected harm from continued use of substance and balancing that against the benefits of continued use.
   a. What sorts of information would you use in making estimates of the projected harm (short-term tests, animal studies, epidemiology, specific tests. . . ?)
   b. What sorts of information would you use in making estimates of the costs of restricting use of substance?
   c. How would you balance a against b?
   d. Whom would you trust to supply you with the information and make the comparison?
2. What components go into determining an unreasonable risk?
   a. How would you weigh each component?
   b. Must the components be quantitative?
3. Is a decision about unreasonable risk tantamount to a cost-benefit or risk-benefit decision?
4. Is there an approachable numerical level for unreasonable risk?
5. Do you think we have gained anything by introduction of the term "unreasonable risk" in decision making?
6. Have you or has your organization ever conducted an exercise that you consider to have a determination of unreasonable risk? If so, we would appreciate your describing it (or we'll be glad to talk to you on the phone, or if it's already printed somewhere, just tell use the reference.)

Table B-1.

The OTA thanks the following individuals who responded to a letter inquiry about unreasonable risk.

John T. Barr,	Air Products and Chemicals, Inc.
Jan Beyea,	Audubon Society
Eula Bingham,	Occupational Safety and Health Administration
Ralph Engel,	Chemical Specialties Manufacturers Association
P. J. Gehring,	Dow Chemical Co.
Harold P. Green,	Fried, Frank, Harris, Shriver, and Kampelman
Fred Hoerger,	Dow Chemical Co,
Peter Hutt,	Covington and Burling
Kenneth L. Johnson,	Clement Associates, Inc.
Lorin E. Kerr,	United Mine Workers of America
Arnold Kuzmack,	Environmental Protection Agency
Linda B. Kiser,	Consumer Products Safety Commission
Lester Lave,	The Brookings Institution
William J. McCarville,	Monsanto Co.
Richard A. Merrill,	University of Virginia
Franklin E. Mirer,	United Auto Workers
F. W. Mooney,	The Proctor & Gamble Co.
Parry M. Norling,	E. I. du Pont de Nemours & Co., Inc.
Glenn Paulson,	Audubon Society
David P. Rall,	National Institute of Environmental Health Sciences
Sheldon W. Samuels	American Federation of Labor/Congress of Industrial Organizations

confident of the precision of quantitative risk assessment and economic analysis.

A representative of the Consumer Product Safety Commission (CPSC) described CPSC interpretation of unreasonable risk:

> The legislative history of the Consumer Product Safety Act (CPSA) indicates that unreasonable risk of injury is to be determined by balancing the probability that the risk will result in harm and the gravity of the harm against a rule's effect on the product's utility, cost, and availability to the consumer. Thus, in addition to an assessment of the risk that a rule will eliminate or reduce, an important component of unreasonable risk of injury is the economic impact of a planned regulatory initiative. The legislative history explains that an unreasonable risk is one which can be prevented or reduced with little or no economic impact; or one where the rule's effect on a product's utility, cost or availability is outweighed by the need to protect consumers from the hazard associated with the product.

One respondent made the point that our knowledge of carcinogenicity forces a balancing approach.

As a policy matter, there is no recognition of a "threshold dose:" the safe haven of a "no effect" level does not exist for carcinogens.

The subjective qualitative approach is exemplified by a lawyer who wrote: "A substance constitutes an 'unreasonable risk' only where the probability and/or the severity of harm are deemed to outweigh its utility." He explained that all pertinent elements, "probability, severity, harm, utility," in that statement are highly subjective, and that their definitions are shaped by participating individuals, who may include: "legislators, regulators, business persons, voters, writers of letters to the editor, interested citizens, etc." This type of balancing emphasizes subjective judgments in qualitative determinations and limits to purely objective determinations.

Another lawyer describes the process of unreasonable risk determinations as:

> . . . paramount to a cost-benefit or risk-benefit decision. In essence, it relies as much on procedure as on substance for correct decisions. The concept is that, if all potentially relevant information is taken into account and all interested parties have an opportunity to contribute to the proceedings, the ultimate decision will be rational and as sound as it possibly can be in an area where there is no certainty. While that is perhaps not acceptable to a mathematician, I see little possibility of improving upon it as long as the concept remains in statutory language.

Another respondent sees the language of TSCA as allowing a broad range of options for regulatory approaches. He suggests that TSCA rulings might follow the pattern of the Food and Drug Administration's development of criteria for drug effectiveness tests, beginning as loose, intuitive, ad hoc decisions, later becoming codified into lengthy regulations. Once that state is reached, it is difficult to depart from the formula.

A variation on this theme came from an industrial executive, who feels that determinations should be qualitative, and decided on a case-by-case basis. However, he calls for explicit criteria to be addressed in balancing, listing as examples:

- level of hazard inherent in exposure to the chemical;
- types of exposure which create the hazard;
- populations likely to be exposed;
- extent of the exposed populations;
- whether the exposure would be voluntary or involuntary;
- availability of substitutes;
- the worth to society of continued availability of the substance;
- cost inherent in various levels of control or elimination;

- nature of the data suggesting the existence of a hazard;
- ability to extrapolate from those data to predict the hazard in other situations; and
- relative importance of regulating the particular chemical in view of the risks presented by other as yet unregulated chemicals.

A chemical trade association representative addressed the issue broadly:

> Many criteria or approaches for one substance will not be appropriate for another. We believe that there is no formula for such an assessment, but that each case must be decided on its own merits. This is not to say that scientific methodology should not be used, but it does say that the foundation and assumptions that lead to the determination of "unreasonable risk" should be clearly identified, along with their limitations, by the regulatory agency on a case-by-case basis and not through a generic approach.

A public interest advocate deplored the high degree of quantification of risks, costs, and benefits emanating from the Environmental Protection Agency (EPA), which are seen as based on methods inadequate to the task. The large areas of uncertainty surrounding these estimates are rarely specified, especially for economic evaluations. Risk estimates, he feels, are good only for the grossest distinctions between the most and least potent carcinogens. Balancing, therefore, should rely heavily on qualitative decisions, in which doubts must be resolved, by the language of the law, in favor of greater protection.

A middle ground position is taken by many respondents, who would like to see all of the available quantitative information enter into the final regulatory decision, but modified by such factors that are less readily and more controversially quantified. Within this group, there are those who feel that eventually all factors will be quantified, and that more energy should be directed at methodologies for reaching that goal. Others feel that certain measures, especially the value of a human life, cannot be converted to monetary terms.

Some industry respondents lean toward quantitative approaches to deciding unreasonable risk. One expressed his belief that risks from hazardous chemicals are overstated, and that regulation probably will not materially benefit health. This respondent places confidence in risk assessment:

> The question of "risk" can be assessed with some certainty. "Unreasonable" is by definition a matter of perception, and would include consideration of the benefits of a substance and the cost to regulate it.

As a part of risk analysis, respondents from across the spectrum advocate risk comparisons of different types. An industry representative thinks it would be useful to compare the risk from exposure to a carcinogenic chemical to other risks we accept willingly in daily life.

A highly quantitative cost-effectiveness approach is promoted by one economist. Measures that achieve the greatest risk reduction, most economically, would be the first to be required. This method requires risk assessments for known carcinogens and identification of carcinogens with exposures that can be reduced. This respondent suggested a 2-stage approach, accepting reductions to an intermediate level which maximize risk reduction for each dollar spent. However, final limits would be set requiring an explicit valuation of life. He acknowledges that an implicit value for life is found abhorrent by some, but, he says: "it is inherent in all toxic substance regulation." This suggested scheme would not allow for a regulation that was less cost effective than an alternative, nor any final regulation which cost more per human life saved than the value placed on a life.

Acceptable Risk and Consumer Choice

Unreasonable risk determinations were not always discussed in the context of a deliberative body making a decision. Individuals, it is pointed out, make risk-benefit decisions continuously, and much might be learned from those behaviors in which individuals decide what risks are acceptable. Some respondents prefer to approach unreasonable risk from a perspective of "acceptable risk."

An industry representative expressed the view :

> . . . this more positive direction of attack is useful in considering prospectively the extent to which regulation should be carried, as opposed to a retrospective review to see if regulatory actions were adequate.

Amplifying, he explains:

> In the long run, acceptable risk is the perceived risk to which informed persons do not object. That statement implies a higher level of knowledge than the general population now has, and acknowledges the emotional issues present in any cancer controversy.

This respondent joins those who call for improvements in present methods of risk and benefit estimation, but adds:

> It seems probable that there is no general answer to acceptable risk, and no numerical value that is correct for all situations.

The issue of whether a risk is taken voluntarily or involuntarily is a major determinant of levels of hazard that are considered acceptable. It is supposed, in general, that higher risk is acceptable for a purely voluntary exposure than for an involuntary one, and different approaches to regulation may be appropriate for different degrees of voluntarism.

A member of the legal community, concerned particularly with consumer products, advocates a "consumer choice" approach:

> . . . under which the Government would assess the risks but would not have authority to ban on the basis of this risk assessment, would be responsible for assuring that information about risk is provided to consumers through product labeling and other educational techniques, and would leave the ultimate risk-benefit judgment to consumers. The uniqueness of this approach is that the consumer, rather than the government, would make the "regulatory" decision of whether human exposure would occur. Some consumers would conclude that their benefits outweigh the risks and would use the product; others would conclude the opposite and would not use it.

Concerning the benefits derived from consumer goods, he explains:

> Most benefits are psychological or in any event nonobjective and nonquantifiable in nature. In the area of food . . . virtually all people eat not for health or nutrition reasons but rather for pleasure. If one eats enough of virtually anything that one likes, one will, after all receive sufficient nutrition. Thus, choice of food—i.e., consumer benefit—is wholly subjective and personal in nature. With the exception of a very few essential nutrients, in our country no food can be said to have any "benefits" in the sense that they are in any way essential or irreplaceable. And if you define "benefits" to include simple consumer desire for pleasure, the term soon becomes meaningless.
>
> I believe this same analysis holds true not just in the area of food, but indeed for all consumer products. And because TSCA deals with chemicals broadly, it ultimately impacts upon all consumer goods.

Opinions Expressed in the Responses Parallel the Diversity of Laws

From banning of carcinogens based only on consideration of risk, to balancing risks, costs, and benefits, to an antiregulatory position of letting the consumer decide, the responses parallel developments and discussions in regulatory law. This range of attitudes is not surprising because many respondents have testified before the legislature or been party to lawsuits about carcinogen regulation. On the other hand, the spectrum of opinion confounds conclusions that environmental laws can be fit into an evolutionary pattern and that some approaches, for instance, zero-risk laws, no longer have adherents.

The evolutionary analysis suggests that more sophisticated laws, such as TSCA, with its balancing, have now displaced risk-only approaches. Overall, responses received by OTA indicate that risk-only regulations are favored by some for the workplace and that "evolution" has not displaced all interest in risk-based regulations. In fact, the responses show

that the breadth of carcinogen regulatory approaches, including the old and the new laws, reflects the spectrum of current thinking. The responses did not produce a "new" approach to determining unreasonable risk. Quantitative risk assessment is an integral part of many of the responses, and its frequent mention reflects the perceived importance of this technique.

The New York Academy of Sciences Meeting

The title of the NYAS meeting, "Workshop on Management of Assessed Risk for Carcinogens," was chosen to show that the focus of the meeting was not risk assessment. The meeting lasted 2½ days. There was some overlap between participants in the meeting and respondents to the OTA letter, and because of that and the inherent problems of capturing a long meeting in a few pages, no attempt will be made here to summarize the meeting. This short description will highlight some points made there that did not arise in any other context in this assessment.

William Ruckelshaus of the Weyerhaeuser Co., a former EPA Administrator, was asked why industry does not remove risks in advance of regulation. His answer had two parts. First, he said, "industry leaders often do not know the extent of the health or environmental problems." Second, a "company that spends money on a problem in advance of regulation may fall behind its competitors who make the same product but do not spend for risk reduction." He suggested that regulations are sometimes welcomed because all competitors are affected.

Peter Preuss described CPSC's approach to regulation of carcinogens. Each of CPSC's actions has originated from a petition asking for agency action. All but one of the chemicals had been regulated by another agency. His analysis of CPSC actions led him to conclude that CPSC has employed no overarching method to settle unreasonable risk questions; each decision was largely independent of the others.

A number of speakers made the point that many chemicals are carcinogens when tested and that there are perhaps hundreds of candidates for regulation. Lively discussions broke out between those who want to order carcinogens on the basis of their potency and those who hold that extrapolation is too imprecise to estimate potency.

Surprisingly enough, there was general agreement about the value of cost effectiveness as a method to plot regulatory strategy. Cost effectiveness involves ordering the risks, estimating the cost of reducing or eliminating the risk, and deciding which expenditure of resources will accomplish the largest reduction in risk. A perhaps essential difference between cost effectiveness which found favor, and benefit-cost analysis which did not, is that cost effectiveness presupposes that risk reduction is a goal, and the method guides efforts toward that goal.

There were few advocates of benefit-cost analysis at the workshop, and many participants attacked the method. It was characterized as expensive and as ignoring values, costs, and benefits that cannot be converted to dollars. And, for those interested in regulation, benefit-cost analysis does not set a goal of reducing risks. Instead, it puts each projected regulation to a test of whether or not it should be promulgated.

Proceedings of the workshop have recently been published. *Management of Assessed Risks for Carcinogens* (276a) is a valuable source of information about approaches to risk management.

Appendix C.—Abbreviations and Glossary of Terms

Abbreviations

2-AAF	2-acetylaminofluorene
ACS	American Cancer Society
AIHC	American Industrial Health Council
B(a)P	benzo(a)pyrene
BAT	best available technology
BPT	best practical technology
CAA	Clean Air Act
CAG	Carcinogen Assessment Group (EPA)
CAI	Carcinogenicity Activity Indicator
CDC	Centers for Disease Control (PHS)
CEQ	Council on Environmental Quality
CIIT	Chemical Industry Institute of Toxicology
CPSA	Consumer Product Safety Act
CPSC	Consumer Product Safety Commission
CSIN	Chemical Substances Information Network (EPA)
CWA	Clean Water Act
DES	diethylstilbestrol
DHEW	Department of Health, Education, and Welfare
DHHS	Department of Health and Human Services
EPA	Environmental Protection Agency
FDA	Food and Drug Administration (PHS)
FDCA	Food, Drug, and Cosmetic Act
FIFRA	Federal Insecticide, Fungicide, and Rodenticide Act
FILS	Federal Information Locator System
FSC	Food Safety Council
g	gram
GAO	General Accounting Office
GRAS	generally recognized as safe
HANES	Health and Nutrition Examination Survey (NCHS)
HCFA	Health Care Financing Administration (DHHS)
HDL	high dose level
HIS	Health Interview Survey (NCHS)
IARC	International Agency for Research on Cancer (WHO)
ICD	International Classification of Diseases (WHO)
IOM	Institute of Medicine (NAS)
IRLG	Interagency Regulatory Liaison Group
ITC	Interagency Testing Committee
kg	kilogram (1,000 g)
LASS	Linked Administrative Statistical Sample
m	meter
mg	milligram (one-thousandth of a gram; 10^{-3} g)
MTD	maximum tolerated dose
NAS	National Academy of Sciences
NCAB	National Cancer Advisory Board
NCHS	National Center for Health Statistics (DHHS)
NCI	National Cancer Institute (NIH)
NCTR	National Center for Toxicological Research (EPA/FDA)
NDI	National Death Index (NCHS)
ng	nanogram (one-billionth of a gram; 10^{-9} g)
NIEHS	National Institute of Environmental Health Sciences
NIH	National Institutes of Health (PHS)
NIOSH	National Institute of Occupational Safety and Health (CDC)
NOHS	National Occupational Hazard Survey (NIOSH)
NORS	National Organics Reconnaissance Survey (EPA)
NRC	National Research Council (NAS)
NRDC	Natural Resources Defense Council
NSF	National Science Foundation
NTP	National Toxicology Program (DHHS)
OECD	Organization for Economic Cooperation and Development
OHRST	Office of Health Research, Statistics, and Technology
OSH Act	Occupational Safety and Health Act
OSHA	Occupational Safety and Health Administration (Department of Labor)
OSTP	Office of Science and Technology Policy
PAH	polycyclic aromatic hydrocarbons
PCBs	polychlorinated biphenyls
PHS	Public Health Service (DHHS)
PMN	premanufacturing notice
RCRA	Resource Conservation and Recovery Act
RPAR	rebuttable presumption against registration
SAB	Scientific Advisory Board (EPA)
SDWA	Safe Drinking Water Act
SEER	Surveillance, Epidemiology, and End Results program (NCI)
SNUR	significant new use rule
SSA	Social Security Administration (DHHS)
TSCA	Toxic Substances Control Act
TSSC	Toxic Substances Strategy Committee
ug	microgram (one-millionth of a gram; 10^{-6} g)
WHO	World Health Organization (United Nations)

Glossary of Terms

Benign tumor: A tumor confined to the territory in which it arises, not invading surrounding tissue or metastasizing to distant organs. Benign tumors can usually be excised by local surgery.

Carcinoma: Cancers of the epithelia, including the external epithelia (mainly skin and linings of the gastrointestinal tract, lungs, and cervix) and the internal epithelia that line various glands (e.g., breast, pancreas, thyroid).

Bioassay: In general, a test in living organisms. As used in this report, a test for carcinogenicity in laboratory animals, generally rats and mice, which includes near-lifelong exposure to the agent under test. Used interchangeably with "animal test."

Carcinogen: A substance that causes cancer.

Epigenetic: As used in reference to cancer, an effect on cancer causation that does not directly involve an interaction with DNA.

Epithelium: The covering of internal and external surfaces of the body, including the lining of vessels and other small cavities.

Incidence: The number of new cases of a disease, usually expressed as a rate:

$$\frac{\text{Number of new cases of a disease occurring in a population during a specified period of time}}{\text{Number of persons exposed to risk of developing the disease during that period of time}}$$

The incidence rate is a direct estimate of the probability, or risk, of developing a disease during a specified period of time.

Initiator: An external stimulus or agent that produces a cell that is "latently premalignant." An initiation event, or more generally, an early event, may be a mutational change in the cell's genetic material, but the change is unexpressed, and it causes no detectable change in the cell's growth pattern. The change is considered to be irreversible.

Leukemia: Cancers of the blood-forming organs, characterized by abnormal proliferation and development of leukocytes (white blood cells) and their precursors in the blood and bone marrow.

Lymphoma: Cancers of cells of the immune system, i.e., the various types of lymphocytes. Hodgkin's disease is included among the lymphomas.

Malignant tumor: A tumor that has invaded neighboring tissue and/or undergone metastasis to distant body sites, at which point the tumor is called a cancer and is beyond the reach of local surgery.

Melanoma: A tumor made up of melanin-pigmented cells. As used in this report, "malignant melanoma."

Mesothelioma: A tumor developing from a cell on the surface of the peritoneum (the membrane lining the abdominal cavity), pericardium (the membrane enclosing the heart), or pleura (the membrane lining each half of the thorax).

Metastasis: The spread of a malignancy to distant body sites by cancer cells transported in blood or lymph circulation.

Morbidity: The condition of being diseased.

Mortality rate: The death rate, often made explicit for a particular characteristic, e.g., age, sex, or specific cause of death. A mortality rate contains three essential elements: 1) the number of people in a population group exposed to the risk of death; 2) a time factor; 3) the number of deaths occurring in the exposed population during a certain time period. For example, the annual U.S. cancer mortality rate is:

$$\frac{\text{Number of deaths from cancer in the United States during 1 year}}{\text{Number of people in the population at midyear}}$$

Mutagen: A chemical or physical agent that interacts with DNA to cause a permanent, transmissible change in the genetic material of a cell.

Myelomatosis: A malignant neoplasm of plasma cells usually arising in the bone marrow. Also called multiple myeloma.

Neoplasm: A new growth of tissue in which growth is uncontrolled and progressive. A tumor.

Nonmelanoma: Skin cancer of two types: basal cell and squamous cell carcinomas. Though these tumors may invade surrounding tissue, and therefore are technically cancers, they seldom metastasize and are usually successfully treated with local surgery. Because they are relatively easily treated, often outside hospitals, cause relatively few deaths, and are not often enumerated, they are usually excluded from cancer statistics.

Prevalence: The number of existing cases of a disease, usually expressed as a rate:

$$\frac{\text{Number of cases of a disease present in the population at (or during) a specified time (period)}}{\text{Number of persons in the populaton at (or during) the specified time}}$$

Promoter: An influence or agent causing an initiated cell to produce a tumor. Promotion events, or more generally, late events, can occur only in "initiated" cells, and are somewht reversible. Discontinuation of exposure to a promoter, if exposure has not yet caused a tumor, may prevent the appearance of a tumor.

Sarcoma: Cancers of various supporting tissues of the body (e.g., bone cells, blood vessels, fibrous tissue cells, muscle).

Short-term test: Tests that take less time to complete than do bioassays. Most of these tests biologically measure interactions between the agent under test and DNA. Agents that have effects in short-term tests are considered more likely to be carcinogens than those that have no effect.

Transformed cell: A cell that has undergone both initiation and promotion, and will eventually give rise to a tumor.

Tumor: A new growth of tissue in which growth is uncontrolled and progressive. A neoplasm.

References

References

1. Abraham, J. L., "Underdiagnosis of Pulmonary Asbestosis," *N. Eng. J. Med.* 302:464, 1980.
2. Adamson, R., National Cancer Institute, personal communication, December 1980.
3. Albert, R. A., "Toward a More Uniform Federal Strategy for the Assessment and Regulation of Carcinogens," a report prepared for OTA, Washington, D.C., 1980.
4. American Bar Association, Commission on Law and the Economy, *Federal Regulation: Roads to Reform*, final report (Washington, D.C.: ABA, 1979).
5. American Cancer Society, *Facts on Testicular Cancer* (New York: ACS, 1978).
6. _____, *Cancer Facts and Figures: 1981* (New York: ACS , 1980).
7. American Federation of Labor and Congress of Industrial Organizations and United Steelworkers of America, "Post-Hearing Brief on OSHA's Proposed Standard on the Identification, Classification, and Regulation of Toxic Substances Posing a Potential Occupational Carcinogenic Risk" (Washington, D.C.: AFL-CIO, 1978).
8. American Industrial Health Council, *AIHC Recommended Alternative to OSHA's Generic Carcinogen Proposal* (Scarsdale, N.Y.: AIHC, 1978).
9. _____, "A Reply to: 'Estimates of the Fraction of Cancer in the United States Attributable to Occupational Factors (Sept. 15, 1978),' " (Scarsdale, N.Y.: AIHC, 1978).
9a. _____, "AIHC Comments on: A Report of the Interagency Regulatory Liaison Group (IRLG) Work Group on Risk Assessment Entitled 'Scientific Bases for Identifying Potential Carcinogens and Estimating Their Risks' " (Scarsdale, N.Y.: AIHC). Draft for review and comment May 5, 1979.
10. _____, "AIHC Proposal for a Science Panel" (Scarsdale, N.Y.: AIHC, 1980).
11. Ames, B. N., "Identifying Environmental Chemicals Causing Mutations and Cancer," *Science* 204:587, 1979.
12. Ames, B. N., and Hooper, K., " 'Does Carcinogenic Potency Correlate With Mutagenic Potency in the Ames Assay?' A Reply," *Nature* 274:19-20, 1979.
13. Ames, B. N., and McCann, J., "Validation of the Salmonella Test: A Reply to Rinkus and Legator," *Cancer Res.*, in press, 1981.
14. Ames, B. N., et al., "Carcinogenic Potency: A Progress Report," in *Banbury Report 5: Ethyl-ene Dichloride: Economic Importance and Potential Health Risks*, B. N. Ames, P. Infante, and R. Reitz (eds.) (Cold Spring Harbor, N.Y.: Cold Spring Harbor Press, 1980).
15. Anderson, D. E., "Some Characteristics of Familial Breast Cancer," *Cancer* 28(6): 1500-1504, 1971.
16. Armstrong, B., and Doll, R., "Bladder Cancer Mortality in England and Wales in Relation to Cigarette Smoking and Saccharin Consumption," *Br. J. Prev. Soc. Med.* 30:151-157, 1974.
17. _____, "Environmental Factors and Cancer Incidence and Mortality in Different Countries, With Special Reference to Dietary Practices," *Int. J. Cancer* 15:617-631, 1975.
18. Ashby, J., and Styles, J. A., "Does Carcinogenic Potency Correlate With Mutagenic Potency in the Ames Assay?" *Nature* 271:452-455, 1978.
19. Baram, M. S., *Regulation of Health, Safety, and Environmental Quality and the Use of Cost-Benefit Analysis*, Final Report to the Administrative Conference of the United States (Washington, D.C.: Administrative Conference, 1979).
20. _____, "The Legal Framework for Determining Unreasonable Risk From Carcinogenic Chemicals," a report prepared for OTA, U.S Congress, Washington, D.C., 1980.
21. Barnard, R. C., "The Emerging Regulatory Dilemma" in *Management of Assessed Risk for Carcinogens*, W. J. Nicholson (ed.) (New York: New York Academy of Sciences, 1981).
22. Bartsch, H., et al., "Bacterial and Mammalian Mutagenicity Tests: Validation and Comparative Studies on 180 Chemicals" in *Molecular and Cellular Aspects of Carcinogen Screening Tests*, R. Montesano, H. Bartsch, and L. Tomatis (eds.) (Lyon, France: International Agency for Research on Cancer, 1980).
23. Beebe, G. W., "Some Aspects of Record Linkage in Epidemiologic Research in the U.S.," paper presented at the Workshop on Computerized Record Linkage in Cancer Epidemiology, Ottawa, Canada, Aug. 8-10, 1979.
24. Berg, J. W., "Diet," in *Persons at High Risk of Cancer: An Approach to Cancer Etiology and Control*, J. F. Fraumeni (ed.) (New York: Academic Press, 1975).
25. Berg, J. W., and Burbank, F., "Correlation Between Carcinogenic Trace Metals in Water Supplies and Cancer Mortality," *Ann. N.Y. Acad. Sci.* 199:249, 1972.

26. Bionetics Research Laboratory, *Evaluation of Carcinogenic, Teratogenic, and Mutagenic Activities of Selected Pesticides and Industrial Chemicals, Vol. I: Carcinogenic Study,* NTIS PB-223-159, August 1968.

27. Blot, W. J., "Changing Patterns of Breast Cancer Among American Women," *Am. J. Pub. Health* 70(8):832-835, 1980.

28. Blot, W. J., and Fraumeni, J. F., "Arsenical Air Pollution and Lung Cancer," *Lancet* 2:142-144, 1975.

29. Blot, W. J., "Developing Clues to Environmental Cancer: A Stepwise Approach With the Use of Cancer Mortality Data," *Env. Health Persp.* 32:53-58, 1979.

30. Boston Collaborative Drug Surveillance Program, "Surgically Confirmed Gallbladder Disease, Venous Thromboembolism, and Breast Tumors in Relation to Postmenopausal Estrogen Therapy," *N. Eng. J. Med.* 290(1):15-19, 1974.

31. Boyland, E., "The Correlation of Experimental Carcinogenesis and Cancer in Man," *Prog. Exp. Tumor Res.* 11:222-234, 1969.

32. Breslow, N. E., and Enstrom, J. E., "Geographic Correlations Between Cancer Mortality Rates and Alcohol-Tobacco Consumption in the United States," *J. Natl. Cancer Inst.* 53(3):631-639, 1974.

33. Breslow, N., et al., "Latent Carcinoma of Prostate at Autopsy in Seven Areas," *Int. J. Cancer* 20:680-688, 1977.

34. Bridges, B. A., "Short-Term Tests and Human Health—The Central Role of DNA Repair," in *Environmental Carcinogenesis,* P. Emmelot and E. Kriech (eds.) (Amsterdam: Elsevier/ North Holland Biomedical Press, 1979).

35. Brown, C. C., "The Statistical Analysis of Dose-Effect Relationships," in *Principles of Ecotoxicology,* C. C. Butler (ed.) (New York: John Wiley & Sons, 1978).

36. Brown, C. C., et al., "Models for Carcinogenic Risk Assessment," *Science* 202:1105, 1978.

37. Burbank, F., Patterns in Cancer Mortality in the United States: 1950-1967, National Cancer Institute Monograph 33, (Bethesda, Md.: National Institute of Health, 1971).

38. Bureau of Radiological Health, *The Selection of Patients for X-Ray Examinations* (Rockville, Md.: Food and Drug Administration, 1980).

39. _____, *The Selection of Patients for X-Ray Examinations* The Pelvimetry Examination, PHS publication (FDA) 80-8128 (Rockville, Md.: Food and Drug Administration, 1980).

40. Burkitt, D., "Related Disease—Related Cause?" *Lancet* 2:1229-1231, 1969.

41. Butterworth, C. E., Jr., "The Concept of Localized Nutrient Deficiency in Target Tissue, With Particular Reference to Folacin: Implications for Carcinogenesis," paper presented at the National Academy of Sciences, Washington, D.C., Nov. 6, 1980.

42. Cairns, J., *Cancer: Science and Society* (San Francisco: W. H. Freeman, 1978).

43. _____, "Cancer: The Case for Preventive Strategies," in *Healthy People: The Surgeon General's Report on Health Promotion and Disease Prevention, Background Papers,* DHEW (PHS) publication No. 79-55071A (Washington, D.C.: Public Health Service, 1979).

44. California, State of, "Occupational Mortality in the State of California, 1959-1961," January 1980.

45. Cambien, F., Ducimetiere, P., and Richard, J., "Total Serum-Cholesterol and Cancer Mortality in a Middle-Aged Male Population," *Am. J. Epidem.* 112:388-394, 1980.

46. Campbell, J. A., "X-Ray Pelvimetry: Useful Procedure or Medical Nonsense," *J. Natl. Med. Assoc.* 68(6):514-520, 1976.

47. Campbell, T. C., "Influence of Nutrition on Metabolism of Carcinogens," in *Advances in Nutritional Research,* H. H. Draper (ed.) (New York: Plenum Press, 1979).

48. Carcinogen Assessment Group, "The Carcinogen Assessment Group's Procedure for Calculating Water Quality Criteria," typescript (Washington, D.C.: Environmental Protection Agency, 1980).

49. Carlborg, F. W., "Dose Response Functions in Carcinogenesis and the Weibull Model," *Food Cosmet. Tox.,* in press, 1981.

50. _____, "2-AAF and the Weibull Model," *Food Cosmet. Tox.,* in press, 1981.

51. _____, "Multistage Dose Response Models and Carcinogenesis," *Food Cosmet. Tox.,* in press, 1981.

52. Carroll, K. K., and Hopkins, G. J., "Dietary Polyunsaturated Fat Versus Saturated Fat in Relation to Mammary Carcinogenesis," *Lipids* 14(2):155-158, 1979.

53. Carroll, K. K., and Khor, H .T., "Effects of Level and Type of Dietary Fat on Incidence of Mammary Tumors Induced in Female Sprague-Dawley Rates by 7, 12-dimethylbenz(α)anthracene," *Lipids* 6(6):415-420, 1971.

54. Cederlöf, R., et al., "Air Pollution and Cancer:

Risk Assessment Methodology and Epidemiologic Evidence," *Env. Health Persp.* 22:1-12, 1978.

55. Center for Disease Control, "Glioblastoma Cluster in a Chemical Plant—Texas," *MMWR* 29(30):359-360, 1980.

56. _____, "Statement of Organization, Functions and Delegations of Authority," *Federal Register* 45:67772, 1980.

57. Chand, N., and Hoel, D. G., "A Comparison of Models for Determining Safe Levels of Environmental Agents," in *Reliability and Biometry: Statistical Analysis of Lifelength* (Philadelphia, Pa.: Society for Industrial and Applied Mathematics, 1974).

58. Cicero, J., National Center for Health Statistics, personal communication, 1981.

59. Clark, T. B., "New Approaches to Regulatory Reform—Letting the Market Do the Job," *Nat. J.* 11:1316-1322, 1979.

60. Clayson, D., "Bladder Carcinogenesis in Rats and Mice: Possibility of Artifacts," *J. Natl. Cancer Inst.* 52:1685-1689, 1974.

61. Clement Associates, Inc., contract report prepared for OTA, U.S. Congress, Washington, D.C., Oct. 31, 1980.

62. Cole, P., "Cancer and Occupation: Status and Needs of Epidemiologic Research," *Cancer* 39:1788-1791, 1977.

63. Committee on Governmental Affairs, U.S. Senate, *Study on Federal Regulations*, vols. 1-4 (Washington, D.C.: U.S. Government Printing Office, 1977, 1978).

64. _____, *Report on the Paperwork Reduction Act of 1980*, report no. 96-930 (Washington, D.C.: U.S. Government Printing Office, 1980).

65. Committee on Interstate and Foreign Commerce, U.S. House of Representatives, *Report on the Toxic Substances Control Act*, report No. 94-1341 (Washington, D.C.: U.S. Government Printing Office, 1976).

66. Conservation Foundation, *Approaches for the Development of Testing Guidelines Under the Toxic Substances Control Act* (Washington, D.C.: The Conservation Foundation, 1978).

67. Cornfield, J., "Carcinogenic Risk Assessment," *Science* 198:691-699, 1977.

68. _____, "Models for Carcinogenic Risk Assessment," *Science* 202: 1107-1109, 1978.

69. Costle, D., "Panel III: Managing the Regulatory Process," *Ad. Law Rev.* 32:256-260, 1980.

70. Council on Environmental Quality, *Environmental Quality (1980): The Eleventh Annual Report of the Council on Environmental Quality* (Washington, D.C.: U.S. Government Printing Office, 1980).

71. Creech, J. L., and Johnson, M. N., "Angiosarcoma of Liver in the Manufacture of Polyvinyl Chloride," *J. Occup. Med.* 16:150, 1974.

72. Crouch, E., and Wilson, R., "Interspecies Comparison of Carcinogenic Potency," *J. Tox. Env. Health* 5:1095-1118, 1979.

73. Crump, K. S., "Models for Carcinogenic Risk Assessment," *Science* 202:1106, 1978.

74. Crump, K. S., and Guess, H. A., *Drinking Water and Cancer: Review of Recent Findings and Assessment of Risks* (Washington, D.C.: Council on Environmental Quality, 1980).

75. Crump, K. S., et al., "Fundamental Carcinogenic Processes and Their Implication for Low Dose Risk Assessment," *Cancer Res.* 36:-2973-2979, 1976.

76. Cutler, L., "Panel III: Managing the Regulatory Process," *Ad. Law Rev.* 32:240-243, 1980.

77. Cutler, S. J., and Young, J. L., *Third National Cancer Survey: Incidence Data*, National Cancer Institute Monograph No. 41, DHEW publication No. (NIH) 75-787 (Washington, D.C.: U.S. Government Printing Office, 1975).

78. Davies, J.C., Gusman, S., and Irvin, F., *Determining Unreasonable Risk Under the Toxic Substances Control Act* (Washington, D.C.: The Conservation Foundation, 1979).

79. de Waard, F., "Premenopausal and Postmenopausal Breast Cancer: One Disease or Two?" *J. Natl. Cancer Inst.* 63(3):549-552, 1979.

80. Deisler, P. F., Jr., "Dealing With Industrial Health Risks: A Step-Wise, Goal-Oriented Concept," in *Risk in the Technological Society*, C. Hohenemser and J. Kasperson (eds.) (Boulder, Colo.: Westview Press, 1981), in press.

81. _____, Shell Oil Co., personal communication, 1981.

82. Department of Health, Education, and Welfare, "Estimates of the Fraction of Cancer in the United States Related to Occupational Factors" (Bethesda, Md.: National Cancer Institute, National Institute of Environmental Health Sciences, National Institute of Occupational Safety and Health, 1978).

83. Department of Health and Human Services, *First Annual Report on Carcinogens* (Washington, D.C.: DHHS, 1980).

84. Devesa, S. S., and Silverman, D. T., "Cancer Incidence and Mortality Trends in the United States: 1935-1974," *J. Natl. Cancer Inst.* 60(3):545-571, 1978.

85. DeVita, V. T., "Opportunities in Cancer Treat-

ment," paper presented at the Science Writers Seminar, American Cancer Society, Daytona Beach, Fla., Mar. 23, 1980.

86. DeVita, V. T., Jr., Henney, J. E., and Hubbard, S. M., "Estimation of the Numerical and Economic Impact of Chemotherapy in the Treatment of Cancer," in *Cancer Achievement, Challenges, and Prospects for the '80's*, J. H. Burchenal, and H. S. Oettgen (eds.) (New York: Grune & Statton, 1981).

87. Devoret, R., "Bacterial Tests for Potential Carcinogens," *Sci. Am.* 241:40-49, 1979.

88. Dickson, D., "More Tests Required on New Chemicals," *Nature* 285:60, 1980.

89. _____, "Melanoma Increase in Radiation Labs?" *Nature* 287:475, 1980.

90. Dieckmann, W. J., et al., "Does the Administration of Diethylstilbestrol During Pregnancy Have Therapeutic Value?" *Am. J. Obstet. Gynecol.* 66(5):1062-1081, 1953.

91. Doll, R., "Atmospheric Pollution and Lung Cancer," *Env. Health. Persp.* 22:23-32, 1978.

92. Doll, R., and Peto, R., "Mortality in Relation to Smoking: 20 Years' Observations on Male British Doctors," *Br. Med. J.* 2(6051):1525-1556, 1976.

93. _____, "The Causes of Cancer: Quantitative Estimates of Avoidable Risks of Cancer in United States Today," *J. Natl. Cancer Inst.* 66:1191-1308, 1981.

94. Doll, R., et al., "Mortality in Relation to Smoking: 22 Years' Observations on Female British Doctors," *Br. Med. J.* 280:967-971, 1980.

95. Doniger, D., Natural Resources Defense Council, personal communication, March 1981.

96. Donovan, P. J., and DiPaolo, J. A., "Caffeine Enhancement of Chemical and Carcinogen-Induced Transformation of Cultured Syrian Hamster Cells," *Cancer Res.* 34:2720-2727, 1974.

97. Economist, The, "Cancer Testing: Chinese Hamsters to the Rescue," *Economist* 111-112, May 26, 1979.

98. Ederer, F., et al., "Cancer Among Men on Cholesterol-Lowering Diets," *Lancet* 2:203-206, 1971.

99. Engel, L. W., et al., "Accuracy of Death Certification in an Autopsied Population With Specific Attention to Malignant Neoplasms and Vascular Diseases," *Am. J. Epidem.* 111(1): 99-112, 1980.

100. Enstrom, J. E., "Cancer Mortality Among Low Risk Populations," *CA* 29(6):352-361, 1979.

101. Environmental Protection Agency, "Interim Procedures and Guidelines for Health Risk and Economic Impact Assessments of Suspected Carcinogens," *Federal Register* 41:-21402-21405, 1976.

102. _____, Pesticide Programs, "Proposed Guidelines for Registering Pesticides in the U.S.: Hazard Evaluation: Humans and Domestic Animals," *Federal Register* 43:37336-37403, 1978.

103. _____, "Response to Interagency Testing Committee Recommendations," *Federal Register* 43:50134-50138, 1978.

104. _____, "Water Criteria Documents. Request for Comments." *Federal Register* 44:15926, 1979.

105. _____, "Toxic Substances Control; Premanufacturing Notification Requirements and Review Procedures; Statement of Interim Policy," *Federal Register* 44:28564, 1979.

106. _____, "Proposed Health Effects Test Standards for Toxic Substances Control Act Test Rules," *Federal Register* 43:37336-37403, 1979.

107. _____, "National Primary Drinking Water Regulations: Control of Trihalomethanes in Drinking Water, Final Rule," *Federal Register* 44:68624, 1979.

108. _____, "Pesticides and Toxic Substances; General Recordkeeping and Reporting Requirements: Preliminary Assessment Information," *Federal Register* 45:13646, 1980.

109. _____, "Toxic Substances Control Act; Records and Reports of Allegations of Significant Adverse Reactions to Health or the Environment," *Federal Register* 45:47008, 1980.

110. _____, "Chloromethane and Chlorinated Benzenes, Proposed Test Rule, Proposed Health Effects Standards Amended," *Federal Register* 45:48524-48566, 1980.

111. _____, "Policy and Procedures for Identifying, Assessing, and Regulating Airborne Substances Posing a Risk of Cancer: Proposed Rule," *Federal Register* 44:58642, 1980.

112. _____, *Economic Impact Analysis of Proposed Test Rule for Chloromethane and Chlorobenzenes* (Washington, D.C.: EPA, 1980).

113. _____, "Pilot Assessment of Ambient Conditions—Action Memorandum," Memorandum from Chairman, Committee on Monitor-

ing and Information Management to the Administrator, Feb. 8, 1980.

114. _____, "New Chemical Substances; Premanufacture Testing Policy," *Federal Register* 46:8986, 1981.

115. Epstein, S. S., "Environmental Determinants of Human Cancer," *Cancer Res.* 34:2425-2435, 1974.

116. Farber, E., "Reversible and Irreversible Lesions in Processes of Cancer Development," in *Molecular and Cellular Aspects of Carcinogen Screening Tests*, R. Montesano, H. Bartsch, and L. Tomatis (eds.) (Lyon, France: International Agency for Research on Cancer, 1980).

117. Fausett, R., Consumer Product Safety Commission, personal communication, 1981.

118. Feldman, J. G., et al., "A Case-Control Investigation of Alcohol, Tobacco, and Diet in Head and Neck Cancer," *Prev. Med.* 4(4):444-463, 1975.

119. Feminella, J. G., Jr., and Lattimer, J. K., "An Apparent Increase in Genital Carcinomas Among Wives of Men With Prostatic Carcinomas: An Epidemiologic Survey," *Pirquet Bull. Clin. Med.* 20:3-10, 1974.

120. Field, R., "Statutory Language and Risk Management," a report prepared for the Committee on Risk and Decision Making, National Research Council, Washington, D.C., 1980.

121. Fishman, J., "Fatness, Puberty, and Ovulation," *N. Eng. J. Med.* 303(1):42-43, 1980.

122. Fong, L. Y. Y., Sevals, A., and Newberne, P. M., "Zinc Deficiency and Methylbenzylnitrosamine-Induced Esophageal Cancer in Rats," *J. Natl. Cancer Inst.* 61:145-150, 1978.

123. Food and Drug Administration, Advisory Committee on Protocols for Safety Evaluation, Panel on Carcinogenesis, "Report on Cancer Testing in the Safety Evaluation of Food Additives and Pesticides," *Toxicol. Appl. Pharmacol.* 20:419-438, 1971.

124. _____, "Polychlorinated Biphenyls (PCB's); Reduction of Tolerances, Final Rule," *Federal Register* 44:37336-37403, 1979.

125. Food Safety Council, *Proposed System for Food Safety Assessment*, Final Report of the Scientific Committee (Washington, D.C.: Food Safety Council, 1980).

126. Fox, A. J., and Adelstein, A. M., "Occupational Mortality: Work or Way of Life?" *J. Epid. Comm. Health* 32:73-78, 1978.

127. Fraser, P., et al., "Nitrate and Human Cancer: A Review of the Evidence," *Intl. J. Epidem.* 9:3-11, 1980.

128. Fraumeni, J. F., and Mason, T. J., "Cancer Mortality Among Chinese Americans 1950-69," *J. Natl. Cancer Inst.* 52:659-665, 1974.

129. Fraumeni, J. F., et al., "Cancer Mortality Among Nuns: Role of Marital Status in Etiology of Neoplastic Disease in Women," *J. Natl. Cancer Inst.* 42(3):455-468, 1969.

130. Fredrickson, D. S., "Chairman's Overview," in *Health Research Activities of the Department of Health, Education, and Welfare: Current Efforts and Proposed Initiatives* (Washington, D.C.: Department of Health, Education, and Welfare, 1979).

131. Freeman, A. M., III., "Technology-Based Effluent Standards: The U.S. Case," *Water Resources Research* 16:21-27, 1980. (Also available as RFF Reprint 178 from Resources for the Future, Washington, D.C.).

132. _____, Bowdoin College, personal communication, March 1981.

133. Friedman, G. D., and Ury, H. K., "Initial Screening for Carcinogenicity of Commonly Used Drugs," *J. Natl. Cancer Inst.* 65(4): 723-733, October 1980.

134. Frisch, R. E., Wyshak, G., and Vincent, L., "Delayed Menarche and Amenorrhea in Ballet Dancers," *N. Eng. J. Med.* 303(1):17-19, 1980.

135. Gabrial, G. N., and Newberne, P. M., "Zinc Deficiency, Alcohol, and Esophageal Cancer," *Trace Substances in Environmental Health— XIII*, D. D. Hemphill (ed.). (Columbia, Mo.: University of Missouri Press, 1979).

136. Gaylor, D. W., National Center for Toxicological Research, personal communication, June 13, 1980.

137. Gaylor, D. W., and Kodell, R. L., "Linear Interpolation Algorithm for Low Dose Risk Assessment of Toxic Substances," *J. Env. Pathol. Toxicol.*, in press, 1981.

138. Gaylor, D. W., and Shapiro, R. E., "Extrapolation and Risk Estimation for Carcinogenesis," in *Advances in Modern Toxicology*, vol. 1, pt. 2 (New York: John Wiley & Sons, 1978).

139. Gehring, P. J., Watanabe, G., and Young, J. D., "The Relevance of Dose-Dependent Pharmacokinetics in the Assessment of Carcinogenic Hazard of Chemicals," in *Origins of Human Cancer*, H. H. Hiatt, J. D. Watson, and J. A. Winsten (eds.) (Cold Spring Harbor, N.Y.: Cold Spring Harbor Laboratory, 1977).

140. General Accounting Office, *Indoor Air Pollution: An Emerging Health Problem* (Washington, D.C.: GAO, 1980).

141. _____, *EPA is Slow To Carry Out Its Responsibilities To Control Harmful Chemicals* (Washington, D.C.: GAO, 1980).

141a. General Electric Co., "General Electric Comments on IRLG Report," typescript, Nov. 13, 1979.

142. Golberg, L., "Rapid Tests in Animals and Lower Organisms as Predictors of Long-Term Toxic Effects," paper presented at the Fourth Conference on Cutaneous Toxicity, Washington, D.C., May 9-11, 1979.

143. _____, paper delivered at the Toxicology Forum: International Update on Short-Term Tests, Washington, D.C., May 30-31, 1979.

144. Gray, G. E., Henderson, B. E., and Pike, M. C., "Changing Ratio of Breast Cancer Incidence Rates with Age of Black Females Compared With White Females in the United States," *J. Natl. Cancer Inst.* 64(3):461-463, 1980.

145. Green, H. P., "The Role of Law in Determining Acceptability of Risk," in *Management of Assessed Risk for Carcinogens,* W. J. Nicholson (ed.) (New York: New York Academy of Sciences, 1981).

146. Griesemer, R. A., and Cueto, C., Jr., "Toward a Classification Scheme for Degrees of Experimental Evidence for the Carcinogenicity of Chemicals for Animals," in *Molecular and Cellular Aspects of Carcinogen Screening Tests,* R. Montesano, H. Bartsch, and L. Tomatis (eds.) (Lyon, France: International Agency for Research on Cancer, 1980).

147. Gross, R. L., and Newberne, P. M., "Role of Nutrition in Physiological Function," *Physiol. Rev.* 60(1):188-302, 1980.

148. Guralnick, L., "Mortality by Occupation and Industry Among Men 20 to 64 Years of Age: U.S., 1950," *Vital Statistics—Special Reports* 53(2):49-92, 1963.

149. _____, "Mortality by Occupation and Cause of Death Among Men 20 to 64 Years of Age: U.S., 1950," *Vital Statistics—Special Reports* 53(3):93-340, 1963.

150. _____, "Mortality by Industry and Cause of Death Among Men 20 to 64 Years of Age: U.S., 1950," *Vital Statistics—Special Reports* 53(4):341-438, 1963.

151. _____, "Mortality by Occupational Level and Cause of Death Among Men 20 to 64 Years of Age: U.S., 1950," *Vital Statistics—Special Reports* 53(5):439-612, 1963.

152. Hammond, E. C., "Tobacco," in *Persons at High Risk of Cancer: An Approach to Cancer Etiology and Control,* J. F. Fraumeni, (ed.), (New York: Academic Press, 1975).

153. _____, "The Long-Term Benefits of Reducing Tar and Nicotine in Cigarettes," in *Banbury Report 3, A Safe Cigarette* (Cold Spring Harbor, N.Y.: Cold Spring Harbor Laboratory, 1980).

154. Hammond, E. C., and Garfinkel, L., "General Air Pollution and Cancer in the United States," *Prev. Med.* 9(2):206-211, 1980.

155. Hammond, E. C., and Seidman, H., "Smoking and Cancer in the United States," *Prev. Med.* 9(2):169-173, 1980.

156. Hammond, E. C., Selikoff, I. J., and Seidman, H., "Asbestos Exposure, Cigarette Smoking and Death Rates," *Ann. N.Y. Acad. of Sci.* 330:473-490, 1979.

157. Hammond, E.C., et al., "Some Recent Findings Concerning Cigarette Smoking," in *Origins of Human Cancer,* H. H. Hiatt, J. D. Watson, and J. A. Winsten (eds.) (Cold Spring Harbor, N.Y.: Cold Spring Harbor Laboratory, 1977).

158. Harris, R. H., Page, T., and Reiches, N. A., "Carcinogenic Hazards of Organic Chemicals in Drinking Waters," in *Origins of Human Cancer,* H. H. Hiatt, J. D. Watson, and J. A. Winsten (eds.) (Cold Spring Harbor, N.Y.: Cold Spring Harbor Laboratory, 1977).

159. Harrison, T. R., *Harrison's Principles of Internal Medicine,* 9th ed., K. J. Isselbacher, et al. (eds.) (New York: McGraw-Hill, 1980).

160. Harsanyi, Z., Granek, I. A., and Mackenzie, D. W. R., "Genetic Damage Induced by Ethyl Alcohol in *Aspergillus nidulans,*" *Mutat.Res.* 48:51-74, 1977.

161. Hegsted, D. M., "Optimal Nutrition," *Cancer* 43(5):1996-2003, 1979.

162. Henderson, B. E., et al., "An Epidemiologic Study of Breast Cancer," *J. Natl. Cancer Inst.* 53(3):609-614, 1974.

163. _____, "Sexual Factors and Pregnancy," in *Persons at High Risk of Cancer: An Approach to Cancer Etiology and Control,* J. F. Fraumeni (ed.) (New York: Academic Press, 1975).

164. Higginson, J., "Present Trends in Cancer Epidemiology," *Proc. Canadian Cancer Conference* 8:40-75, 1969.

165. Higginson, J., and Muir, C. S., "The Role of Epidemiology in Elucidating the Importance of Environmental Factors in Human Cancer," *Cancer Det. Prev.* 1:79-105, 1976.

166. _____, "Guest Editorial: Environmental Car-

cinogenesis: Misconceptions and Limitations to Cancer Control," *J. Natl. Cancer Inst.* 63:1291-1298, 1979.

167. Hirayama, T., "Non-Smoking Wives of Heavy Smokers Have a Higher Risk of Lung Cancer: A Study from Japan," *Br. Med. J.* 282:183-185, 1981.

168. Hodgson, T. A., National Center for Health Statistics, personal communication, December 1980.

169. Hoel, D. G., and Crump, K. S., "Scientific Evidence of Risks From Water-Borne Carcinogens," paper presented at the Conference on the Scientific Basis of Health and Safety Regulations, Brookings Institution, Washington, D.C., Nov. 8-9, 1979.

170. Hoel, D. G., et al., "Estimation of Risks of Irreversible, Delayed Toxicity," *J. Toxicol. Env. Health* 1:133-151, 1975.

171. Hogan, M. D., and Hoel, D. G., "Estimated Cancer Risk Associated With Occupational Asbestos Exposure," *Risk Analysis*, in press, 1981.

172. Hollstein, M., et al., "Short-Term Tests for Carcinogens and Mutagens," *Mutat. Res.* 65:133-226, 1979.

173. Hoover, R., and Fraumeni, J. F., "Drug-Induced Cancer," *Cancer*, in press, 1981.

174. Hoover, R. N., and Strasser, P. H., "Artificial Sweeteners and Human Bladder Cancer," *Lancet* 1:837-840, 1980.

175. Howe, G. R., et al., "Artificial Sweeteners and Human Bladder Cancer," *Lancet* 2:578-581, 1977.

176. Innes, J. R. M., et al., "Bioassay of Pesticides and Industrial Chemicals for Tumorigenicity in Mice: A Preliminary Note," *J. Natl. Cancer Inst.* 42:1101-1114, 1969.

177. Institute of Medicine, *Reliability of Hospital Discharge Abstracts* (Washington, D.C.: National Academy of Sciences, 1977).

178. _____, *Alcoholism and Related Problems: Opportunities for Research* (Washington, D.C.: National Academy of Sciences, 1980).

179. _____, *Costs of Environment-Related Health Effects: A Plan for Continuing Study* (Washington, D.C.: National Academy Press, 1981).

180. Interagency Regulatory Liaison Group, "Scientific Bases for Identification of Potential Carcinogens and Estimation of Risks," *Federal Register* 44:39858-39879, 1979 and *J. Natl. Cancer Inst.* 63:241-268, 1979.

181. _____, *Documentation Guidelines for Epidemiologic Studies* (Washington, D.C.: IRLG, 1979).

182. Interagency Task Force on the Health Effects of Ionizing Radiation, *Report of the Work Group on Exposure Reduction* (Washington, D.C.: Department of Health, Education, and Welfare, 1979).

182a. _____, *Report of the Work Group on Records and Privacy* (Washington, D.C.: Department of Health, Education, and Welfare, 1979).

183. Interagency Testing Committee, *Initial Report of the TSCA Interagency Testing Committee to the Administrator* (Washington, D.C.: Environmental Protection Agency, 1978).

184. International Agency for Research on Cancer, *Cancer Incidence in Five Continents*, J. Waterhouse, et al. (eds.) (Lyon, France: IARC, 1976).

185. _____, *Chemicals and Industrial Processes Associated With Cancer in Humans, IARC Monographs Supplement 1* (Lyon, France: IARC, 1979).

186. _____, "An Evaluation of Chemicals and Industrial Processes Associated With Cancer in Humans Based on Human and Animal Data: IARC Monographs Volumes 1 to 20," *Cancer Res.* 40:1-12, 1980.

187. _____, *Long-Term and Short-Term Screening Assays for Carcinogens: A Critical Appraisal* (Lyon, France: IARC, 1980).

188. International Program for the Evaluation of Short-Term Tests for Carcinogenicity, transcript of Public Information Meeting, Bethesda, Md., Dec. 3, 1979.

189. Ip, C., "Factors Influencing the Anticarcinogenic Efficacy of Selenium in Dimethylbenz (α) anthracene-induced Mammary Tumorigenesis in Rats," *Cancer Res.* 41, in press, 1981.

190. Ip, C., and Sinha, D. K., "Enhancement of Mammary Tumorigenesis by Dietary Selenium Deficiency in Rats With a High Polyunsaturated Fat Intake," *Cancer Res.* 41:31-34, 1981.

191. Jablon, S., and Bailar, J. C., III., "The Contribution of Ionizing Radiation to Cancer Mortality in the United States," *Prev. Med.* 9(2):219-226, 1980.

192. Jellinek, S. D., paper presented at Fuji Techno Systems Seminar on the Impact of Regulatory Requirements on Chemical Substances, Tokyo, Japan, Oct. 30, 1980.

193. Jensen, O. M., "Cancer Morbidity and Causes of Death Among Danish Brewery Workers," *Int. J. Cancer* 23:454-463, 1979.

194. Jick, H., Walker, A. M., and Rothman, K. J., "The Epidemic of Endometrial Cancer: A Commentary," *Am. J. Pub. Health* 70(3):264-267, 1980.

195. Jose, D. G., "Dietary Deficiency of Protein, Amino Acids, and Total Calories on Development and Growth of Cancer," *Nutr. Cancer* 1(3):58-63, 1979.

196. Kaplan, D. L., Parkhurst, E., and Whelpton, P. K., "The Comparability of Reports on Occupation From Vital Records and the 1960 Census," *Vital Statistics—Special Reports* 53(1), 1961.

197. Kellermann, C., Shaw, C. R., and Luyten-Kellerman, M., "Aryl Hydrocarbon Hydroxylase Inducibility and Bronchogenic Carcinoma," *N. Eng. J. Med.* 289(18):934-937, 1973.

198. Kelly, K. M., et al, "The Utilization and Efficacy of Pelvimetry," *Am. J. Roentg. Rad. Ther. Nuc. Med.* 125(1):66-74, 1975.

199. Keys, A., "Alpha Lipoprotein (HDL) Cholesterol in the Serum and the Risk of Coronary Heart Disease and Death," *Lancet* 1:603-606, 1980.

200. Kilss, B., and Scheuren, F., "Planning for a Linked Administrative Statistical Sample," staff paper, Statistical Analysis and Survey Implementation Branch, Division of Economic Research, Social Security Administration, November 1979.

201. Knudson, A. G., "Genetic Predisposition to Cancer", in *Origins of Human Cancer*, H. H. Hiatt, J. D. Watson, and J. A. Winsten (eds.) (Cold Spring Harbor, N.Y.: Cold Spring Harbor Laboratory, 1977).

202. Kozlowski, L.T., "Tar and Nicotine Delivery of Cigarettes. What a Difference a Puff Makes," *J.A.M.A.* 245(2):758-759, 1981.

203. Kraybill, H. F., "Evaluation of Public Health Aspects of Carcinogenic/Mutagenic Biorefractories in Drinking Water," *Prev. Med.* 9: 212-218, 1980.

204. Lave, L. B., *Quantitative Analyses of Proposed Social Regulations"* (Washington, D.C.: The Brookings Institution, in press, 1981).

205. Lawther, P. J. and Waller, R. E., "Trends in Urban Air Pollution in the United Kingdom Relation to Lung Cancer Mortality," *Env. Health Persp.* 22:71-74, 1978.

206. Levin, R. W., "Judicial Review and the Bumpers Amendment," report prepared for the Committee on Judicial Review of the Administrative Conference of the United States, November 1979.

207. Lew, E. A., and Garfinkel, L., "Variations in Mortality by Weight Among 750,000 Men and Women," *J. Chron. Dis.* 32:563-576, 1979.

208. Li, F. P., and Fraumeni, J. F., "Testicular Cancers in Children: Epidemiologic Charac-

209. Li, M., et al., "Formation of Carcinogenic N-nitroso Compounds in Corn-Bread Inoculated With Fungi," *Scientia Sinica* 22(4):471-477, 1979.

210. Lilienfeld, A. M., *Foundations of Epidemiology* (New York: Oxford University Press, 1976).

211. Lin, H. J., et al., "Zinc Levels in Serum, Hair, and Tumors From Patients With Esophageal Cancer," *Nutr. Rep. Int.* 15(6):635-643, 1977.

212. Linsell, C. A., and Peers, F. G., "Field Studies on Liver Cell Cancer," in *Origins of Human Cancer*, H. H. Hiatt, J. D. Watson, and J. A. Winsten (eds.) (Cold Spring Harbor, N.Y.: Cold Spring Harbor Laboratory, 1977).

213. Littlefield, N. A., et al., "Effects of Dose and Time in a Long-Term, Low-Dose Carcinogenic Study," *J. Env. Pathol. Toxicol.* 3:17-34,1979.

214. Lloyd, W., "Cancer Epidemiology," paper presented at the 18th Annual Medical-Legal Industrial Symposium, Mt. Sinai Medical Center, Milwaukee, Wis., Nov. 9, 1979.

215. MacGregor, J. T., "Natural Plant Constituents and Products Formed During Food Processing as Possible Contributors to Dietary Carcinogenesis," paper presented at National Academy of Sciences, Washington, D.C., Nov. 6, 1980.

216. MacMahon, B., "Prenatal X-Ray Exposure and Childhood Cancer," *J. Natl. Cancer Inst.* 28(5):1173-1191, 1962.

217. _____, "Overview: Environmental Factors," in *Persons at High Risk of Cancer: An Approach to Cancer Etiology and Control*, J. F. Fraumeni (ed.) (New York: Academic Press, 1975).

218. MacMahon, B., and Pugh, T. F., *Epidemiology: Principles and Methods* (Boston: Little, Brown, 1970).

219. MacMahon, B., Cole, P., and Brown, J., et al., "Etiology of Human Breast Cancer: A Review," *J. Natl. Cancer Inst.* 50(1):21-42, 1973.

220. MacMahon, B., et al., "Coffee and Cancer of the Pancreas," *N. Eng. J. Med.* 304(11): 630-633, 1981.

221. Magee, P. N., Montesano, R., and Preussmann, R., "N-Nitroso Compounds and Related Carcinogens," in *Chemical Carcinogenesis*, ACS Monograph #173, C. E. Searle (ed.) (Washington, D.C.: American Chemical Society, 1976).

222. Markey, H. T., "Statement" in *Risk/Benefit Analysis in the Legislative Process*, Subcom-

teristics," *J. Natl. Cancer Inst.* 48(6): 1575-1581, 1972.

mittee on Science, Research, and Technology, U.S. House of Representatives (Washington, D.C.: U. S. Government Printing Office, 1979).

223. Mason, T. J., *Atlas of Cancer Mortality for U.S. Counties: 1950-1969*, DHEW publication no. (NIH) 75-780 (Bethesda, Md.: National Cancer Institute, 1975).

224. Maugh, T. H., "Chemical Carcinogens: How Dangerous Are Low Doses?" *Science* 202: 37-41, 1978.

225. Mausner, J. S., and Bahn, A. K., *Epidemiology: An Introductory Text* (Philadelphia: W. B. Saunders, 1974).

226. McCann, J., and Ames, B. N., "The Salmonella/Microsome Mutagenicity Test: Predictive Value for Animal Carcinogenicity," in *Origins of Human Cancer*, H. H. Hiatt, J. D. Watson, and J. A. Winsten (eds.) (Cold Spring Harbor, N.Y.: Cold Spring Harbor Laboratory, 1977).

227. McCann, J., "Detection of Carcinogens as Mutagens in the Salmonella/Microsome Test: Assay of 300 Chemicals," *Proc. Nat. Acad. Sci. USA* 72:5135-5139, 1975.

228. McCarran, P. A., Debate in the Senate, recorded in *Congressional Record*, Mar. 12, 1946.

229. McGaughey, C., "Models for Carcinogenic Risk Assessment," *Science* 202:1106, 1978.

230. McGaughy, R. E., Environmental Protection Agency, personal communication, Aug. 19, 1980.

231. McGowan, C., "Congress, Court, and Control of Delegated Power," *Colum. Law Rev.* 77: 1119, 1977.

232. _____, "Panel III: Managing the Regulatory Process," *Ad. Law Rev.* 32:280, 1980.

233. McMahon, R. E., Cline, J. C. and Thompson, C. Z., "Assay of 855 Test Chemicals in Ten Tester Strains Using a New Modification of the Ames Test for Bacterial Mutagens," *Cancer Res.* 39:682-693, 1979.

234. Menck, H. R., "Cancer Incidence in the Mexican American," in *Epidemiology and Cancer Registries in the Pacific Basin*, NCI Monograph # 47: DHEW publication No. (NIH) 77-1223 (Bethesda, Md.: NCI, 1977).

235. Meselson, M., and Russell, K., "Comparisons of Carcinogenic and Mutagenic Potency," in *Origins of Human Cancer*, H. H. Hiatt, J. D. Watson, and J. A. Winsten (eds.) (Cold Spring Harbor, N.Y.: Cold Spring Harbor Laboratory, 1977).

236. Milham, S., *Occupational Mortality in Wash-ington State, 1950-1971* (Olympia, Wash.: Washington State Department of Social and Health Services, 1979).

237. Miller, A. B., "Nutrition and Cancer," *Prev. Med.* 9(2):189-196, 1980.

238. Miller, A. B., and Bulbrook, R. D., "The Epidemiology and Etiology of Breast Cancer," *N. Eng. J. Med.* 303(21):1246-1248, 1980.

239. Miller, J. A., and Miller, E. C., "Perspectives on the Metabolism of Chemical Carcinogens," in *Environmental Carcinogenesis*, P. Emmelot and E. Kriek (eds.) (Amsterdam: Elsevier/North Holland Biomedical Press, 1971).

240. Montesano, R., Bartsch, H., and Tomatis, L. (eds.), *Molecular and Cellular Aspects of Carcinogen Screening Tests*, IARC Scientific publication No. 27. (Lyon, France: International Agency for Research on Cancer, 1980).

241. Morgan, K. Z., "Cancer and Low Level Ionizing Radiation," *Bul. Atomic Sci.* 30-40, September 1978.

242. Morgan, R. W., "Analysis of Cancer Incidence and Mortality," typescript (Washington, D.C.: American Industrial Health Council, 1980).

243. Muir, W., affidavit presented in the U.S. District Court, Southern District of New York, 79 Civ. 2411, July 11, 1979.

244. Nahmias, J., Naib, Z. M., and Josey, W. E., "Epidemiological Studies Relating Genital Herpetic Infection to Cervical Carcinoma," *Cancer Res.* 34:1111-1117, 1974.

245. National Cancer Advisory Board, "General Criteria for Assessing the Evidence for Carcinogenicity of Chemical Substances: Report of the Subcommittee on Environmental Carcinogensis, National Cancer Advisory Board," *J. Natl. Cancer Inst.* 58:461, 1977.

246. _____, "Report of the Subcommittee on Environmental Carcinogenesis: The Relation of Bioassay Data on Chemicals to the Assessment of the Risk of Carcinogens for Humans Under Conditions of Low Exposure," typescript draft, 1979.

247. National Cancer Institute, *Cancer Patient Survival: Report Number 5*, L. M. Axtell, A. J. Asire, and M. H. Myers (eds.) DHEW publication No. (NIH) 77-992, (Bethesda, Md.: NCI, 1976.)

248. _____, *SEER Program: Cancer Incidence and Mortality in the United States: 1973-1976*, J. L. Young, Jr., A. J. Asire, and E. S. Pollack (eds.), DHEW publication No. (NIH) 78-1837 (Bethesda, Md: NCI, 1978).

249. National Cancer Institute and National Tox-

icology Program, *Carcinogenesis Testing Program: Chemicals on Standard Protocol* (Bethesda, Md: NCI, 1980).

250. National Cancer Institute, *Incidence of Nonmelanoma Skin Cancer in the United States, 1977-1978: Preliminary Report*, DHEW publication No. (NIH) 80-2154 (Bethesda, Md.: NCI, 1980).

251. _____, *Cancer Patient Survival Experience*, NIH publication No. 80-2148 (Bethesda, Md.: NCI, 1980).

252. National Center for Health Statistics, *Environmental Health: A Plan for Collecting and Coordinating Statistical and Epidemiologic Data*, DHHS publication No. (PHS) 80-1248 (Washington, D.C.: DHHS, 1980).

253. _____, *Data Systems of the National Center for Health Statistics*, DHEW publication No. (PHS) 80-1247 (Hyattsville, Md.: Office of Health Research, Statistics, and Technology, 1980).

254. _____, *Monthly Vital Statistics Report*, (29):1, 1980.

255. _____, published and unpublished U.S. Vital Statistics Data, 1933-1978.

256. National Center for Toxicological Research, "Innovations in Cancer Risk Assessment (ED01 Study)," *J. Env. Pathol. Toxicol.* 3:1-246, 1980.

257. National Institute on Alcohol Abuse and Alcoholism, *Third Special Report to the U.S. Congress on Alcohol and Health* (Washington, D.C.: U.S. Government Printing Office, 1978).

258. National Institutes of Health, *DES Task Force Summary Report*, DHEW publication No. 79-1688 (Washington, D.C.: U.S. Government Printing Office, 1978).

259. National Research Council, *Evaluating the Safety of Food Chemicals* (Washington, D.C.: National Academy of Sciences, 1970).

260. _____, *Particulate Polycyclic Organic Matter* (Washington, D.C.: National Academy of Sciences, 1972).

261. _____, *Safety of Saccharin and Sodium Saccharin in the Human Diet* (Washington, D.C.: National Academy of Sciences, 1974).

262. _____, *Pest Control: An Assessment of Present and Alternative Technologies* (Washington, D.C.: National Academy of Sciences, 1975).

263. _____, *Principles for Evaluating Chemicals in the Environment* (Washington, D.C.: National Academy of Sciences, 1975).

264. _____, *Halocarbons: Effects on Stratospheric Ozone*, Panel on Atmospheric Chemistry, Assembly of Mathematics and Physical Sciences (Washington, D.C.: National Academy of Sciences, 1976).

265. National Research Council/National Academy of Sciences, *Drinking Water and Health* (Washington, D.C.: National Academy of Sciences, 1977).

266. National Research Council, *Drinking Water and Health* (Washington, D.C.: National Academy of Sciences, 1977).

267. _____, *Pesticides*, draft (Washington, D.C.: National Academy of Sciences, 1980).

268. _____, Committee on the Biological Effects of Ionizing Radiation, *The Effects on Populations of Exposure to Low Levels of Ionizing Radiation* (Washington, D.C.: National Academy of Sciences, 1980).

269. National Research Council/Institute of Medicine, *Food Safety Policy: Scientific and Societal Considerations* (Washington, D.C.: National Academy of Sciences, 1979).

270. National Research Council, *Drinking Water and Health*, vol. 3 (Washington, D.C.: National Academy Press, 1980).

271. National Toxicology Program, *Annual Plan: Fiscal Year 1979* (Washington, D.C.: Department of Health, Education, and Welfare, 1979).

272. _____, *Fiscal Year 1980 Annual Plan*, publication No. NTP-79-7 (Washington, D.C.: Department of Health, Education, and Welfare, 1980).

273. _____, *NTP Technical Bulletin* 1(3):1-2, 1980.

274. Nature, "Inflexibility of Delaney Clause Criticised," *Nature* 84:205, 1980.

275. Neustadt, R., "The Administration's Regulatory Reform Program: An Overview," Also in *Ad. Law Rev.* 32:129-163, 1980.

276. Neyman, J., "Models for Carcinogenic Risk Assessment," *Science* 202:1106-1107, 1978.

276a. Nicholson, W. J. (ed.), "Management of Assessed Risk for Carcinogens," *Ann. N.Y. Acad. Sci.* 363 (New York: New York Academy of Sciences, 1980).

277. Obe, G., and Ristow, H., "Mutagenic, Carcinogenic and Teratogenic Effects of Alcohol," *Mutat. Res.* 65:229-259, 1979.

278. Occupational Safety and Health Administration, "Identification, Classification and Regulation of Toxic Substances Posing a Potential Occupational Carcinogenic Risk," *Federal Register* 42:54148-54247, 1977.

279. _____, "Identification, Classification and Regulation of Potential Occupational Carcinogens," *Federal Register* 45:5001-5296, 1980.

279a. _____, personal communication letter, Jan. 14, 1981.

280. Office of Management and Budget, *Improving Government Regulation: Current Status and Future Directions* (Washington, D.C.: Executive Office of the President, 1980).

281. Office of Science and Technology Policy, *Identification, Characterization, and Control of Potential Human Carcinogens: A Framework for Federal Decision-making* (Washington, D.C.: Executive Office of the President, 1979). Also in *J. Natl. Cancer Inst.* 64:169-176, 1980.

282. Office of Technology Assessment, U.S. Congress, *Cancer Testing Technology and Saccharin* (Washington, D.C.: U.S. Government Printing Office, 1977).

283. _____, *Selected Topics in Federal Health Statistics* (Washington, D.C.: U.S. Government Printing Office, 1979).

284. _____, *Environmental Contaminants in Food* (Washington, D.C.: U.S. Government Printing Office, 1979).

285. _____, *The Implications of Cost-Effectiveness Analysis of Medical Technology* (Washington, D.C.: U.S. Government Printing Office, 1980).

286. Office on Smoking and Health, *Smoking and Health: A Report of the Surgeon General*, DHEW publication No. (PHS) 79-50066 (Washington, D.C.: Public Health Service, 1979).

287. _____, *The Health Consequences of Smoking for Women: A Report of the Surgeon General* (Washington, D.C.: Public Health Service, 1980).

288. Omenn, G., Office of Science and Technology Policy, personal communication, 1980.

289. Paffenbarger, R. S., Kampert, J. B., and Chang, H. G., "Characteristics That Predict Risk of Breast Cancer Before and After the Menopause," *Am. J. Epidem.* 112(2):258-268, 1980.

290. Pearce, M. L., and Dayton, S., "Incidence of Cancer in Men on a Diet High in Polyunsaturated Fat," *Lancet* 1:464-467, 1971.

291. Percy, C., Stanek, E., and Gloeckler, L., "Accuracy of Cancer Death Certificates and Its Effect on Cancer Mortality Statistics," *Am. J. Pub. Health* 71(3):242-250, 1981.

292. Peto, R., et al., "Can Dietary Beta-Carotene Materially Reduce Human Cancer Rates?" *Nature* 290:201-208, 1981.

293. Phillips, R. L., Kuzma, J. W., and Lotz, T. M., "Cancer Mortality Among Comparable Members Versus Nonmembers of the Seventh-day Adventist Church," in *Cancer Incidence in Defined Populations*, J. Cairns, J. L. Lyon, and M. Skolnick (eds.) (Cold Spring Harbor, N.Y.: Cold Spring Harbor Laboratory, 1980).

294. Pike, M. C., et al., "Air Pollution," in *Persons at High Risk of Cancer: An Approach to Cancer Etiology and Control*, J. F. Fraumeni, Jr. (ed.) (New York: Academic Press, 1975).

295. Pollack, E. S., "Cancer Incidence Trends in the United States: Some Methodological Problems," paper presented at UICC Symposium on Trends in Cancer Incidence, Oslo, Norway, Aug. 6, 1980, proceedings in press.

296. Pollack, E. S., and Horm, J. W., "Trends in Cancer Incidence and Mortality in the United States, 1969-1976," *J. Natl. Cancer Inst.* 64(5):1091-1103, 1980.

297. Pradhan, S. N., et al., "Potential Carcinogens: I. Carcinogenicity of Some Plant Extracts and Their Tannin-Containing Fractions in Rats," *J. Natl. Cancer Inst.* 52(5):1579-1582, 1974.

298. Public Health Service, *Survey of Compounds Which Have Been Tested for Carcinogenic Activity*, PHS publication No. 149 (Washington, D.C.: Department of Health, Education, and Welfare, 1951; Supplement 1, 1957; Supplement 2, 1969; 1961-1967 Volume, 1969; 1968-1969 Volume, 1971; 1970-1971 Volume, 1974; 1972-1973 Volume, 1975).

299. _____, *Healthy People: The Surgeon General's Report on Health Promotion and Disease Prevention, 1979*, DHEW, PHS, Office of the Assistant Secretary for Health and Surgeon General, DHEW (PHS) publication No. 79-55071 (Washington, D.C.: U.S. Government Printing Office, 1979).

300. Purchase, I. F., "Inter-species Comparisons of Carcinogenicity," *Br. J. Cancer* 41:454-468, 1980.

301. Purchase, I. F. H., et al., "Evaluation of Six Short Term Tests for Detecting Organic Chemical Carcinogens and Recommendations for Their Use," *Nature* 264:624-627, 1976.

302. Radman, M., and Kinsella, A. R., *Chromosomal Events in Carcinogenic Initiation and Promotion: Implications for Carcinogenicity Testing and Cancer Prevention Strategies* (Lyon, France: International Agency for Research on Cancer, 1980).

303. Rall, D., Director, National Toxicology Program, personal communication, May, 1980.

304. Rapp, F., "Virology and Cancer," *Prev. Med.* 9(2):244-251, 1980.

305. Reddy, B. S., et al., "Effect of Quality and Quantity of Dietary Fat and Dimethylhydrazine in Colon Carcinogenesis in Rats,"

Proc. of the Soc. for Experimental Biol. and Medicine 151:237-239, 1976.

306. Regulatory Council, *Regulation of Chemical Carcinogens* (Washington, D.C.: Regulatory Council, 1979).

307. Rettig, R., *Cancer Crusade: The Story of the National Cancer Act of 1971* (Princeton, N.J.: Princeton University, 1977).

308. Rice, D. P., and Hodgson, T. A.,"Social and Economic Implications of Cancer in the United States," paper presented to the Expert Committee on Cancer Statistics of the World Health Organization and International Agency for Research on Cancer, Madrid, Spain, June 20-26, 1978.

309. Rinkus, S. J., and Legator, M. S., "Chemical Characterization of 465 Known or Suspected Carcinogens and Their Correlation With Mutagenic Activity in the *Salmonella Typhimurium* System," *Cancer Res.* 39:3289-3318, 1979.

310. Robbins, J. H., "Xeroderma Pigmentosum: An Inherited Disease With Sun Sensitivity, Multiple Cutaneous Neoplasms, and Abnormal DNA Repair," *Ann. Int. Med.* 80(2):221-248, 1974.

311. Rogers, A. E., and Newberne, P. M., "Dietary Effects on Chemical Carcinogenesis in Animal Models for Colon and Liver Tumors," *Cancer Res.* 35:3427-3431, 1975.

312. Rogot, E., and Murray, J. L., "Smoking and Causes of Death Among Veterans: 16 Years of Observation," *Pub. Health Rep.* 95(3):213-222, 1980.

313. Rothman, K. J., "The Proportion of Cancer Attributable to Alcohol Consumption," *Prev. Med.* 9(2):174-179, 1980.

314. _____, "Comments on, 'Trends in Cancer Incidence and Mortality, 1969-76' by Pollack and Horm," typescript, undated.

315. Rothman, K., and Keller, A., "The Effect of Joint Exposure to Alcohol and Tobacco on Risk of Cancer of the Mouth and Pharynx," *J. Chron. Dis.* 25:711-716, 1972.

316. Rowe, W. D., "Regulation of Toxic Chemicals Within the Limits of Knowledge," a report submitted to OTA , U.S. Congress, 1980.

317. Rubin, H., "Is Somatic Mutation the Major Mechanism of Malignant Transformation?" *J. Natl. Cancer Inst.* 64:995-1000, 1980.

318. Sandler, H. M., and Fishman, S. A., "Underdiagnosis of Occupational Illnesses," *N. Eng. J. Med.* 303(11):644.

319. Scherer, E., and Emmelot, P., "Models for Carcinogenic Risk Assessment," *Science* 202:1107, 1978.

320. Schneiderman, M. A., statement before the Subcommittee on Health and Scientific Research of the Senate Committee on Human Resources, Mar. 5, 1979.

321. _____, "What's Happening to Cancer in our Advanced Industrial Society? Have the Risks Been Overstated?" paper presented at the meeting of the Society for Occupational and Environmental Health, Washington, D.C., Dec. 3, 1979.

322. Schottenfeld, D., *Cancer Epidemiology and Prevention: Current Concepts* (Springfield, Ill.: Charles C. Thomas, 1975).

323. _____, "Alcohol as a Co-factor in the Etiology of Cancer," *Cancer* 43(5):1962-1966, 1979.

324. Schottenfeld, D., and Berg, J., "Incidence of Multiple Primary Cancers. IV. Cancers of the Female Breast and Genital Organs," *J. Natl. Cancer Inst.* 46(1):161-170, 1971.

325. Secretary's Committee on Pesticides and Their Relationship to Environmental Health, report to the Secretary of Health, Education, and Welfare, (Washington, D.C.: Department of Health, Education, and Welfare, 1969).

326. Severs R. K., "Air Pollution and Health," in *Environment and Health*, N. M. Tarieff (ed.) (Ann Arbor, Mich.: Ann Arbor Science, 1980).

327. Shiono, P. H., Chung, C. S., and Myrianthopoulos, N. C., "Preconception Radiation, Intrauterine Diagnostic Radiation, and Childhood Neoplasia," *J. Natl. Cancer Inst.* 65(4):681-686, 1980.

328. Shubik, P., "Food Additives, Contaminants and Cancer," *Prev. Med.* 9(2): 197-201, 1980.

329. Sinclair, W., "The Scientific Basis for Risk Quantification," paper presented at the Annual Meeting of the National Council on Radiation Protection and Measurement, Washington, D.C., Apr. 2, 1980, to be published in the Proceedings of the Annual Meeting.

330. Sontag, J. M., "Carcinogenicity of Substituted-Benzenediamine (Phenylenediamines) in Rats and Mice," *J. Natl. Cancer Inst.* 66(3):591-602, 1981.

331. Sontag, J. M., Page, N. P., and Saffiotti, U., *Guidelines for Carcinogenic Bioassay in Small Rodents* (Bethesda, Md.: National Cancer Institute, 1976).

332. Stallones, R. A., and Downs, T., "A Critical Review of: 'Estimates of the Fraction of Cancer

in the United States Related to Occupational Factors,' " typescript, 1978.

333. Stewart, A., Webb, J., and Hewitt, D., "A Survey of Childhood Malignancies," *Br. Med. J.* 1:1495-1508, 1958.

334. Subcommittee on Oversight and Investigation, House Committee on Interstate and Foreign Commerce, *Cost-Benefit Analysis: Word, Tool or Mirage*, Committee Print 96-IFC62 (Washington, D.C.: U.S. Government Printing Office, 1980).

335. Sugimura, T., et al., "A Critical Review of Submammalian Systems for Mutagen Detection" in *Progress in Genetic Toxicology*, D. Scott, B. A. Bridges, and F. H. Sobles (eds.) (Amsterdam: Elsevier/North Holland Biomedical Press, 1977).

336. _____, "Mutagen-Carcinogens in Food, With Special Reference to Highly Mutagenic Pyrolytic Products in Broiled Foods," in *Origins of Human Cancer*, H. H. Hiatt, J. D. Watson, and J. A. Winsten (eds.) (Cold Spring Harbor, N.Y.: Cold Spring Harbor Laboratory, 1977).

337. Supreme Court of the United States, "Industrial Union Department, AFL-CIO v. American Petroleum Institute, et al.," argued Oct. 10, 1979, decided July 2, 1980, No. 78-911, 1980.

338. Tamura, G., et al., "Fecalase: A Model for the Activation of Dietary Glycosides to Mutagens by Intestinal Flora," *Proc. Natl. Acad. Sci. USA*, 77:4961-4965, 1980.

339. Task Force on Environmental Cancer and Heart and Lung Disease, *First Annual Report to Congress* (Washington, D.C.: Environmental Protection Agency, 1978).

340. _____, *Environmental Cancer and Heart and Lung Disease: Third Annual Report to Congress, 1980* (Washington, D.C.: Environmental Protection Agency, 1980).

341. Tomatis, L., "The Value of Long-term Testing for the Implementation of Primary Prevention," in *Origins of Human Cancer*, H. H. Hiatt, J. D. Watson, and J. A. Winsten (eds.) (Cold Spring Harbor, N.Y.: Cold Spring Harbor Laboratory, 1977).

342. _____, "The Predictive Value of Rodent Carcinogenicity Tests in the Evaluation of Human Risk," *Ann. Rev. Pharmacol. Toxicol.* 19:511-530, 1979.

343. Tomatis, L., Partensky, C., and Montesano, R., "The Predictive Value of Mouse Liver Tumor Induction in Carcinogenicity Testing: A Literature Survey," *Int. J. Cancer* 12:1-20, 1973.

344. Tomatis, L., et al., Evaluation of the Carcinogenicity of Chemicals: A Review of the Monograph Program of the International Agency for Research on Cancer," *Cancer Res.* 38:877-885, 1978.

345. Toxic Substances Strategy Committee, *Toxic Chemicals and Public Protection*, report to the President (Washington, D.C.: U.S. Government Printing Office, 1980).

346. Tulinius, H., et al., "Reproductive Factors and Risk for Breast Cancer in Iceland," *Int. J. Cancer* 21:724-730, 1978.

347. Tuyns, A. J., "Alcohol and Cancer," *Alcoh. Health Res.* 2:20-31, 1978.

348. _____, "Epidemiology of Alcohol and Cancer," *Cancer Res.* 39:2840-2843, 1979.

349. U.S. Bureau of the Census, *1970 Census of Population and Housing: Estimates of Coverage of Population by Sex, Race, and Age: Demographic Analysis*, Evaluation and Research Program PHC(E)-4 (Washington, D.C.: U.S. Government Printing Office, 1973).

350. _____, *The Methods and Materials of Demography*, third printing (rev.) (Washington, D.C.: U.S. Government Printing Office, 1975).

351. _____, *Bureau of the Census Statistical Abstract of the United States: 1978, 99th ed.* (Washington, D.C.: U.S. Government Printing Office, 1978).

352. Union Carbide, *The Vital Consensus: American Attitudes on Economic Growth* (New York: Union Carbide Corporate Communications Department, 1980).

353. Upton, A., testimony before the Subcommittee on Nutrition of the Committee on Agriculture, Nutrition, and Forestry, U.S. Senate, 96th Cong., Oct. 1, 1979 (Washington, D.C.: U.S. Government Printing Office, 1980).

354. Urbach, F., "Ultraviolet Radiation and Skin Cancer in Man," *Prev. Med.* 9(2):227-280, 1980.

355. Verkuil, P. R., "The Emerging Concept of Administrative Procedure," *Colum. Law Rev.* 78:258-329, 1978.

356. Vitale, J. J., " Possible Role of Nutrients in Neoplasia," *Cancer Res.* 35:3320-3325, 1975.

357. Waters, M. D., "Gene-Tox Program," *Banbury Report 2. Mammalian Cell Mutagenesis: The Materializaton of Test Systems*, A. Hoie, J. P. On'Neill, and V. K. McElheny (eds.) (Cold Spring Harbor, N.Y.: Cold Spring Harbor Laboratory, 1979).

358. Weinstein, I. B., 1979. Quoted in reference 302.

359. Weisburger, J. H., Cohen, L. A., and Wynder, E. L., "On the Etiology and Metabolic Epidemi-

ology of the Main Human Cancers," in *Origins of Human Cancer*, H. H. Hiatt, J. D. Watson, and J. A. Winsten (eds.) (Cold Spring Harbor, N.Y.: Cold Spring Harbor Laboratory, 1977).

360. Weiss, N.S., and Sayvetz, T. A., "Incidence of Endometrial Cancer in Relation to the Use of Oral Contraceptives," *N. Eng. J. Med.* 302(10):552-554, 1980.

361. Williams, R. R., et al., "Cancer Incidence by Levels of Cholesterol," *J.A.M.A.* 245(3): 247-252, 1981.

362. Wilson, R. E., Department of Physics, Harvard University, personal communication, January, 1981.

363. Winn, D.M., et al., "Snuff Dipping and Oral Cancer Among Women in the Southern United States," *N. Eng. J. Med.* 304(13):745-749, 1981.

364. World Health Organization, *Prevention of Cancer*, report of a WHO Expert Committee, Technical Report No. 276, (Geneva: WHO, 1964).

365. _____, *Smoking and Its Effects on Health*, Technical Report No. 568 (Geneva: WHO, 1975).

366. _____, *Steroid Contraception and the Risk of Neoplasia*, Technical Report No. 619 (Geneva: WHO, 1978).

367. Wynder, E. L., and Bross, I. J., "A study of Etiological Factors in Cancer of the Esophagus," *Cancer* 14:389-413, 1961.

368. Wynder, E. L., and Gori, G. B., "Guest Editorial: Contribution of the Environment to Cancer Incidence: an Epidemiologic Exercise," *J. Natl. Cancer Inst.* 58:825-832, 1977.

369. Yamasaki, E., and Ames, B. N., "Concentration of Mutagens From Urine by Adsorption With the Non-polar Resin, XAD-2: Cigarette Smokers Have Mutagenic Urine," *Proc. Nat. Acad. Sci. USA* 74:35555-3559, 1977.

370. Yeh, S., *"Skin Cancer in Chronic Arsenicism," Human Path.* 4(4):469-485, 1973.